The Critical Care Drug Handbook
Second edition

W9-CAJ-697

The Critical Care Drug Handbook
Second edition

GARY P. ZALOGA, MD, FCCM, FCCP
Professor of Anesthesia/Critical Care and
Medicine
Bowman Gray School of Medicine
Wake Forest University
Winston-Salem, North Carolina

DREW MACGREGOR, MD
Assistant Professor of Anesthesia,
Critical Care, and Medicine (Pulmonary)
Bowman Gray School of Medicine
Wake Forest University
Winston-Salem, North Carolina

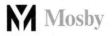 Mosby

St. Louis Baltimore Boston Carlsbad Chicago Naples New York
Philadelphia Portland London Madrid Mexico City Singapore
Sydney Tokyo Toronto Wiesbaden

Mosby

Dedicated to Publishing Excellence

A Times Mirror Company

Publisher: Anne S. Patterson
Senior Editor: Laurel Craven
Developmental Editor: Kimberley Cox
Project Manager: Chris Baumle
Production Editor: Michelle R. Fitzgerald
Design Manager: Nancy McDonald
Manufacturing Supervisor: Bill Winneberger

Second edition

Page composition by Compset, Inc.
Printing/binding by Malloy Printing

Copyright © 1997 Mosby-Year Book, Inc.

Mosby–Year Book, Inc.
11830 Westline Industrial Drive
St. Louis, MO 63146

Library of Congress Cataloguing-in-Publication Data

The critical care drug handbook / [edited by] Gary P. Zaloga, Drew
  MacGregor. — 2nd. ed.
    p. cm.
  Includes bibliographical references and index.
  ISBN 0-8151-9892-2
  1. Critical care medicine—Handbooks, manuals, etc.   2. Drugs
—Handbooks, manuals, etc.   I. Zaloga, Gary P.   II. MacGregor, Drew.
  [DNLM: 1. Drugs—handbooks.   2. Critical Care—handbooks.   QV 39
C934   1996]
  RC86.8.C75   1996
  616′.028—dc20
  DNLM/DLC   96-38859
  for Library of Congress   CIP

CONTRIBUTORS

David Bowton, MD
Associate Professor of Anesthesia/Critical Care and Medicine (Pulmonary)
Bowman Gray School of Medicine
Wake Forest University
Winston-Salem, North Carolina

Richard Browder, MD
Fellow, Critical Care Medicine and Nephrology
Bowman Gray School of Medicine
Wake Forest University
Winston-Salem, North Carolina

Randy Carpenter, MD
Associate Professor of Anesthesia
Bowman Gray School of Medicine
Wake Forest University
Winston-Salem, North Carolina

Jeffrey Kelly, MD
Assistant Professor of Anesthesia/Critical Care and Emergency Medicine
Bowman Gray School of Medicine
Wake Forest University
Winston-Salem, North Carolina

Daniel Kennedy, MD
Assistant Professor of Anesthesia/Critical Care
Bowman Gray School of Medicine
Wake Forest University
Winston-Salem, North Carolina

Drew MacGregor, MD
Assistant Professor of Anesthesia/Critical Care and Medicine
*   (Pulmonary)*
Bowman Gray School of Medicine
Wake Forest University
Winston-Salem, North Carolina

Samuel Pegram, MD
Professor of Medicine (Infectious Disease)
Bowman Gray School of Medicine
Wake Forest University
Winston-Salem, North Carolina

Richard Preilipp, MD
Associate Professor of Anesthesia/Critical Care
Bowman Gray School of Medicine
Wake Forest University
Winston-Salem, North Carolina

Roger Royster, MD
Professor of Anesthesia/Critical Care and Medicine (Cardiology)
Bowman Gray School of Medicine
Wake Forest University
Winston-Salem, North Carolina

Phillip Scuderi, MD
Associate Professor of Anesthesia/Critical Care
Bowman Gray School of Medicine
Wake Forest University
Winston-Salem, North Carolina

Kenton O. Smitherman, MD
Fellow, Critical Care Medicine
Bowman Gray School of Medicine
Wake Forest University
Winston-Salem, North Carolina

Gary P. Zaloga, MD
Professor of Anesthesia/Critical Care, and Medicine
*   (Endocrinology)*
Bowman Gray School and Medicine
Wake Forest University
Winston-Salem, North Carolina

Dedicated to all those who have contributed to improving the care of critically ill patients. Far and away the best reward that life offers is the chance to improve the life of another.

PREFACE

Drug administration is a vital component in the care of the critically ill patient. Most patients admitted to an intensive care unit receive between 3 and 10 drugs during their stay. Optimal care requires that the clinician understand the specific pharmacologic actions of these drugs, their adverse effects, and the interactions between agents. Only with adequate knowledge of drug action and adverse effects can the clinician choose the best drug for treating a problem and balance the beneficial effects of the drug against its possible adverse actions.

Extensive information on drug action is available in both the literature and large pharmacology texts. Unfortunately, this information is seldom readily accessible at the bedside. The first edition of this handbook was well received as a handy, quick reference guide for physicians, nurses, and other health care providers. Using suggestions from our readers, we increased the number of drugs included herein and eliminated some of the agents which have become obsolete in the intensive care environment. The result is an improved handbook designed to provide important prescribing information on drugs used in the critical care setting. The information is presented in a standard, compact, and easy-to-use format that can be quickly accessed at the bedside. We highly recommend use of computer searches, medical literature, and pharmacology textbooks when more extensive information on a drug is needed.

We have included in this book the most common drugs used in a multidisciplinary intensive care unit. Experts in various subspecialty areas, such as pulmonary medicine, cardiology, internal medicine, endocrinology, infectious disease, nephrology, and anesthesiology, reviewed each drug and formulated the material in the text. The recommendations for treatment in this handbook may at times differ from those in other texts and the *Physicians' Desk Reference*, because the treatments are based upon doses used in clinical practice. When discrepancies arise between your experience and those suggested here, we recommend that you consult the *Physicians' Desk Reference* and other pharmacologic texts.

The book is organized into three basic sections to assist in drug administration. The first section lists common clinical problems and the drugs used to treat those problems. The second section lists drugs in alphabetical order, so that they can be accessed quickly. A large number of appendixes are also included to aid in drug administration. A complete index allows for ready access to drug information. Each drug is presented in a similar format and includes trade names, drug actions, indications, dosages and pharmacokinetic parameters, adverse effects, drug interactions, drug monitoring, and selected references.

An extensive amount of work went into the preparation of this book. We thank all of the contributors for their hard work, dedication to accuracy, and thoughtful review. We believe that the goal of producing a small, compact, and easy-to-access book for use at the bedside has been met.

Gary P. Zaloga, MD, FCCM
Drew MacGregor, MD

CONTENTS

PROBLEMS

1

Problems

Acidosis
  See Metabolic acidosis
Adrenal insufficiency
  Glucocorticoids
  Mineralocorticoids
Agitation
  Phenothiazines
  Benzodiazepines
  Narcotics
  Barbiturates
  Paraldehyde
  Chloral hydrate
Alcohol withdrawal
  Benzodiazepines
  Paraldehyde
  β-adrenergic blockers
  Clonidine
  Haloperidol
Alkalosis
  See Metabolic alkalosis
Allergic reaction
  See Anaphylactic reaction
Altitude sickness
  Acetazolamide
  Glucocorticoids
Analgesia
  Salicylates
  Nonsteroidal anti-inflammatory drugs (NSAIDs)
  Acetaminophen
  Narcotics
Anaphylactic reaction
  Epinephrine
  Diphenhydramine
  Glucocorticoids
  Hydroxyzine

Anemia
  Erythropoietin
Anesthesia
  Narcotics
  Benzodiazepines
  Etomidate
  Propofol
  Barbiturates
  Ketamine
Aneurysm
  See Aortic aneurysm
Angina pectoris
  Nitrates
  β-adrenergic blockers
  Calcium channel blockers
  Narcotics
Anticholinesterase
  Edrophonium
  Neostigmine
  Physostigmine
  Pyridostigmine
Anticoagulants
  See Thrombosis
Antiemetics
  See Nausea/vomiting
Anti-inflammatory
  See Inflammation
Antiplatelet
  Salicylates
  Dipyridamole
  Ticlopidine
Anxiety
  Benzodiazepines
  Narcotics
  Barbiturates
  Paraldehyde
  Chloral hydrate
Aortic aneurysm
  β-adrenergic antagonist
  Calcium channel blocker

Trimethaphan
Vasodilator (use with β-blocker or calcium channel blocker)
Nitroprusside
Nitroglycerine

Arrhythmia: Cardiac
Magnesium
Potassium
Lidocaine (group II; ventricular); Tocainide
Quinidine (group I; ventricular, supraventricular)
Procainamide (group I; ventricular, supraventricular)
Bretylium (group IV; ventricular)
Amiodarone (group III; ventricular, supraventricular)
β-adrenergic antagonists (supraventricular, ventricular)
Calcium channel blockers
Digoxin (rate control for atrial fibrillation/flutter)
Phenytoin (especially for tricyclic antidepressant overdose)

Arthritis
See Inflammation

Asthma
See Bronchospasm

Bacterial infection
See Appendix A: Treatment of Specific Infections
See Appendix B: Tetanus Prophylaxis
See Appendix E: Prevention of HIV—Associated Opportunistic
Infections
See Appendix G: Metabolic Alkalosis
See Appendix I: Selected Serum/Plasma Drug Levels
See Appendix J: Comparison of Muscle Relaxants
See Appendix K: Nucleoside Analogue Antiretrovirals
Amikacin
Gram-negative aerobes (*Pseudomonas*): staphylococci
Amoxicillin
Gram-negative aerobes (*H. influenzae, Escherichia coli,*
Proteus mirabilis, Neisseria gonorrhoeae)
Gram-positive aerobes (streptococci, enterococci, non–
penicillinase-producing staphylococci)
Amoxicillin/clavulanic acid (Augmentin)
Spectrum similar to amoxicillin, plus
β-lactamase staphylococci

Ampicillin
    Gram-positive staphylococci (non–penicillinase-producing)
    Gram-negative aerobes (non-β-lactamase-producing)
    Gram-negative anaerobes (not *Bacteroides*)
    Active against enterococci when combined with aminoglyco-
        side
    Listeria monocytogenes
Ampicillin/sulbactam (Unasyn)
    Increases activity of ampicillin to include β-lactamase-
        producing staphylococci, *Haemophilus influenzae,* gono-
        cocci, and *Bacteroides fragilis*
Azlocillin
    Gram-positive staphylococci (non–penicillinase-producing)
    Gram-negative aerobes and anaerobes (*Pseudomonas aerugi-
        nosa, Proteus, Enterobacter, Klebsiella, B. fragilis*)
Aztreonam
    Gram-negative aerobes (*P. aeruginosa*)
Carbenicillin
    Non–β-lactamase-producing gram-positive aerobes (*Strepto-
        coccus;* not *Staphylococcus*)
    Gram-negative aerobes (*P. aeruginosa;* not *Klebsiella*)
    Gram-negative anaerobes (*B. fragilis*)
Cefaclor
    Gram-positive aerobes (*Staphylococcus aureus*)
    Gram-negative aerobes (*H. influenzae*)
Cefazolin
    Gram-positive aerobes (staphylococci; not enterococci)
    Gram-negative aerobes (*P. aeruginosa, Proteus*)
Cefoperazone
    Gram-positive and gram-negative aerobes and anaerobes
Cefotaxime
    Gram-positive aerobes (not enterococci or methicillin-
        resistant *S. aureus* [MRSA])
    Gram-negative aerobes (Enterobacteriaceae, *H. influenzae;*
        not *P. aeruginosa*)
Cefotetan
    Gram-positive and gram-negative aerobes and anaerobes
        (not enterococci, MRSA, *P. aeruginosa;* active against
        B. fragilis)

Cefoxitin
  Gram-positive and gram-negative aerobes and anaerobes
    (not enterococci, MRSA, *P. aeruginosa;* active against
    Bacteroides)
Ceftazidime
  Gram-positive and gram-negative aerobes and anaerobes
    (not enterococci, MRSA, *Bacteroides*)
Ceftizoxime
  Gram-positive and gram-negative aerobes and anaerobes
    (not enterococci, MRSA, *P. aeruginosa;* active against
    Bacteroides)
Ceftriaxone
  Gram-positive and gram-negative aerobes and anaerobes
    (not enterococci, MRSA, *P. aeruginosa, Bacteroides*)
Cefuroxime
  Gram-positive and gram-negative aerobes and anaerobes
    (not enterococci, MRSA, *P. aeruginosa, Bacteroides*)
Cephalexin
  Gram-positive and gram-negative aerobes and anaerobes
    (not enterococci, MRSA, *P. aeruginosa, Bacteroides*)
Cephradine
  Gram-positive and gram-negative aerobes and anaerobes
    (not enterococci, MRSA, *P. aeruginosa, Bacteroides*)
Chloramphenicol
  Gram-positive and gram-negative aerobes and anaerobes
    (not *P. aeruginosa*)
  Rickettsiae, chlamydiae
Ciprofloxacin
  Staphylococci (MRSA)
  Gram-negative aerobes (*P. aeruginosa*)
Clindamycin
  Gram-positive aerobes (not enterococci or MRSA)
  Anaerobes (not *Clostridium difficile*)
Doxycycline
  Many aerobes and anaerobes
  Mycoplasma pneumoniae, chlamydiae, rickettsiae
Erythromycin
  Gram-positive aerobes
  Legionella, Mycoplasma, chylamydiae, *Bordetella pertussis,*
    Campylobacter, Corynebacterium diphtheriae

Ethambutol
Mycobacterium
Gentamicin
Staphylococci
Enterococci (use with penicillin or vancomycin)
Gram-negative aerobes
Imipenem/cilastatin
Most aerobes and anaerobes
Campylobacter, Yersinia, Nocardia, Mycobacterium
Not active against *Pseudomonas maltophilia, Pseudomonas cepacia*
Isoniazid
Mycobacterium
Methicillin
Staphylococcus
Metronidazole
Anaerobes
C. difficile
Mezlocillin
Gram-positive aerobes (not β-lactamase–producing *Staphylococcus*)
Gram-negative aerobes (*P. aeruginosa*)
Gram-negative anaerobes (*Bacteroides*)
Nafcillin
Staphylococcus
Norfloxacin
Gram-positive aerobes (*Staphylococcus*)
Gram-negative aerobes (*P. aeruginosa*)
Oxacillin
Staphylococcus
Penicillin
Gram-positive aerobic cocci (*Streptococcus, Pneumococcus,* enterococci with aminoglycoside; not penicillinase-producing *Staphylococcus*)
Anaerobes (*Actinomyces;* not *Bacteroides*)
Spirochetes, meningococci (*Neisseria meningitidis*)
Piperacillin
Gram-positive aerobes (non–β-lactamase-producing)
Gram-negative aerobes (*P. aeruginosa*)
Gram-negative anaerobes (*Bacteroides*)

Rifampin
    Mycobacterium
    Gram-positive aerobes (*Staphylococcus*)
    Gram-negative aerobes (*Neisseria, H. influenzae*)
    Legionella
    Chlamydiae, *C. difficile*
Silver sulfadiazine (topical)
    Gram-negative and gram-positive organisms
Streptomycin
    Mycobacterium
    Yersinia pestis, Francisella tularensis, Brucella
Sulfonamides
    Gram-positive and gram-negative aerobes
    Chlamydiae
Tetracycline
    Gram-positive and gram-negative bacteria
    Rickettsiae
    Mycoplasma
Ticarcillin
    Gram-positive aerobes (non–β-lactamase-producing)
    Gram-negative aerobes (*P. aeruginosa;* not *Klebsiella*)
    Anaerobes (*Bacteroides*)
Ticarcillin/clavulanic acid
    Expands spectrum of ticarcillin to β-lactamase–producing
        bacteria (*Staphylococcus*)
Tobramycin
    Staphylococcus
    Enterococcus (with penicillin or vancomycin)
    Gram-negative aerobes (*P. aeruginosa*)
Trimethoprim/sulfamethoxazole
    Gram-positive and gram-negative aerobes (not
        P. aeruginosa)
Vancomycin
    Gram-positive bacteria (*Staphylococcus, Streptococcus,
        Enterococcus* with another antibiotic)
    C. difficile
Bleeding
    dDAVP (especially von Willebrand disease, hemophilia A, ure-
        mia, postcardiac surgery)

Vasopressin (varices)
Aminocaproic acid
Protamine
Vitamin K
Bradycardia
Atropine
β-adrenergic agonists
Glucagon (especially β-blocker and calcium blocker induced)
Bronchospasm
β-adrenergic agonists
Ipratropium
Theophylline compounds
Glucocorticoids

Cardiac arrhythmia
See Arrhythmia: Cardiac
Cardiogenic shock
Combined α and β-adrenergic agonists
Epinephrine, norepinephrine, dopamine
α-adrenergic agonists
Phenylephrine
β-adrenergic agonists
Dobutamine, isoproterenol
Cerebral edema
Glucocorticoids (dexamethasone)
Mannitol
Barbiturates
Congestive heart failure
Morphine
Nitrates
Inotropic Agents
β-adrenergic agonists: epinephrine, dobutamine, dopamine, isoproterenol
Phosphodiesterase inhibitors: amrinone, milrinone
Digoxin
Vasodilators
Hydralazine, angiotensin converting enzyme inhibitors, nitroprusside
Diuretics

Constipation
  Laxatives/stool softeners
    Bulking agents
    Emollients
    Lubricants
    Magnesium-containing agents
    Stimulants
    Hyperosmotic agents
Coronary vasospasm
  Nitrates
  Calcium channel blockers
Cough
  Narcotics
  Antihistamines
Cryptococcus
  Flucytosine
  Amphotericin B
  Ketoconazole

Delirium
  See Sedation and Alcohol withdrawal syndrome
Depression
  Tricyclic antidepressants
  Monoamine oxidase inhibitors
  Selective serotonin reuptake inhibitors
Diabetes insipidus (DI)
  dDAVP
  Chlorpropamide (partial DI)
  Vasopressin
  Prostaglandin inhibitors: nonsteroidals (nephrogenic DI)
Diabetes mellitus
  See Hyperglycemia
Diarrhea
  Narcotics
  Diphenoxylate/atropine (Lomotil), loperamide (Imodium),
    paregoric, belladonna alkaloids, morphine, codeine
  Pectin
  Bismuth subsalicylate
  Activated attapulgite

Octreotide
Lactobacillus acidophilus
Disseminated intravascular coagulation (DIC)
Heparin
Antithrombin III
Diuresis
See Oliguria
Ductus arteriosus
Alprostadil

Eclampsia
See Hypertension
Magnesium
Edema
See Fluid overload
Embolism
See Thrombosis
Emesis induction
Apomorphine
Ipecac
Emesis control
See Nausea/vomiting
Esophageal foreign body (meat impaction)
Glucagon
Esophageal spasm
Nitrates
Calcium channel blockers
Ethanol withdrawal
See Alcohol withdrawal
Expectorant
Iodide

Fever
Salicylates
Nonsteroidal anti-inflammatory drugs
Acetaminophen
Fluid overload
Diuretics
Loop diuretics: furosemide, ethacrynic acid, bumetanide,
thiazides, torsemide
Carbonic anhydrase inhibitors: acetazolamide

Metolazone
Spironolactone
Fungal infection
Amphotericin B
Flucytosine
Ketoconazole

Gastroesophageal reflux
Antacids
Histamine H$_2$ receptor antagonists
Sucralfate
Promotility agents
Gastroparesis
Promotility agents
Glaucoma: Acute angle closure
Mannitol
Acetazolamide
Goiter: Nontoxic
Thyroid hormone
Gout
Allopurinol
Colchicine
Nonsteroidal anti-inflammatory agents
Growth deficiency
Growth hormone

Heart block
See Bradycardia
Heart failure
See Congestive heart failure
Hepatic encephalopathy
Neomycin
Lactulose
Bromocriptine
Levodopa
Hiccup
Chlorpromazine
Hyperammonemia
See Hepatic encephalopathy

Hypercalcemia
Diuretics
Calcitonin
Etidronate, panidronate
Plicamycin (mithramycin)
Glucocorticoids (especially vitamin D–mediated)
Hyperglycemia
Insulin
Sulfonylureas
Hyperkalemia
Calcium
Loop diuretics
Insulin/glucose
Sodium polystyrene sulfonate (Kayexalate)
Sodium bicarbonate
Hypermagnesemia
Calcium
Diuretics
Hyperparathyroidism
See Hypercalcemia
Hyperphosphatemia
Amphojel, ALternaGEL, Basaljel
Hypertension
Diuretics
β-adrenergic antagonists
α-adrenergic antagonist
Combined α- and β-adrenergic antagonists
Angiotensin converting enzyme inhibitors
Nitrates
Nitroprusside
Calcium channel blockers
Trimethaphan
Vasodilators
Clonidine
Methyldopa
Hypertension: Intracranial
See Cerebral edema
Hyperthermia
See Malignant hyperthermia; Fever

Hyperthyroidism
  Propylthiouracil
  Methimazole
  Iodide
  Lithium
  β-adrenergic antagonists
Hypertrophic obstructive cardiomyopathy
  β-adrenergic antagonists
  Calcium channel blockers
Hyperuricemia
  Allopurinol
  Mannitol
Hypoaldosteronism
  Fludrocortisone
Hypocalcemia
  Calcium
  Vitamin D
Hypoglycemia
  Glucose
  Glucagon
  Diazoxide (insulinoma)
Hypokalemia
  Potassium salts
Hypomagnesemia
  Magnesium
Hyponatremia
  See Syndrome of inappropriate antidiuretic hormone
Hypoparathyroidism
  See Hypocalcemia
Hypophosphatemia
  Phosphorus
Hypotension
  α-adrenergic agonists
  Combined α- and β-adrenergic agonists
Hypothyroidism
  Thyroid hormone (thyroxine, T_4)
Hypotonic agents
  Glucagon
  Narcotics (*See* Diarrhea)

Hypovolemia
  Dextran
  Albumin, hetastarch

Infection
  See Bacterial infection
  See Viral infection
  See Fungal infection

Inflammation
  Salicylates
  Nonsteroidal anti-inflammatory drugs
  Glucocorticoids

Inotropic agents
  See Congestive heart failure

Insomnia
  See Sedation

Intracranial hypertension
  See Cerebral edema

Ketoacidosis
  Insulin

Labor: Premature
  Selective β-agonists
  Magnesium

Malabsorption
  Pancreatic enzymes
  Lactase replacement preparations

Malignant hyperthermia
  Dantrolene

Manic depressive illness
  Lithium

Metabolic acidosis
  Carbicarb
  Sodium bicarbonate
  Tris-hydroxymethyl-amino methane (Tham)

Metabolic alkalosis
  See Appendix G: Metabolic Alkalosis
  Potassium
  Acetazolamide
  Ammonium chloride
  Hydrochloric acid

Loop diuretics
    Furosemide, ethacrynic acid, bumetanide, torsemide
Metolazone
Potassium-sparing diuretics
    Spironolactone (inhibits aldosterone)
Dopamine

Opioid antagonists
Naloxone

Organ transplantation: Immunosuppression
Glucocorticoids
Cyclosporine

Organophosphate poisoning
See Appendix H: Antidotes to Poisoning/Overdose
Atropine
Pralidoxime

Orthostatic hypotension
Fludrocortisone

Osteomalacia
Vitamin D
Calcium

Osteoporosis
Calcium
Calcitonin

Overdose
See Appendix H: Antidotes to Poisoning/Overdose
See Poisoning

Paget's disease of bone
Calcitonin
Diphosphonates
Etidronate, pamidronate

Pain
See Analgesia

Panic attack
Benzodiazepines
Tricyclic antidepressants
Monoamine oxidase inhibitors
Selective serotonin reuptake inhibitors

Parkinsonism
Amantadine
Levodopa

Peptic ulcer
  Antacids
  Histamine H_2 receptor blockers
  Sucralfate
  See Proton pump inhibitors
Proton pump inhibitors
  Omeprazole
Prostaglandin analogs
  Misoprostol
Peristaltic stimulation
  Vasopressin
  Promotility agents
  Metoclopramide
  Cisapride
  Bethanechol
Pheochromocytoma
  α-adrenergic antagonists
  β-adrenergic antagonists (only after α-antagonist)
  Combined α- and β-adrenergic antagonists
  Magnesium
Poisoning
  See Appendix H: Antidotes to Poisoning/Overdose
  Activated charcoal
  Acetylcysteine (acetaminophen)
  Cholinesterase inhibitors (tricyclics, anticholinesterases)
  Atropine (organophosphates)
  Digoxin immune Fab (digoxin)
Preeclampsia
  See Eclampsia
Premature labor
  See Labor: Premature
Protozoan infection
  Metronidazole
    Trichomoniasis, amebiasis, giardiasis, American mucocuta-
      neous leishmaniasis
  Pyrimethamine
    Malaria, toxoplasmosis
  Sulfonamides
    Toxoplasmosis

Pentamidine
Pneumocystis carinii, Trypanosoma
Trimethoprim/sulfamethoxazole
P. carinii
Pruritus
Antihistamines
Psychosis
Phenothiazines
Butyrophenomes
Haloperidol
Lithium
Combined treatment with benzodiazepines
See Agitation
Pulmonary edema
See Congestive heart failure
Diuretics
See Fluid overload
Narcotics
Pulmonary hypertension
Isoproterenol
Calcium channel blockers
Nitrates
Amrinone (inotropic agent/vasodilator)
Hydralazine
Prostaglandin E_1

Rabies
See Appendix C: Rabies Prevention
Respiratory depression
Doxapram

Secretions
Iodine
Atropine
Sedation
See Agitation
Narcotics
Antihistamines
Ketamine
Etomidate
Benzodiazepines

Tricyclic antidepressants
Barbiturates
Paraldehyde
Buspirone
Chloral hydrate
Zolpidem

Seizures
Benzodiazepines
Phenytoin (especially tonic-clonic, partial complex, complex absence seizures)
Ethosuximide (especially absence seizures, myoclonic seizures)
Valproic acid (especially myoclonic, tonic-clonic, partial, absence seizures)
Gabapentin (especially partial, focal seizures)
Primidone (especially partial, tonic-clonic seizures)
Felbamate (especially partial seizures)
Carbamazepine (especially partial, tonic-clonic seizures)
Paraldehyde (especially abstinence seizures)
Barbiturates
Magnesium

Shivering
Meperidine

Sleep
See Sedation

Spasticity
Dantrolene
Benzodiazepines

Status epilepticus
See Seizures

Stress ulcer
See Peptic ulcer

Syndrome of inappropriate antidiuretic hormone (SIADH)
Diuretics
Furosemide/sodium replacement
Lithium
Demeclocycline

Tachycardia
Adenosine
Amiodarone

Calcium channel blockers
β-adrenergic blockers
Digoxin (atrial tachyarrhythmias)
See Arrhythmia: Cardiac

Tetanus
See Appendix B: Tetanus Prophylaxis
See Sedation

Thrombosis
Dextran
Heparin
Low molecular weight heparin
Heparin/dihydroergotamine (Embolex)
Warfarin
Thrombolytics
Antiplatelet agents

Thyroid nodule
Thyroid hormone (thyroxine, T_4)

Thyrotoxicosis
See Hyperthyroidism

Transplantation
See Organ transplantation: Immunosuppression

Ulcer
See Peptic ulcer

Urticaria
See Pruritus

Variceal bleeding
Vasopressin
β-blockers
Octreotide

Vasodilators
Nitroprusside
Nitrates
Angiotensin converting enzyme inhibitors
Calcium channel blockers
Hydralazine
Prazosin
α-adrenergic antagonists
Phosphodiesterase inhibitors
Isoproterenol

Vasopressors
  α-adrenergic agonists
  Calcium
  Vasopressin
Vasospasm
  Nitrates
  Calcium channel blockers
Vertigo
  See Nausea/vomiting
Viral infection
  See Appendix C: Rabies Prevention
  See Appendix D: Prophylaxis of Viral Hepatitis
  See Appendix A: Treatment of Specific Infections
  Acyclovir
    Herpes simplex virus, varicella-zoster virus
  Amantadine
    Prophylaxis and treatment of influenza A virus
  Zidovudine (AZT)
    Retroviruses (AIDS)
  Ribavirin
    Respiratory syncytial virus
Vomiting
  See Nausea/vomiting

DRUGS

2

Drugs

ACETAMINOPHEN

Trade Names: *Aspirin Free Anacin-3, Datril, Tempra, Tylenol,* among others.

Drug Action: Acetaminophen has analgesic and antipyretic properties similar to aspirin but weak anti-inflammatory activity. The antipyretic action of acetaminophen, like that of aspirin, is probably mediated by decreased prostaglandin levels in the hypothalamus; however, unlike aspirin, acetaminophen has little effect peripherally on prostaglandin synthesis. The drug does not affect platelet function.

Indications: Arthritic pain, myalgias, neuralgias, dysmenorrhea, pain associated with minor surgical procedures, fever. Acetaminophen is useful in patients with a history of peptic ulcer disease or clotting disorders, because there is no gastric irritation or potential for ulceration, and platelet function is not altered.

Pharmacokinetics:

1. **Absorption:** Rapid and nearly complete after PO administration; variable rectal absorption.
2. **Distribution:** Throughout most body fluids, variable plasma protein binding, but not usually significant with therapeutic doses.
3. **Metabolism:** Greater than 98%; hepatic microsomal metabolism; conjugated predominately with glucuronide, sulfate, and to a lesser extent cysteine; small amounts hydroxylated and deacetylated. Less frequent dosing is needed in severe liver disease, and prolonged use should be avoided.
4. **Excretion:** Renal.
5. **Half-life:** 2 hr.

Drug Preparations: Multiple drug forms and strengths are made; the following are most commonly used:

> *Tablets:* 80, 160, 325, 500 mg.
> *Capsules:* 325, 500 mg.
> *Drops:* 100 mg/l mL.
> *Elixir/Syrup:* 160 mg/5 mL.
> *Suppositories:* 125, 325, 650 mg.

Dosage:

1. **Adult:** 325–1000 mg q 4–6 hr.
2. **Pediatric:** Approximately 60 mg/kg/24 hr in divided doses q 4–6 hr.

Adverse Effects: Fewer than with aspirin; include skin rash, drug fever, thrombocytopenia, rarely methemoglobinemia, and with prolonged abuse, nephrotoxicity. Overdose causes hepatic failure.

Drug Interactions: Metoclopramide may speed intestinal absorption.

Monitoring: Acetaminophen serum levels are of great significance when treating poisoning or overdose but are of no real value in routine clinical practice.

BIBLIOGRAPHY

McEvoy GK (ed): *AHFS Drug Information 89* Bethesda, 1988, American Society of Hospital Pharmacists.
AMA Drug Evaluations, ed 6, Philadelphia, 1986, WB Saunders.
Chernow B (ed): *The Pharmacologic Approach to the Critically Ill Patient,* ed 2, Baltimore, 1988, Williams & Wilkins.

ACETAZOLAMIDE

Trade Names: *Diamox, Diamox Sequels, Acetazolam, AK-Zol, Dazamide.*

Drug Action:

1. **Carbonic anhydrase inhibition:** Noncompetitive inhibition of the enzyme carbonic anhydrase decreases formation in the

renal tubules of hydrogen and bicarbonate ions from carbon dioxide and water.

2. **Diuresis:** Reduction of hydrogen ion concentration in the renal tubules increases excretion of sodium, potassium, water, and bicarbonate (alkaline diuresis).

Indications:

1. **Metabolic alkalosis:** Inhibition of carbonic anhydrase activity decreases formation in the renal tubules of hydrogen and bicarbonate ions from carbon dioxide and water, resulting in a net loss of bicarbonate in the urine and reduction in serum bicarbonate.
2. **Edematous states:** Increased excretion of sodium, potassium, water, and bicarbonate causes an alkaline diuresis.
3. **Glaucoma:** Acetazolamide decreases production of aqueous humor, probably by decreasing the bicarbonate concentration in ocular fluid. This is independent of the diuretic action.
4. **Epilepsy:** The mechanism of anticonvulsant activity is unclear.
5. **Altitude Sickness:** Acetazolamide produces a metabolic acidosis that results in increased respiratory drive and arterial oxygenation. Diuresis may reduce the risk of pulmonary and cerebral edema.

Pharmacokinetics:

1. **Metabolism:** None.
2. **Excretion:** Renal; 90% excreted unchanged within 24 hr.
3. **Volume of distribution:** Throughout body; highest concentration in erythrocytes and renal cortex.
4. **Protein binding:** 93%.
5. **Plasma Half-Life:** 10–15 hr (tablets).
6. **Compatibilities:** Increased risk of toxicity from high doses of salicylates.

Drug Preparations:

1. **Parenteral:**
   Vial: 500 mg dry powder reconstituted with at least 5 mL sterile water.
2. **Oral:**
   Tablets: 125, 250 mg.
   SR Capsules: 500 mg.
   Suspension: 50, 100 mg/mL.

Dosage:

1. **Adult:**
   a. **Metabolic alkalosis:** 250 mg IV/PO bid–qid until alkalosis resolves (usually 2–4 days).
   b. **Edematous states:** 5 mg/kg qd in AM, may be given for 2 days, followed by 1 day off.
   c. **Glaucoma:** 250 mg q d–qid initially, then titrated to patient response. Acute closed angle glaucoma, 500 mg IV followed by 250 mg q 4 hr.
   d. **Epilepsy:** 8–30 mg/kg/day in four divided doses.
   e. **Altitude sickness:** 250 mg q d–qid initiated 24–48 hr prior to ascent and continued for, 48 hr to control symptoms.
2. **Pediatric:** 8–30 mg/kg in divided doses.
   a. **Glaucoma:** usually 10–15 mg/kg in divided doses.
   b. **Anticonvulsant:** 8–30 mg/kg/day in divided doses.

Adverse Effects:

1. **Common:** Malaise, anorexia, weight loss, fatigue, headache, weakness, nervousness, loss of libido, impotence, paresthesia, lethargy, depression, gastric distress, nausea, vomiting, diarrhea, troublesome diuresis, hypokalemia.
2. **Uncommon:** Severe metabolic acidosis, confusion, ataxia, tremor, tinnitus, renal calculi, gout, increased toxicity from high-dose salicylates.

Drug Interactions: May interact adversely with the following drugs:

1. **Increased hypokalemia:** Adrenocorticoids, amphotericin B, diuretics, urea, mineralocorticoids, mannitol.
2. **Decreased effectiveness:** Insulin, oral hypoglycemics.
3. **Increased toxicity:** Salicylates, digitalis.
4. **Increased efficacy/increased risk of toxicity:** Carbamazepine, primidone, phenytoin, ephedrine, nondepolarizing neuromuscular blocking agents.

Monitoring:

1. **Serum electrolyte and bicarbonate determinations** prior to therapy and at periodic intervals, especially in cases where electrolyte imbalance (e.g., hypokalemia) would be detrimental.

2. **Blood pH** can be monitored by arterial blood gas determinations. Can be used to monitor the course of therapy in treatment of metabolic alkalosis.
3. **Urologic examination** to detect crystalluria or renal calculi.
4. CBC with platelet count.

BIBLIOGRAPHY

Agents used to treat glaucoma. In *AMA Drug Evaluations,* Annual 1995, American Medical Association, 1995, pp 376, 842, 2232, 2242.

Carbonic anhydrase inhibitors: diuretics and cardiovasculars. In *Drug Facts and Comparisons,* New York, 1996, JB Lippincott, pp 664–667.

Carbonic anhydrase inhibitors. In *Drug Information for the Health Care Provider,* Rockville, 1995, US Pharmacopeial Convention, pp. 658–664.

Weiner IM, Mudge GH: Diuretics and other agents employed in the mobilization of edema fluid. In Gilman A, Goodman L, Rall T, et al (eds): *Goodman and Gilman's The Pharmacologic Basis of Therapeutics,* ed 7, New York, 1985, Macmillan, pp 890–892.

ACETYLCYSTEINE

Trade Names: *Mucomyst, Mucosil.*

Drug Action:

1. **Mucolytic:** cleaves disulfide bonds in mucoprotein secretions.
2. Repletes hepatic stores of glutathione in the setting of acetaminophen overdose.

Indications:

1. Mucolytic agent.
2. Acetaminophen overdose.

Pharmacokinetics:

1. **Absorption:** Well absorbed from GI tract, but significant first pass effects result in limited (10%–30%) bioavailability; may be given by inhalation; IV administration has been described but is experimental.
2. **Metabolism:** Liver.
3. **Excretion:** Unknown.

Drug Preparations:

Solution: 10%, 20%.

Dosage:

1. **Direct tracheal instillation:** 1–2 mL 10% or 20% solution q 1–4 hr.
2. **Nebulizer:** 3–5 mL 20% solution q 2–3 hr.
3. **For acetaminophen toxicity:**
   a. **Oral:** Dilute to a 5% solution with fruit juice or soft drink. Initial dose 140 mg/kg, then 70 mg/kg q 4 hr for 17 doses (most effective if given within 8 hr of ingestion). The patient should receive a full course of therapy regardless of subsequent acetaminophen levels.
   b. **Intravenous (experimental and not FDA–approved):** Can be given simultaneously with activated charcoal. Load with 150 mg/kg in 200 mL D_5W over 15 min, then 50 mg/kg in 500 mL D_5W over 4 hr, followed by 100 mg/kg in 100 mL D_5W over 16 hr. An alternative IV regimen is 140 mg/kg loading dose followed by 70 mg/kg IV q 4 hr $\times$ 17 doses.

Adverse Effects:

1. **Respiratory:** Rhinorrhea, hemoptysis, bronchospasm.
2. **Gastrointestinal:** Nausea, vomiting, stomatitis.
3. **CNS:** Drowsiness.
4. **Skin:** Rash, urticaria.
5. **Other:** Fever, anaphylaxis (IV only).

Drug Interactions:

1. **GI absorption** decreased by activated charcoal but not to a clinically significant degree.

2. **Incompatible** with tetracyclines, ampicillin, erythromycin, amphotericin B.

Monitoring: No specific monitoring required when used for inhalation/mucolytic therapy.

1. **Acetaminophen overdose:** Monitor one acute acetaminophen serum levels ($\geq$4 hr postingestion) and serial liver function tests.

BIBLIOGRAPHY

Howland MA, Smilkstein MJ, Weisman RS. *N*-Acetylcysteine. In Goldfrank LR, Flomenbaum NE, Lewin NA, et al (eds): *Toxicologic Emergencies,* ed 5, Norwalk, 1990, Appleton & Lange, p 498.

Committee on Injury and Poison Prevention. *Handbook of Common Poisonings in Children,* ed 3, 1994, American Academy of Pediatrics, p 36.

Facts and Comparisons Loose-Leaf Drug Information Service, 1995, p 182c.

ACTIVATED CHARCOAL

Trade Names: *Activated Charcoal Powder, Actidose-Aqua, Actidose with Sorbitol, Charcoaid, Liqui-Char, Superchar.*

Drug Action:

1. **Antidote:** Adsorbs toxins and inhibits their GI absorption.
2. **Antidiarrheal:** Adsorbs toxic and nontoxic irritants.

Indications:

1. Poisoning
2. Diarrhea due to toxins.

Pharmacokinetics:

1. **Absorption:** None from GI tract.
2. **Metabolism:** None.
3. **Excretion:** Feces.

4. **Half-life:** None.
5. **Maximal drug adsorbed:** 100–1000 mg/g charcoal.

Drug Preparations:

Powder: 15, 30, 40, 120, 240 g.
Liquid Suspension: 4, 4.8, 5, 8, g/mL.

Dosage:

1. Insoluble in water, GI transit time decreased by coadministration of a cathartic such as 70% sorbitol.
2. **For poisoning** (adult/pediatric):
   a. **Initial:** 1 g/kg. Enterally; ≥10 : 1 charcoal:drug ratio when known amount of ingested toxin.
   b. **Maintenance:** ("multidose charcoal"—see below): 0.75–1.0 g/kg enterally q 4 hr until the patient is stable and out of danger.

Adverse Effects: Contraindicated: bowel obstruction, ileus, toxins unaffected/not adsorbed.

Constipation, diarrhea, nausea, vomiting, black stools, aspiration, bowel obstruction/perforation.

Drug Interactions:

1. Can inactivate and absorb most PO and some IV medications used therapeutically. Multidose activated charcoal is particularly effective for drugs that undergo enterohepatic circulation (e.g., theophylline, digitoxin, glutethimide), enteroenteric circulation (e.g., phencyclidine, phenobarbital, tricyclic antidepressants), or sustained release/enteric coated preparations.
2. Ineffective for poisoning due to ions (cyanide, iron, lithium), caustics, alcohols, hydrocarbons.
3. Adsorptive capacity diminished by milk, ice cream.

Monitoring: No specific monitoring other than ongoing airway patency and protection.

1. Follow specific drug levels for overdose as clinically indicated.

BIBLIOGRAPHY

Flomenbaum NE, Goldfrank LR, Weisman RS, et al: General management of the poisoned or overdosed patient. In Goldfrank LR,

Flomenbaum NE, Lewin NA, et al: *Toxicologic Emergencies,* ed 5, Norwalk, 1994, Appleton & Lange, p 25.

Smilkstein MJ, Flomenbaum NE: Techniques used to prevent absorption of toxic compounds. In Goldfrank LR, Flomenbaum NE, Lewin NA, et al: *Toxicologic Emergencies,* ed 5, Norwalk, 1994, Appleton & Lange, p 47.

Committee on Injury and Poison Prevention: Handbook of common poisonings in children, ed. 3, 1994, American Academy of Pediatrics, p 8.

Facts and Comparisons loose-leaf drug information service, 1995, p 713c.

Charcoal, activated. In *Drug Facts and Comparisons,* New York, 1989, JB Lippincott, pp 2185–2186.

ACYCLOVIR

Trade Name: *Zovirax.*

Drug Action:

1. Converted into monophosphate by cells containing viral-coded thymidine kinase; then as triphosphate, interferes with herpesvirus DNA polymerase, inhibiting viral DNA replication.
2. Active against herpes simplex virus (HSV) types 1 and 2 and varicella-zoster virus (VZV).
3. Not clinically useful against cytomegalovirus (CMV), Epstein-Barr virus (EBV), or human herpesvirus 6 (HHV).

Indications:

1. **Immunocompromised patients:**
   a. **HSV infections:** Given PO or IV, prevents reactivation in transplant recipients, patients with leukemia; treats active infections, including AIDS (e.g., perianal or CNS disease).
   b. **VZV infections:** Beneficial when given IV within 72 hr of outbreak; prevents complications of pneumonitis, hepatitis, thrombocytopenia.

2. **Normal hosts:**
   a. **HSV infections:**
      (1) **HSV encephalitis:** Drug of choice and superior to vidarabine.
      (2) **HSV genital, labial, perianal, rectal infection:** Useful in first episode (IV if severe) and recurrent disease.
      (3) (?) **Herpes zoster:** Controversial, but may be considered if ophthalmic branch of trigeminal nerve involved (high dose PO or IV).

Pharmacokinetics:

1. **Absorption:** Slow, variable, and incomplete (bioavailability 15%–30%).
2. **Distribution:** Into all tissues (kidney highest, CNS lowest).
3. **Excretion:** Renal.
   a. **Hemodialysis:** Readily hemodialysable, and 60% of drug is removed during single 6-hr course. No data on peritoneal dialysis but should work.
4. **Plasma half-life:** 3.3 hr with normal renal function; approximately 20 hr with anuria.

Drug Preparations:

Zovirax Capsules: 200 mg.
Zovirax Ointment: 5% in 15-g tube.
Zovirax Sodium for IV infusion: 500 mg/10 mL.

Dosage:

1. *Oral:*
   a. Treatment of initial genital herpes: 200 mg five times per day for 10 days.
   b. Chronic suppressive therapy for recurrent HSV disease: 200 mg tid for up to 6 mo (patients have taken for, e.g., 4 yr without identified adverse effect).
   c. Intermittent therapy for recurrent HSV disease: 200 mg five times per day for 5 days, initiated at the earliest sign or symptom (prodrome) of recurrence.
   d. Herpes zoster: 800 mg five times per day for 5–10 days, begun as early as possible.
2. *Ointment:* Reserved for immunocompromised hosts with mucocutaneous HSV. Inferior to PO or IV.

3. *Intravenous:*
   a. **Normal renal function:**

Infection	Dose (q 8 hr)	Duration (day)
Immunocompromised:		
HSV (prophylaxis)	250 mg/m^2	Duration
HSV (treatment)	250 mg/m^2	7
VZV (herpes zoster or varicella)	500 mg/m^2	7
Nonimmunocompromised:		
HSV encephalitis	10 mg/kg	10
Primary HSV genital infection	5 mg/kg	5
VZV (rarely indicated)	5 mg/kg	≥5

   b. **Renal insufficiency:**

Creatinine clearance (mL/min/1.73m^2)	Dose (q 8 hr)	Dosing Interval (hr)
>50	5	8
25–50	5	12
10–25	5	24
0–10	2.5	24

Adverse Effects:

1. **Phlebitis and IV site irritation** (high pH).
2. **Renal dysfunction** (reversible and related to IV use and crystallization).
3. **Liver enzyme elevation.**
4. **Neurotoxicity:** CNS toxicity (e.g., delirium tremens, abnormal EEG).

Drug Interactions:

1. *Probenecid:* Inhibits renal clearance.
2. *Methotrexate:* Decreased elimination with higher levels.

ADENOSINE

Trade Name: *Adenocard.*

Drug Action: Slows conduction time through AV node; can interrupt reentry pathways.

Indications: Paroxysmal supraventricular tachycardia secondary to AV node re-entry and accessory pathways (including Wolff-Parkinson-White syndrome).

Contraindications: Second- or third-degree AV block, sick sinus syndrome, atrial flutter/fibrillation, ventricular tachycardia/fibrillation.

Pharmacokinetics:

1. Must be given IV.
2. Taken up by erythrocytes and vascular endothelial cells; metabolized to inosine and adenosine monophosphate.
3. Serum half-life <10 sec.
4. Not affected by renal/hepatic disease.

Drug Preparations:

   Vial: 6 mg/2 mL

Dosage: Adults. 3, 6, 9, 12 mg IV (fast injection).

Adverse Effects:

1. May cause transient AV block, bradycardia.
2. Bronchospasm rarely.
3. Facial flushing, headache, sweating, palpitations, chest pain, rare hypotension.
4. Dyspnea, shortness of breath, hyperventilation.
5. Lightheadedness, tingling, numbness, blurred vision, neck/back pain.
6. Nausea, metallic taste, throat tightness.

Drug Interactions:

1. Antagonized by methylxanthines such as caffeine and theophylline.
2. Potentiated by dipyridamole.
3. Higher degrees of heart block with carbamazepine.

Monitoring: ECG, blood pressure, heart rate.

BIBLIOGRAPHY

DiMarco JP, Miles W, Akhtar M, et al: Adenosine for paroxysmal supraventricular tachycardia: dose ranging and comparison with verapamil, *Ann Intern Med,* 1990, 113:104–110.

ALCOHOL WITHDRAWAL SYNDROME MEDICATIONS

Trade Names:
  Benzodiazepines:
    Chlordiazepoxide: *Librium.*
    Diazepam: *Valium.*
    Oxazepam: *Serax.*
    Midazolam: *Versed.*
  Paraldehyde: *Paral.*
  Atenolol: *Tenormin.*
  Haloperidol
    See haloperidol
  Clonidine:
    See clonidine

Drug Action:

1. **Benzodiazepines** are CNS depressants. Their anxiolytic and anticonvulsant properties are mediated via facilitation or enhancement of the inhibitory neurotransmitter γ-aminobutyric acid (GABA). Additional properties of benzodiazepines (muscle relaxation, amnesia, anticonvulsant) ameliorate the symptoms of alcohol withdrawal.
2. **Paraldehyde** is a nonspecific CNS depressant.
3. **Atenolol** is a β_1-selective adrenergic receptor blocker.

Indications: All the above agents are used in managing alcohol withdrawal syndrome. Both paraldehyde and the benzodiazepines are anxiolytics and anticonvulsants. Intravenous benzodiazepines are used to gain control in acute alcohol withdrawal. Atenolol is indicated in alcohol withdrawal because it is thought to block the stress response associated with increased serum catecholamines (e.g., hypertension, arrhythmias, angina).

Pharmacokinetics: *See* Table 1.

Drug Preparations: *See* Table 2.

Dosage: *See* Table 3.

Adverse Effects:

1. **Benzodiazepines** cause mental status depression, clumsiness, weakness, fatigue, amnesia.
2. **Paraldehyde** causes drowsiness, characteristic "fruity" breath odor, clumsiness, dizziness, nausea/vomiting. Hepatitis can occur with prolonged use.
3. **Atenolol** can cause bronchoconstriction in patients with reactive airway disease, hypotension, bradycardia, constipation, or diarrhea. β-blockers can mask symptoms of hypoglycemia.

Drug Interactions:

1. **Benzodiazepines** are additive with other CNS depressants. They can potentiate antihypertensives. Cimetidine delays elimination of benzodiazepines. Carbamazepine and rifampin enhance elimination of benzodiazepines by induction of hepatic microsomal enzyme activity.
2. **Paraldehyde** is additive with other CNS depressants. Disulfiram decreases paraldehyde metabolism, resulting in increased levels.
3. **Atenolol** potentiates the antihypertensive effects of other medications. Cimetidine increases atenolol blood levels. Pronounced bradycardia can occur with concomitant administration of cardiac glycosides and/or calcium channel blockers.
4. **Clonidine**—Hypotension, sedation.

Comments and Recommendations: Alcohol withdrawal is a serious and potentially life-threatening disorder that still has a 5%–15% mortality rate. The signs and symptoms of acute withdrawal are usually noted within the first 36 hours following abstinence and include agitation, confusion, hallucinations, anxiety, tachycardia, hypertension, tremor, insomnia, fever, and reduction of the seizure threshold. Delirium tremens or major withdrawal that includes severe agitation with disorientation and hallucination

TABLE 1.
Pharmacokinetics

Drug	Absorption	Metabolism	t½ (hr)	Duration (hr)	Excretion
Benzodiazepines					
Chlordiazepoxide	Good	Hepatic	5–30	Long	Renal/hepatic
Diazepam	Good	Hepatic	20–70	Long	Renal/hepatic
Oxazepam	Good	Hepatic	5–15	Short	Renal/hepatic
Lorazepam	Good	Hepatic	4–8	Medium	Renal/hepatic
Midazolam	Give IV/IM	Hepatic	2–6	1–4	Renal
Paraldehyde	Good	Hepatic	—	8	Hepatic
Atenolol	50%	Hepatic	6–7	Long	Renal

TABLE 2.
Drug Preparations

Drug	Tabs/Caps	Syrup	Parenteral
Benzodiazepines			
Chlordiazepoxide	5, 10, 25 mg	—	100 mg/2 mL
Diazepam	2, 5, 10 mg	—	5 mg/mL
Oxazepam	10, 15, 30 mg	—	—
Lorazepam	0.5, 1, 2 mg	—	2, 4 mg/ml
Midazolam	—	—	1, 5 mg/mL
Paraldehyde	—	5, 30 mL	5, 30 mL
Atenolol	50, 100 mg	—	—

TABLE 3.
Drug Dosage

Drug	Oral	Parenteral
Benzodiazepines*		
Chlordiazepoxide	50, 100 mg tid/qid up to 300 mg/day	50–100 mg IM/IV q2–4h
Diazepam	10 mg tid/qid × 24 hr	10 mg, then 5–10 mg q3–4h
Oxazepam	15–30 mg tid/qid	—
Lorazepam	2–10 mg/day bid–qid	1–4 mg IV
Midazolam	—	1–4 mg IV/IM
Paraldehyde*†	5–10 mL q4–6h to 60 mL/day	5 mL IM q4–6h to 30 mL/day
Atenolol	50–100 mg/day	—

*With the benzodiazepines and paraldehyde there is dosage reduction after 24 hours of therapy to avoid oversedation. A good general rule is that the initial total daily dose is reduced 25%–33% and divided q6–8h. This same reduction is continued on subsequent days (*see* Comments and Recommendations).

†Paraldehyde 5–10 mL can be diluted with 1 or 2 parts olive oil, cottonseed oil, or normal saline solution and administered rectally.

occurs in only 5% of patients. Many times the clinician is alerted to the potential for alcohol withdrawal because the patient presents with an alcohol-related disease (e.g., gastritis, pancreatitis, aspiration pneumonia). In some cases, such as acute myocardial infarction or traumatic injury, a patient's physical dependence on alcohol may not be readily recognized; therefore, a high index of suspicion must be maintained.

General supportive management includes IV hydration, correction of electrolyte disturbances (particularly potassium and magnesium), and thiamine replacement (100 mg IM or slow IV infusion). The patient should be kept under close supervision in a quiet setting.

Benzodiazepines are the cornerstone of specific pharmacotherapy. There is no evidence that one is better than another. Chlordiazepoxide and diazepam are longer-acting agents with active metabolites; therefore, therapy can be complicated by their cumulation. Once withdrawal symptoms are acutely controlled with careful titration of an IV preparation, this initial total daily dose can be given orally and reduced each subsequent day by 25%–33% and given in divided doses q 6–8 hr (e.g., chlordiazepoxide: day 1, 400 mg; day 2, 300 mg; day 3, 200 mg; day 4, 100 mg, . . .). Occasionally, very high doses, usually IV diazepam, are required to gain control in a patient with acute withdrawal. In such situations, more rapid reduction in PO dosage on subsequent days is recommended. Oxazepam has a shorter half-life; hence, accumulation is less likely.

Paraldehyde is useful in alcohol withdrawal but is more toxic and less effective than the benzodiazepines. The large-volume (5 mL) IM injections are painful and associated with sterile abscesses. Rectal administration is impractical in the agitated alcoholic and has been associated with proctitis.

Atenolol can be used in patients with resting heart rate >50 bpm, with benzodiazepines added if necessary. Atenolol therapy is associated with a shorter hospital course and less benzodiazepine requirement.

Clonidine may have a role in amelioration of central hyperadrenergic symptoms.

Alcohol withdrawal seizures occur up to 48 hours after cessation of drinking. They are usually nonfocal and generalized, can occur two or three times, and are self-limited. Acute treatment with IV benzodiazepines, usually diazepam or lorazepam, is indicated.

BIBLIOGRAPHY

Goldfrank LR, Delaney KA, Flomenbaum NE: Substance withdrawal. In Goldfrank LR, Flomenbaum NE, Lewin NA, et al (eds): *Toxicologic Emergencies,* ed 5, Norwalk, 1986, Appleton & Lange, p 905.

Drug Information for the Health Care Provider, ed 6, Rockville, 1986, US Pharmacopeial Convention.

Kraus M, Gottlieb L, Horwitz R, et al: Randomized clinical trial of atenolol in patients with alcohol withdrawal, *N Engl J Med* 1985, 313:905–909.

Physicians Desk Reference, ed 42, Oradel, NJ, 1988, Medical Economics Co.

Sellers E, Kalant H: Alcohol: intoxication and withdrawal, *N Engl J Med* 1976, 294:757–762.

Thompson W, Johnson A, Maddrey W: Diazepam and paraldehyde for treatment of severe delirium tremens, *Ann Intern Med* 1975, 82:175–180.

ALLOPURINOL

Trade Names: *Zyloprim, Lopurin;* several generic drugs.

Drug Action: The end product of purine metabolism is uric acid, which when present in large amounts in the glomerular filtrate or joint fluid can precipitate out of solution and form crystals. The final result is renal tubular damage and joint inflammation.

Allopurinol is a structural analog of hypoxanthine and is converted to oxipurinol (alloxanthine) by xanthine oxidase. Both allopurinol and oxipurinol inhibit xanthine oxidase, thus decreasing the production of uric acid. Hypoxanthine and xanthine may then be reutilized in purine biosynthesis. Hypoxanthine and xanthine are more soluble than uric acid and may be renally excreted with less propensity to produce crystals.

Indications:

1. **Hyperuricemia in gout.** Prevention of gouty arthritis and nephropathy.
2. **Hyperuricemia resulting from tumor lysis.** After chemotherapy for a variety of cancers, especially lymphomas and leukemias, large quantities of nucleic acids are released and metabolized to uric acid. If enough uric acid is produced, urinary crystals form. In large quantities the urate crystals can result in nephron injury, with the potential for acute renal failure. Allopurinol added to the chemotherapy regimen can avert this process. Other therapeutic measures include adequate hydration and diuresis as well as alkalinization of urine.
3. Prevention of recurrent calcium oxalate calculi.

Pharmacokinetics

1. **Absorption:** Rapid, nearly complete after PO administration. Decreases in uric acid occur within 1–2 days with peak effect in 1–2 wk.
2. **Distribution:** In total body water, not plasma protein bound. Secreted in breast milk.
3. **Metabolism:** Converted to oxipurinol.
4. **Excretion:** Approximately 20% may be excreted unchanged in urine.
5. **Half-life:** Elimination t½ is 1–2 hr for allopurinol, 18–24 hr for oxipurinol; both drugs are cleared by glomerular filtration, but oxypurinol is reabsorbed in the tubules. Half-life is prolonged by renal insufficiency. Both allopurinol and oxypurinol are dialyzable.

Drug Preparations:

Tablets: 100, 300 mg.

Dosage:

1. Adults: 200–800 mg/day in two to four divided doses. Children: 10 mg/kg/day in two to three divided doses.
2. **Impaired renal function:** Dosage must be reduced in proportion to the reduction in glomerular filtration; 100 mg/day or 300 mg twice weekly is often satisfactory.

Adverse Effects: Various skin disorders may occur in 1%–3% of patients and include urticaria, various rashes, exfoliative lesions, and vasculitides. Stevens-Johnson syndrome, hepatotoxicity, bone marrow depression, thrombocytopenia, leukopenia, and pancytopenia (especially when the drug is used in conjunction with chemotherapeutic agents) are other serious adverse effects. Drowsiness, headache, neuritis, nausea/vomiting, diarrhea, gastrointestinal upset, fever, and chills also are occasionally seen. The presence of any of these conditions requires that allopurinol therapy be discontinued, or at least that therapy with the drug be seriously evaluated.

Drug Interactions: Dosage of 6-mercaptopurine and azathioprine should be reduced (metabolism inhibited) by 25%–33% of that normally used when given in conjunction with allopurinol. Also, allopurinol prolongs the half-life of PO anticoagulants, theophylline and chloropropamide.

Monitoring: Serum uric acid level should be frequently assessed and kept below 6–8 mg/dL, the upper limit of normal. Also, liver and renal function and blood counts should be periodically assessed and therapy evaluated as needed.

BIBLIOGRAPHY

Insel PA: Analgesic-antipyretics and antiinflammatory agents: drugs employed in the treatment of rheumatoid arthritis and gout. In Gilman AG et al (eds): *The Pharmacological Basis of Therapeutics,* 8th ed, New York, 1993, McGraw-Hill, pp 676–679.

Day RD, Birkett DJ, Hicks M, et al: New uses for allopurinol, *Drugs* 1994, 48:339–344.

Conaghan PG, Day RO: Risks and benefits of drugs used in the management and prevention of gout, *Drug Safety* 1994, 11:252–258.

ALPRAZOLAM

Trade Name: *Xanax.*

Drug Action: 1, 4-benzodiazepine class.

Anxiety reduction, sedation, anticonvulsant, muscle relaxation, amnesia, antipanic, antidepressant (?).

Indications: Anxiety and panic disorder.

Pharmacokinetics:

1. **Metabolism:** Hepatic oxidation.
2. **Half-life:** 12 hr (mean). Longer in elderly patients.
3. **Excretion:** α-OH-metabolites excreted by kidneys.
4. **Dialyzable:** Limited.
5. **Renal failure:** Monitor for sedation.
6. **Hepatic failure:** Reduce dose and monitor for sedation.

Dosage: 0.25, 0.5, 1.0, 2.0 mg tablets.

1. **Antianxiety:** Initial dose 0.25–0.5 mg tid; may be titrated to 2 mg tid.
2. **Panic disorder:** usually responds to doses of 3–6 mg/day in divided doses.

Adverse Effects: Sedation, psychomotor impairment, depression, amnesia, impaired concentration, weakness, impaired sexual function, paradoxical agitation.

Drug Interactions: Oral contraceptives increase half-life of alprazolam. Additive effect with other CNS depressants.

Monitoring: Monitor for excess sedation vs. therapeutic effect.

BIBLIOGRAPHY

Drugs used for anxiety and sleep disorders. In *AMA Drug Evaluations,* ed 6, Philadelphia, 1986, WB Saunders, pp 81–110.
Sussman N: The benzodiazepines: selection and use in treating anxiety, insomnia, and other disorders, *Hosp Formul* 1985, 20:298–305.

ALPROSTADIL

Trade Name: *Prostin VR Pediatric.*

Drug Action:

1. Prostaglandin E_1.
2. Relaxes and dilates vascular smooth muscle.

3. Inhibits platelet aggregation.
4. Stimulates intestinal and uterine smooth muscle.

Indications: Maintain patency of ductus arteriosus.

Pharmacokinetics:

1. **Absorption:** Give IV continuously.
2. **Metabolism:** Lung.
3. **Excretion:** Urine.
4. **Plasma half-life:** <1 min.

Drug preparations:

Injection: 500 μg/mL.

Dosage:

1. **Initial:** 0.05–0.1 μg/kg/min IV.
2. **Maintenance:** Once therapeutic effect seen, attempt to taper dose (by 0.01 μg/kg/min) to lowest effective dose.

Adverse Effects:

1. **Respiratory:** Bronchospasm, respiratory distress, tachypnea, apnea, respiratory depression.
2. **Cardiovascular:** Hypotension, flushing, tachycardia, edema, bradycardia, heart block, arrhythmias.
3. **GI:** Diarrhea, esophageal reflux, hyperbilirubinemia.
4. **CNS:** Apnea, seizures, fever, cerebral bleeding, lethargy, hypothermia, stiffness, hyperirritability.
5. **Hematologic:** Anemia, thrombocytopenia, bleeding, disseminated intravascular coagulation (DIC).
6. **Other:** Hypokalemia, hyperkalemia, hypoglycemia, sepsis, cortical hyperostosis (long-term infusion).

Drug Interactions: Unknown.

Monitoring:

1. Blood pressure, heart rate, respiratory rate.
2. Respiratory status.
3. Serum potassium, bilirubin.
4. Arterial oxygenation, blood pH.
5. Blood cell counts.
6. Prothrombin time (PT), partial thromboplastin time (PTT).

BIBLIOGRAPHY

Alprostadil. In *Drug Facts and Comparisons,* New York, 1989, JB Lippincott, p 22–23.

Alprostadil. In *AMA Drug Evaluations,* ed 6, Philadelphia, 1986, WB Saunders, p 483.

AMANTADINE

Trade Names: *Amantadine hydrochloride, Symmetrel.*

Drug Action:

1. **Mechanism of action:** (?) Inhibits uncoating and release of RNA.
2. **Spectrum of activity:** Clinically inhibits **only influenza A viruses,** not influenza B or parainfluenza viruses.

Indications:

1. **Prophylaxis of influenza A:**
   a. **Alone without vaccine:** High-risk groups for entire epidemic when unable to take vaccine secondary to allergy to egg products or hypersensitivity to vaccine.
   b. **With vaccine:** Short-term (10–14 days) use until antibodies develop.
   c. Use seasonally, postexposure, or for control of institutional outbreak when influenza A is suspected or known to be involved.
2. **Treatment of influenza A:**
   a. Start within 48–72 hr; associated with shortening of duration of fever, symptoms, selected pulmonary function abnormalities, and viral shedding.
   b. Use in high-risk patients (elderly, those with diabetes mellitus and pulmonary, cardiac, or neuromuscular disease).
3. **Treatment of parkinsonism.**

Pharmacokinetics:

1. **Metabolism:** Small (10%).
2. **Excretion:** Renal.

3. **Absorption:** 85%–95% after PO administration.
4. **Plasma half-life:** 15 hr with normal renal function.

Drug Preparations:

Capsules/Tablets: 100 mg.
Liquid: 50 mg/mL.

Dosage:

1. **Normal renal function:**
   a. **Prophylaxis of influenza A:** 200 mg/day, either as single dose or split bid to decrease side effects. Daily during influenza outbreak or for 10 days after contact.
   b. **Treatment of influenza A:** 200 mg/day as soon as possible after onset of signs and symptoms (preferably within 24–48 hr), continued for 24–48 hr after disappearance of signs and symptoms.
2. **Impaired renal function:**

Creatinine Clearance (mL/min/1.73 m2)	Dosage
30–50	200 mg first day, and 100 mg daily thereafter
15–29	200 mg first day, then 100 mg on alternate days
<15	200 mg q 7 days

Adverse Effects:

1. **CNS:** Occur in 5%–10% of patients, with increased incidence in elderly and patients with renal insufficiency.
   a. Difficulty in thinking, confusion, lightheadedness, anxiety, insomnia, rarely hallucinations.
2. **Anticholinergic-like** effects, e.g., dry mouth, urinary retention.
3. **(?) Teratogenic potential;** avoid in pregnancy.
4. **Nausea.**

Drug Interactions: Anticholinergic drugs when administered with amantadine may result in increased adverse effects due to cholinergic blockage.

AMIKACIN

Trade Name: *Amikin.*

Drug Action:

1. Bactericidal inhibition of protein biosynthesis through binding to specific receptor sites on the 30S (sedimentation coefficient) ribosomes.
2. Primarily active against **gram-negative aerobes,** including *Pseudomonas aeruginosa.*
3. Active against staphylococci but **not** pneumococci and strepto-cocci.
4. **No** antianaerobic activity.
5. Active against *Mycobacterium avium-intracellulare* and *Nocardia asteroides.*

Indications:

1. Treatment of serious infections caused by susceptible organisms:
   a. Primarily against **gram-negative aerobic** infections.
   b. Almost never used alone outside of urinary tract:
      (1) Often combined with antipseudomonal penicillin or cephalosporin for synergy.
   c. Decreased penetration and effectiveness in respiratory and CNS infections.

Pharmacokinetics:

1. **Excretion:** Unchanged in urine.
2. **Penetration:** Only 10%–20% of serum level in CNS without inflammation; does not penetrate into biliary tree in presence of obstruction.
3. **Peak serum levels:** 15–30 μg/mL.

Drug Preparations:

Amikacin sulfate for IM/IV use: 50, 250 mg/mL.

Dosage:

1. **Normal renal function:** 15 mg/kg/day divided in two or three equal doses administered at equal intervals (e.g., 7.5 mg/kg q 12 hr or 5 mg/kg q 8 hr IM/IV.

2. **Impaired renal function:**

Dose	Creatinine Clearance	Interval (hr)
5–7.5 (mg/kg)	>80	8–12
	80–50	12
	50–10	24–36
	<10 (anuria)	36–48

3. **Dialysis:**
   a. **Hemodialysis:** 2.5–3.75 mg/kg after each dialysis.
   b. **Peritoneal dialysis:** 3–4 mg/2 L dialysate removed.

Adverse Effects:

1. **Nephrotoxicity** (proximal tubular necrosis).
2. **Ototoxicity** (risk factors include renal insufficiency, high drug levels, aging, concomitant use of loop-inhibiting diuretics such as furosemide).
   a. Avoid in blind or elderly, if possible, and in persons with certain occupations (e.g., pilots).
   b. Loss of acuity at 4000–8000 cycles typically occurs before subjective hearing loss (high-frequency hearing first to go).
3. **Neuromuscular blockage effect.**
   a. May be clinically important in patients being weaned from mechanical ventilation; with myasthenia gravis, parkinsonism, botulism; in children with low calcium; in adults with low magnesium; or in patients massively transfused with citrated blood.

Drug Interactions:

1. Inactivated if mixed with antipseudomonal penicillins in IV administration system. Also, decreased aminoglycoside effect occurs with high antipseudomonal penicillin concentration *in vivo.*
2. Increased nephrotoxicity with amphotericin B, cephalothin (? other cephalosporins), polymyxins, furosemide.
3. Increased ototoxicity with loop diuretics (e.g., furosemide, ethacrynic acid).

4. Increased neuromuscular blockage with magnesium sulfate, polymyxins, neuromuscular blocking agents.

Monitoring: Peak (<25–30 μg/kg) and trough (<5 μg/kg) serum levels.

AMILORIDE

Trade Name(s): *Midamor.*

Drug Actions: Potassium sparing diuretic that inhibits aldosterone action on the cortical collecting tubule, thereby increasing sodium excretion and decreasing potassium excretion.

Indications:

1. Edema.
2. Hypertension.
3. Hypokalemia, when other measures are inadequate.

Pharmacokinetics:

1. Absorption: Incomplete (15%–20%)
2. Onset of action: Within 2 hr
3. Metabolism: Not metabolized
4. Excretion: Renal 20%–50% (unchanged), fecal 40%
5. Half-life: 6–9 hr
6. Therapeutic level:

Drug Preparations:

Tablets: 5 mg.

Dosage: 5–10 mg once daily.

Adverse Effects: Hyperkalemia, particularly when used with ACE inhibitors, salt substitutes.

Drug Interactions:

1. Antihypertensives may be potentiated.
2. Hyperkalemia may result when combined with ACE inhibitors, salt substitutes.

Monitoring: Serum electrolytes, BUN, creatinine, blood pressure.

BIBLIOGRAPHY

Diuretics. In *Drug Information for the Health Care Provider,* vol 1, ed 15, Rockville, 1995, US Pharmacolopeial Convention, pp 1152–1157.

Potassium sparing diuretics. In *Drug Facts and Comparisons,* New York, 1996, JB Lippincott, pp 616–619.

AMIODARONE

Trade Name(s): *Cordarone.*

Drug Actions:

1. Class III antiarrhythmic agent with Na^+, K^+, and Ca^{++} channel blocking properties that prolong action-potential duration.
2. Competitive α- and β-receptor blockade.

Indications:

1. Ventricular tachyarrhythmias refractory to other antiarrhythmic therapy.
2. Rapid conversion of acute atrial fibrillation/flutter to sinus rhythm.

Pharmacokinetics:

1. **Absorption:** PO 33%–65%
2. **Onset of action:** PO (days), IV (min to hr)
3. **Metabolism:** Hepatic.
4. **Excretion:** Biliary excretion.
5. **Half-life:** 20–47 days (PO and IV).
6. **Therapeutic level:** Not established.

Drug Preparations:

IV: ampules of 3 mL, 50 mg/mL.
Oral: 200-mg tablets.

Dosage: IV: 150-mg loading dose followed by 1 mg/min infusion for 6 hr, then reduce to 0.5 mg/min. Oral: 800- to 1600-mg loading dose for 1–3 wk, then 600–800 mg/day in divided doses.

Adverse Effects:

1. Hypotension.
2. Myocardial depression.
3. Bradycardia, AV block.
4. Hepatic necrosis.
5. Pulmonary fibrosis.
6. Thyroid dysfunction.
7. Nausea and vomiting.
8. Tremor, gait problem.
9. Corneal microdeposits.
10. Skin discoloration.
11. Can worsen arrhythmia, prolong QT interval.

Drug Interactions:

1. Elevates cyclosporin levels.
2. Increases β-adrenergic receptor antagonist, digoxin, flecainide, quinidine, phenytoin, procainamide levels.
3. Potentiates warfarin, dosage must be reduced.
4. Additive depressant effects with calcium channel blockers and β-blockers on AV conduction, heart rate, and contractility.

Monitoring:

1. ECG monitoring.
2. Prolonged therapy requires liver and thyroid function studies periodically.

BIBLIOGRAPHY

Bigger JT, Hoffman BF: Antiarrhythmic drugs. In Gilman AG, et al (eds): *The Pharmacological Basis of Therapeutics,* ed 8, New York, 1993, McGraw-Hill, pp 866–869.

Symposium Amiodarone: basic concepts and clinical applications, *Am Heart J* 1983, 106(4 Pt 2):788–797.

AMINOCAPROIC ACID

Trade Name: *Amicar.*

Drug Action:

1. Inhibits plasminogen activation.
2. Inhibits fibrinolysis.

Indications:

1. Bleeding secondary to excessive fibrinolysis.
2. Reversal of excessive thrombolysis due to streptokinase or urokinase.
3. Coagulopathy associated with promyelocytic leukemia in patients with low α_2-plasmin inhibitor.

Contraindications: Active intravascular clotting (e.g., DIC).

Pharmacokinetics:

1. **Absorption:** Rapid and complete from GI tract.
2. **Metabolism:** Minimal.
3. **Excretion:** 40%–60% unchanged in urine.
4. **Duration of action** in plasma <3 hr.
5. **Half-life:** Short; give by continuous IV infusion or repeated PO doses.

Drug Preparations:

> *Tablets:* 500 mg.
> *Syrup:* 250 mg/mL.
> *Injection:* 250 mg/mL.

Dosage:

1. **Adult:** 4–5 g IV over 1 hr, followed by continuous IV infusion of 1 g/hr until bleeding controlled (max. 30 g/24 hr). For chronic bleeding give 5–30 g/day PO in divided doses q 3–6 hr. Reduce dose by 25% in patients with renal failure.
2. **Pediatric:** 100 mg/kg IV over first hour, followed by continuous infusion of 33 mg/kg/hr (max. 18 g/m^2/day).

Adverse Effects:

1. **Cardiovascular:** Hypotension, bradycardia, arrhythmias, infarction, angina, thrombosis.

2. **GI:** Nausea, vomiting, diarrhea, cramps, hepatic failure.
3. **GU:** Dysuria, polyuria, red-brown urine, inhibition of ejaculation, glomerular capillary thrombosis, clots in renal pelvis, urinary tract obstruction (from clots), renal failure.
4. **CNS:** Dizziness, headache, seizures, malaise, delirium.
5. **Musculoskeletal:** Myopathy, rhabdomyolysis.
6. **Other:** Rash, tinnitus, nasal congestion, conjunctival suffusion, thrombosis, hyperkalemia.

Drug Interactions:

1. Increased risk of hypercoagulable state with estrogens.
2. Antagonizes effects of anticoagulants.

Monitoring:

1. Clotting studies.
2. ECG, blood pressure, heart rate.
3. Serum potassium, creatine kinase, alanine aminotransferase, aspartate aminotransferase, bilirubin.

BIBLIOGRAPHY

Aminocaproic acid. In *Drug Facts and Comparisons,* New York, 1989, JB Lippincott, p 241.
Aminocaproic acid. In *AMA Drug Evaluations,* ed 6, Philadelphia, 1986, WB Saunders, p 652.

AMLODIPINE

Trade Name(s): *Norvasc.*

Drug Actions: Dihydropyridine slow calcium channel blocker (vascular effect > cardiac effect), peripheral vasodilator, negative inotropic effect, inhibits coronary vasospasm.

Indications: Hypertension, chronic angina pectoris, vasospastic angina.

Pharmacokinetics:

1. **Absorption:** Oral, 60%–90% bioavailability peak levels 6–12 hr.
2. **Onset of action:** 3–6 hr.

3. **Metabolism:** Hepatic.
4. **Excretion:** 10% unchanged in urine, metabolite exacted in urine.
5. **Half-life:** Terminal half life 30–50 hr.
6. **Therapeutic level:** Decreased clearance with hepatic disease.

Drug Preparations:

Tablets: 2.5, 5, 10 mg.

Dosage: Initial 2.5–5 mg once daily (max 10 mg daily) PO.

Adverse Effects: Cardiovascular: negative inotropic effect (minimal at normal doses), hypotension, arrhythmias, bradycardia, chest pain, orthostasia, tachycardia, headache, edema, dizziness, flushing, palpitations, fatigue, nausea, abdominal pain, somnolence, anorexia, constipation, diarrhea, dysphagia.

Drug Interactions: None reported.

Monitoring: Blood pressure, heart rate.

BIBLIOGRAPHY

Haria M, Wagstaff AJ: Amlodipine—a reapproval of its pharmacological properties and therapeutic use in cardiovascular disease, *Drugs* 1995;50:560–586.

Zidek W, Sprecker C, Knaup G, et al: Comparison of the efficacy and safety of nifedipine coat-core versus amlodipine in the treatment of patients with mild-to-moderate essential hypertension, *Clin Therap* 1995, 17:686–700.

AMMONIUM CHLORIDE

Generic Drug: *Ammonium chloride.*

Drug Action:

1. Acidifying agent.
2. Expectorant.

Indications:

1. Metabolic alkalosis.
2. Urinary acidification.

Contraindications: Severe liver/kidney dysfunction.

Pharmacokinetics:

1. **Absorption:** Rapid from GI tract.
2. **Metabolism:** Liver to urea, H^+, Cl^-.
3. **Excretion:** Urine.
4. One gram provides 18.7 mEq chloride.

Dosage:

1. **Metabolic alkalosis:** 0.9–1.3 mL/min 2.14% solution based on chloride deficit. Estimated need (mEq) = ECF (20% body weight in kg) $\times$ serum chloride deficit (mEq/L). Administer one half calculated needs and recheck pH.
2. **Urine acidification:**
   a. **Adult:** 4–12 g/day PO in divided doses q 4–6 hr.
   b. **Pediatric:** 75 mg/kg PO in four divided doses.

Drug Preparations:

Tablets: 500 mg.
Injection: 2.14% (0.4 mEq/mL), 26.75% (5 mEq/mL) solution.

Adverse Effects:

1. **Respiratory:** Apnea, irregular breathing.
2. **Cardiovascular:** Bradycardia, arrhythmias.
3. **GI:** Nausea, vomiting, anorexia, diarrhea.
4. **GU:** Diuresis, glycosuria.
5. **Metabolic:** Hyperchloremia, hypokalemia, hyperglycemia, hyponatremia, hypomagnesemia, hypocalcemia, metabolic acidosis.
6. **CNS:** Headache, confusion, drowsiness, coma, hyperventilation, muscle twitching, tetany, asterixis, hyperreflexia, seizures.
7. **Other:** Pain at injection site, rash, pallor.
8. **Ammonium toxicity:** Pallor, sweating, irregular breathing, vomiting, bradycardia, arrhythmias, twitching, seizures, coma.

Drug Interactions:

1. Increased risk of acidosis with spironolactone or carbonic anhydrase inhibitors.
2. Incompatible with milk or alkaline solutions.

3. Increased urinary excretion of basic drugs (e.g., amphetamines, quinidine).

Monitoring:

1. Blood pH, Pco_2, HCO_3.
2. Urine pH.
3. Serum potassium, sodium, magnesium, calcium, chloride.

BIBLIOGRAPHY

Ammonium chloride. In *Drug Facts and Comparisons,* New York, 1989, JB Lippincott, pp 164, 3223.

Ammonium chloride. In *AMA Drug Evaluations,* ed 6, Philadelphia, 1986, WB Saunders, p 1636.

AMOXICILLIN

Trade Names: *Amoxil, Trimox, Wymox.*

Drug Action:

1. Interferes with cell wall synthesis.
2. Active against gram-positive (but **not** β-lactamase–producing staphylococci) and many gram-negative (but **not** *Pseudomonas, Klebsiella, Enterobacter, Serratia,* etc.) aerobes, plus anaerobes (but **not** *Bacteroides fragilis*).

Indications:

1. **Infections caused by sensitive organisms:**
   a. Gram-negative aerobes (*Haemophilus influenzae, Escherichia coli, Proteus mirabilis, Neisseria gonorrhoeae*) not producing β-lactamases.
   b. Gram-positive aerobes (streptococci, enterococci, nonpenicillinase staphylococci).

Pharmacokinetics:

1. **Absorption:** 80% absorbed PO; food has no effect on absorption.
2. **Excretion:** Unchanged in urine.
3. **Half-life:** 1 hr.

Drug Preparations:

Capsules: 250, 500 mg.
Tablets (+ chewable): 125, 250 mg.
Suspension: 125, 250 mg/5 mL.

Dosage:

1. **Normal renal function:** 250–500 mg q 8 hr PO.
2. **Impaired renal function:**

Dose (mg)	Creatinine Clearance	Interval (hr)
250–500	>80	8
	80–50	8
	50–10	12
	<10 (anuria)	12–24

Adverse Effects:

1. **Hypersensitivity, neurotoxicity** at high doses, diarrhea (including pseudomembranous colitis), transaminitis.
2. **Maculopapular rash** in patients with infectious mononucleosis or lymphocytic leukemia, or in those taking allopurinol.
3. Nausea/vomiting, interstitial nephritis, pancytopenia.

Drug Interactions: Rash with allopurinol.

AMOXICILLIN AND CLAVULANIC ACID

Trade Name: *Augmentin.*

Drug Action:

1. Amoxicillin inhibits cell wall synthesis; clavulanate potassium acts as a β-lactamase inhibitor.
2. Fixed combination increases spectrum of action of amoxicillin to include β-lactamase–producing organisms, including staphylococci, *H. influenzae,* gonococci.

Indications: Infections caused by susceptible organisms.

Pharmacokinetics:

1. **Absorption:** 80% absorbed PO food has no effect on absorption.
2. **Excretion:** Unchanged in urine.
3. **Half-life:** 1 hr.

Dosage: 250–500 mg q 8 hr PO.

Drug Preparations:

> *Tablets:* 250, 500 mg.
> *Chewable tablets:* 125, 250 mg.
> *PO Suspension:* 125, 250 mg/5 mL.

Both 250 and 500 mg tablets contain the same amount of clavulanic acid (125 mg); therefore, two 250-mg tablets are not equivalent to one 500-mg tablet.

Adverse Effects: Same as for amoxicillin, clavulanate adds no significant new side effects.

Drug Interactions: Same as for amoxicillin.

AMPHOTERICIN B

Trade Name: *Fungizone.*

Drug Action:

1. Interferes with cellular membranes (sterol binding with alteration of permeability, leakage, and cell lysis).
2. Active against most fungi. Includes *Candida* spp., *Histoplasma capsulatum, Cryptococcus neoformans, Aspergillus* spp.

Indications: Systemic fungal infections.

Pharmacokinetics:

1. **Metabolism:** Unknown in humans.
2. **Elimination:** Through biliary tract; not affected by renal dysfunction.
3. **Half-life, biphase:** initial 15–48 hr, terminal 15 days.

4. **Compatibilities:** Can be mixed only in D_5W; IV bottle does not need to be shielded from light.

Drug Preparations:

Vial: (50 mg) Reconstitute with sterile water. To be used IV or as bladder washout.

Cream/ lotion/ointment.

Dosage:

1. Variable (up to 1 mg/kg/day or 1.5 mg/kg qod) IV in adults.
   a. May give 1 mg dose over 2 hr; if tolerated, give 5 mg in D_5W. Give dose in 250–500 mL D_5W. Increase by 5–10 mg/day as tolerated. Duration of therapy depends on severity and nature of the infection. Total dose 1–4 g over 4–10 wks.
   b. As bladder washout (50 mg in 1000 mL D_5W/day) per Foley catheter.
2. Dosage same despite initial renal function; may be adjusted if cause of renal insufficiency is amphotericin B.
3. No change in dosage after hemodialysis.

Adverse Effects: Occur in 80%–100% of patients; usually reversible.

1. **Fever and rigors:** Common in first week. Control with salicylates, antihistamines, meperidine, hydrocortisone.
2. **Gastrointestinal upset:** Anorexia, nausea, vomiting, acute liver injury.
3. **Nephrotoxicity:** Major limiting toxicity that requires careful monitoring.
   a. Distal tubular damage, renal tubular necrosis, decrease in glomerular filtration rate (GFR), hypokalemia.
   b. Returns to normal in most patients, but may become permanent.
   c. Toxicity decreased by saline loading (i.e., 1 L normal saline) before drug administration.
4. **Anemia:** Occurs in 75% of patients, with normochromic, normocytic picture secondary to bone marrow depression. Hematocrit drops 22%–35%, but usually no need for iron or blood transfusion. Leukopenia, thrombocytopenia.

5. **Hypokalemia/Hypomagnesemia:** Develops in 25% of patients. Renal tubular defect with need for supplements.
6. **Phlebitis:** Decrease with slow administration of heparin.
7. **Cardiotoxicity:** Arrhythmias with rapid IV administration, hypotension, hypertension, flushing.
8. **Pulmonary reactions** when combined with leukocyte transfusions.
9. **CNS:** Headache, delirium, seizures.

Drug Interactions:

1. Increased nephrotoxicity when used with other nephrotoxic drugs.
2. Precipitates in fluid other than D_5W.
3. Hypokalemia may increase digitalis toxicity or neuroblocking effect of neuromuscular blocking agents.

Monitoring: Serial creatinine, electrolytes (including magnesium), hematocrit, blood pressure, heart rate. Therapeutic range 1–2 μg/mL.

AMPHOTERICIN B LIPID COMPLEX

Trade Name(s): *Abelcet* (other preparations to be marketed).

Drug Actions:

1. Amphotericin B binds to sterols in fungal cell membranes, causing changes in permeability.
2. The lipid complex formulation consists of amphotericin B complexed with two phospholipids in a 1:1 drug-to-lipid ratio. This allows delivery of greater amounts of amphotericin B and also continued amphotericin B administration in some patients who have developed nephrotoxicity on conventional amphotericin B therapy.
3. Spectrum of activity: *Aspergillus* and *Candida* spp.

Indications: Treatment of aspergillosis in patients who are refractory to or intolerant of conventional amphotericin B therapy.

Pharmacokinetics:

1. **Absorption:** IV.
2. **Metabolism:** Has larger volume of distribution and high clearance rate from blood (compared with amphotericin B desoxycholate), probably reflecting greater uptake by tissues.
3. **Half-life:** 173.4 hr (versus 91.1 hr for amphotericin B desoxycholate).

Drug Preparations:

Vials: 100 mg in 20 mL suspension.

Dosage: 5.0 mg/kg/day as a single administration. Infusion rate should not exceed 2.5 mg/kg/hr.

Adverse Effects:

1. Chills (16%), fever (12%), increased serum creatinine (11%), nausea (8%), hypotension (7%), and others. Multiple organ failure (10%), respiratory failure (9%), and sepsis (7%) were also reported, but the patients in the study groups had serious underlying illnesses.
2. One case of anaphylaxis has occurred with amphotericin B lipid complex.

Drug Interactions:

1. Potential for nephrotoxicity may be increased when amphotericin B is given concurrently with aminoglycosides, cyclosporine, and pentamidine.
2. Hypokalemia associated with amphotericin B administration may potentiate digitalis toxicity or enhance effects of skeletal muscle relaxants (e.g., tubocurarine).
3. Acute pulmonary toxicity has been reported in patients receiving amphotericin B and leukocyte transfusions.

Monitoring: Serial creatinine, electrolyte (including magnesium), and hematocrit determinations. Blood pressure and heart rate should be monitored during drug administration.

BIBLIOGRAPHY

Abelcet product information pamphlet, Princeton, 1995, Liposome Co.

AMPICILLIN

Trade Names: *Omnipen, Principen.*

Drug Action:

1. Inhibition of cell wall synthesis.
2. Active against gram-positive (but **not** penicillinase-producing staphylococci) and gram-negative (non–β-lactamase–producing strains of *H. influenzae* and gonococci) aerobes and anaerobes (but **not** *Bacteroides* family).
3. Active against enterococci when combined with aminoglycosides (gentamicin best).
4. Drug of choice against *Listeria monocytogenes* infections (with/without gentamicin).

Indications: Infections caused by susceptible organisms.

Pharmacokinetics:

1. **Absorption:** 42% absorbed after PO dose; decreased by food.
2. **Excretion:** Renal.
3. **Metabolism:** Partial.
4. **Half-life:** 1–1.5 hr.

Drug Preparations:

Capsules: 250, 500 mg.
Suspension: 125, 250 mg/5mL.
Vial: 125, 250, 500, 1,000, 2,000 mg for IV use.

1. Available in combination with probenecid (3.5 g ampicillin, 1 gm probenecid) as single-dose therapy for non–penicillinase-producing gonococcal infections.

Dosage:

1. **Normal renal function:** 500–2000 mg q 4–6 hr PO/IM/IV.
2. **Impaired renal function:**

Dose (g)	Creatinine Clearance	Interval (hr)
1–2	>80	4–6
	80–50	6
	50–10	8
	<10	12

Adverse Effects: Same as for amoxicillin.

Drug Interactions: Same as for amoxicillin.

AMPICILLIN AND SULBACTAM

Trade Name: *Unasyn.*

Drug Action: Sulbactam acting as a β-lactamase inhibitor increases the spectrum of activity of ampicillin to include β-lactamase–producing strains of staphylococci, *H. influenzae,* gonococci, other gram-negative organisms, and anaerobes, including *Bacteroides fragilis.*

Indications: Infections caused by susceptible organisms; often used in mixed aerobic-anaerobic infections (e.g., intraabdominal and pelvic) where resistant organisms (e.g., *Pseudomonas aeruginosa*) not suspected.

Pharmacokinetics:

1. **Absorption:** Give IV/IM.
2. **Metabolism:** 15%–25%.
3. **Excretion:** Renal.
4. **Half-life:** 1 hr; prolonged in renal failure.

Drug Preparations:

Vials: 1.5 g (a 1.0 g ampicillin as sodium salt and 0.5 g sulbactam as sodium salt), 3.0 g (2 g ampicillin/1 g sulbactam).

Dosage: 1.5–3 g q 6 hr IV/IM.

Adverse Effects: Same as for ampicillin; include nausea/vomiting, diarrhea, pseudomembranous, colitis, dermatitis, anemia, thrombocytopenia, leukopenia, thrombophlebitis, hypersensitivity, interstitial nephritis.

Drug Interactions: Same as for ampicillin. Probenecid decreases excretion. Ampicillin causes *in vitro* inactivation of aminoglycosides.

AMRINONE

Trade Name: *Inocor.*

Drug Action:

1. Inhibition of phosphodiesterase III at cellular membrane results in higher cAMP level, resulting in increased inward calcium flux; no receptor effect.
2. Increased contractility.
3. Arterial and venodilation.
4. Lower myocardial O_2 demand by decreased wall tension despite increased contractility.
5. Enhanced AV nodal conduction.

Indications:

1. Congestive heart failure (CHF).
2. As an adjunct to other inotropes. In CHF or other states of prolonged high levels of circulating catecholamines, the β-receptors may become downregulated. Downregulation can occur during treatment of CHF. Because of the different mechanism of action of amrinone, combinations of this drug and β-agents such as dobutamine have been found to be synergistic.
3. Right ventricular failure.
4. Pulmonary hypertension.

Pharmacokinetics:

1. **Metabolism:** Hepatic.
2. **Excretion:** 80% renal, 20% hepatic.
3. **Plasma half-life:** 6 hr.
4. **Protein binding:** 20%–50%.
5. **Onset of action:** Almost immediate with loading dose.

Drug Preparations:

Ampules: 100 mg/20 mL.

Dosage: Bolus 0.75–3 mg/kg over 2–3 min, followed by infusion of 2.5–20 μg/kg/min.

Adverse Effects:

1. **Thrombocytopenia** with prolonged treatment.
2. **GI:** Nausea, vomiting, abdominal pain.

3. **Hepatic toxicity.**
4. **Arrhythmias.**
5. **Hypotension.**

Drug Interactions: Disopyramide and amrinone may produce severe hypotension.

Monitoring:

1. Blood pressure may decrease due to vasodilation.
2. PA catheter for hemodynamic effects.

BIBLIOGRAPHY

Colucci WS, Wright RF, Braunwald E: New positive inotropic agents in the treatment of congestive heart failure, *N Engl J Med* 1986, 314:349–358.

DiSesa VJ: The rational selection of inotropic drugs in cardiac surgery, *J Cardiac Surg* 1987, 2:385–406.

Gage J, Rutman H, Lucido D, et al: Additive effects of dobutamine and amrinone on myocardial contractility and ventricular performance in patients with severe heart failure, *Circulation* 1986, 74:367–373.

ANGIOTENSIN CONVERTING ENZYME INHIBITORS

Trade Names:

    Benazepril: *Lotensin.*
    Captopril: *Capoten.*
    Lisinopril: *Prinivil, Zestril.*
    Enalapril: *Vasotec.*
    Enalaprilat: *Vasotec IV.*

Drug Action:

1. Blocks conversion of angiotensin I to angiotensin II.
2. Vasodilation.
3. Decreases aldosterone secretion.

Indications:

1. Antihypertensive.
2. Vasodilation (e.g., CHF).

Pharmacokinetics:

1. **Absorption:** Absorbed from GI tract: captopril, 75% (reduced by food); enalapril, 60%; lisinopril, 25%; benazepril, 37%.
2. **Metabolism:** Captopril, 50% liver; lisinopril, not metabolized; enalapril, deesterified in liver to active form, enalaprilat; benazepril, converted in liver to active metabolite benazeprilat.
3. **Excretion:** Captopril, primarily urine; lisinopril, unchanged in urine; enalapril, urine and feces; benazepril, urine and feces.
4. **Onset** (PO): Captopril, 1/4 hr; lisinopril, 1 hr; enalapril, 1 hr; benazepril, 1–2 hr.
5. **Half-Life:** Captopril, <2 hr (increased in renal failure); enalapril, 1.3 hr (enalaprilat is an active metabolite with halflife of 35 hr); lisinopril, 12 hr (prolonged in renal failure); benazepril, 0.6 hr (benazeprilat, 2–4 hr).
6. **Time to peak effect** (PO): Captopril, 0.5–1.5 hr; enalapril, 0.5–1.5 hr; lisinopril, 7 hr.
7. **Duration:** Captopril 2–6 hr (increased in renal failure); enalapril, 24 hr; lisinopril, 24 hr.

Drug Preparations:

Tablets:
Benazepril: 5, 10, 40 mg
Captopril: 12.5, 25, 50, 100 mg.
Lisinopril: 5, 10, 20 mg.
Enalapril: 5, 10, 20 mg.
IV injection: 1.25 mg/mL (Enalaprilat).

Dosage: Reduce dosage in renal insufficiency; patients taking diuretics are more sensitive to drugs.

1. **Hypertension:**
   a. Captopril: **Adult:** Initially 12.5–25 mg PO two to three times/day; increase by 25 mg tid to max. of 150 mg tid (increase dose every 1–2 wk).
   b. Lisinopril: **Adult:** Initially 10 mg PO once/day; increase to 20–40 mg/day as single dose.

   c. Enalapril: **Adult:** Initially 2.5–5 mg PO once/day; increase
     to 10–40 mg/day.
   d. Benazepril: **Adult:** Initially 10 mg PO once/day, increase to
     20–40 mg/day (max 80 mg/day).
     (1) Intravenous enalapril: 1.25 mg q 6 hr (give over 5 min);
        onset 15 min, peak effect 1–4 hr; may increase dose to
        5 mg q 6 hr.
   e. Enalaprilat: 0.625–1.25 mg IV q 6–8 hr.
2. **Congestive Heart Failure:**
   a. Captopril: **Adult:** Initially 6.25–25 mg tid; increase to max.
     of 150 mg tid.
   b. Enalapril, lisinopril, benazepril: Same as for hypertension.

Adverse Effects:

1. **Cardiovascular:** Hypotension, tachycardia, bradycardia,
   angina, myocardial infarction (from hypotension), pericarditis,
   arrhythmias.
2. **Respiratory:** Cough.
3. **GI:** Anorexia, nausea/vomiting, diarrhea, constipation.
4. **GU:** Proteinuria, nephrotic syndrome, membranous glomeru-
   lopathy, renal failure, urinary frequency.
5. **Hematologic:** Leukopenia, neutropenia, agranulocytosis, pancytopenia.
6. **CNS:** Dizziness, syncope, headache, fatigue, insomnia, paresthesias, somnolence, anxiety.
7. **Dermatologic:** Rash, pruritus, hypersensitivity reactions.
8. **Other:** Hyperkalemia, fever, angioedema, nasal congestion.

Drug Interactions:

1. Nonsteroidal anti-inflammatory drugs decrease antihypertensive effect.
2. Antacids decrease effect (decrease absorption).
3. Additive antihypertensive effects when used with diuretics and
   other antihypertensive drugs (especially sympathetic blockers).
4. Hyperkalemia with potassium-sparing diuretics or potassium
   supplements.
5. Increased risk of hypersensitivity reaction when given with allopurinol.

6. May elevate digoxin levels by decreasing renal clearance. Increases effect of allopurinol and lithium.
7. Renal excretion decreased by probenecid (increases antihypertensive action).
8. Drug effect increased by phenothiazines.

Monitoring:

1. Blood pressure, heart rate.
2. Serum potassium.
3. Serum creatinine, liver enzymes, blood cell counts.

BIBLIOGRAPHY

Burris JF: The expanding role of angiotensin converting enzyme inhibitors in the management of hypertension, *J Clin Pharmacol* 1995, 35:337–342.

Pitt B: Importance of angiotensin-converting enzyme inhibitors in myocardial infarction and congestive heart failure: implications for clinical practice, *Cardiology* 1995, 86(suppl):41–45.

ANTACIDS

Trade Names:

Magnesium/aluminum combinations: *Algicon, Camalox, Gelusil, Maalox, Mylanta, Riopan, Simeco.*

Aluminum only: *ALternaGEL, Amphojel, Alu-Cap, Basaljel, Dialume, Rolaids.*

Calcium-containing: *Tums.*

Sodium bicarbonate: *Alka-Seltzer.*

Alginic acid: *Gaviscon.*

Drug Action:

1. Neutralizes gastric acid.
2. Increases lower esophageal sphincter tone.
3. Magnesium-containing antacids have an osmotic laxative effect.
4. Aluminum-containing antacids function as phosphate binders, which is useful in renal failure and in struvite stone formers.

5. Alginic acid forms a floating layer on gastric contents, acting as a barrier to gastroesophageal reflux (GER).

Indications:

1. Treatment of peptic ulcer disease.
2. Treatment of GER disease.
3. Stress ulcer prophylaxis.
4. Laxative (magnesium-containing).
5. Elevated phosphate level in patients with end-stage renal disease (aluminum-containing)

Pharmacokinetics:

1. Magnesium-containing: 10% of Mg^{2+} absorbed.
2. Aluminum-containing: Only small amounts of Al^{2+} absorbed.
3. Calcium-containing: 10% of Ca^{2+} absorbed.
4. Alginic acid: Not absorbed.

Dosage: The most frequent error is incorrect timing. Antacids are most effective when given 30 min–2 hr postprandially and at night, because food acts to neutralize gastric acid at mealtimes. After a meal, rebound hyperacidity occurs after 30 min–2 hr, depending on gastric emptying rates.

1. **Peptic ulcer disease:** General guidelines for selected products:
   Maalox: 1–2 tabs or 1–2 tsp (5–10 mL) 1 hr pc and qhs.
   Mylanta: 1–2 tabs or 1–2 tsp (5–10 mL) 1 hr pc and qhs.
   Riopan: 1–2 tabs or 1–2 tsp (5–10 mL) 1 hr pc and qhs.
   AL*terna*GEL: 1–2 tsp (5–10 mL) 30 min–1 hr pc and qhs.
   Basaljel: 2 caps/tabs or 1 tsp (5 mL) qid.
   Gaviscon: 2–3 tabs or 1–2 tbs (15–30 mL) 30 min–1 hr pc and qhs.
   Gelusil: 2 tabs or 2 tsp (10 mL) 1 hr pc and qhs.
2. **Stress ulcer prophylaxis:** Dosage is somewhat variable, depending on the product. Generally, 10–30 mL high-potency antacid is given NG q 1–2 hr. Gastric aspirate pH is determined q 1–2 hr. If pH is <3.5, standard dose is doubled to 20–60 mL.

Potency: *See* Figure 1.

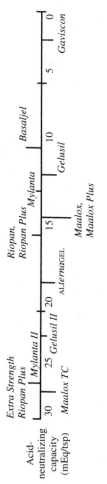

FIG. 1.
Potency of various antacids.

Sodium Content:

High ⟵————————⟶ Low		
Rolaids	Riopan	TUMS
Digel	Maalox	Camalox
Amphojel	Mylanta	Alka-Seltzer
	Basaljel	

Adverse Side Effects:

1. Magnesium-containing:
   a. Diarrhea.
   b. Magnesium intoxication (weakness, fatigue, decreased deep tendon reflexes) in patients with chronic renal failure.
2. Aluminum-containing:
   a. Constipation.
   b. Aluminum toxicity (dementia, osteodystrophy) in patients with chronic renal failure.
3. Calcium-containing antacids coupled with excessive consumption of dairy products in compliance with a bland diet can cause milk-alkali syndrome (hypercalcemia, alkalosis, nephrocalcinosis).
4. Sodium-containing products can exacerbate salt-retaining conditions (CHF, cirrhosis, nephrosis) and can cause milk-alkali syndrome.

All antacids used chronically can predispose to nephrolithiasis. As urinary pH increases, so does the ionization of phosphate, which predisposes to calcium phosphate stone formation. In addition, calcium-containing antacids promote stone formation due to hypercalciuria.

Drug Interactions: Antacids can bind tetracycline and decrease absorption, and also decrease absorption of H_2 blockers and interfere with the effectiveness of sucralfate. Therefore, these drugs should not be administered concomitantly with antacids.

BIBLIOGRAPHY

Agents used in disorders of the upper gastrointestinal tract. In *AMA Drug Evaluations,* ed 6, Philadelphia, 1986, WB Saunders, pp 946–952.

Clearfield HR: Changes in acid/peptic disorders: A symposium overview, *Alim Pharmacol Therap* 1991, 5(suppl 1):1–4.

Drake D, Hollander D: Neutralizing capacity and cost effectiveness of antacids, *Ann Intern Med* 1981, 94:215–217.

Tryba M, Zevounou F, Torok M, et al: Prevention of acute stress bleeding with sucralfate, antacids, or cimetidine, *Am J Med* 1985, 79(suppl 2C):55–61.

ANTICHOLINESTERASES

Trade Names:

Edrophonium: *Tensilon.*
Neostigmine: *Prostigmin, Neostigmine.*
Physostigmine: *Eserine, Isopto Eserine.*
Pyridostigmine: *Mestinon, Regonol.*

Drug Action:

1. Inhibits hydrolysis of acetylcholine by cholinesterase. Facilitates transmission of impulses across myoneural junction.
2. Improves muscle contraction.
3. Reduces intraocular pressure.

Indications:

1. Anticholinergic poisoning.
2. Myasthenia gravis.
3. Nondepolarizing muscle relaxant antagonist (e.g., curariform drugs).
4. Tricyclic antidepressant overdose.
5. Open-angle glaucoma.
6. Ileus.
7. Bladder atony.

Pharmacokinetics:

1. **Absorption:** Poorly absorbed from GI tract.
2. **Metabolism:** Physostigmine and neostigmine are hydrolyzed by cholinesterase; pyridostigmine is not hydrolyzed by cholinesterase.

3. **Excretion:** Urine.
4. **Onset of action:**
   a. Neostigmine: 45–75 min after PO administration; 10–30 min after IM; 4–8 min after IV.
   b. Physostigmine: 1–5 min after IV.
   c. Pyridostigmine: 30–30 min after PO administration; 2–5 min after IV; 15 min after IM.
5. **Duration of action:**
   a. Neostigmine: 2–4 hr after PO/IV/IM.
   b. Physostigmine: 1–2 hr after IV.
   c. Pyrisostigmine: 3–6 hr after PO dose; 2–3 hr after IV/IM.

Drug Preparations:

1. Neostigmine:
   Tablets: 15 mg.
   Injection: 0.25, 0.5, 1 mg/mL.

2. Physostigmine:
   Injection: 1 mg/mL.

3. Pyridostigmine:
   Tablets: 60, 180 mg sustained release.
   Syrup: 60 mg/5 mL.
   Injection: 5 mg/ml (2, 5 mL vial).

Dosage:

1. **Nondepolarizing muscle relaxant antagonist:**
   a. Neostigmine: **Adult:** 0.5–2.5 mg slow IV (give 0.6–1.2 mg atropine IV before neostigmine).
   b. Pyridostigmine: **Adult:** 10–30 mg IV (preceded by atropine 0.6–1.2 mg IV).
2. **Myasthenia gravis:**
   a. Neostigmine: **Adult:** 15–50 mg PO tid or 0.5–2 mg IM/IV q 1–3 hr; taper dose to desired effect. **Pediatric:** 2 mg/kg/day PO in three to four divided doses.
   b. Pyridostigmine: **Adult:** 60–180 mg PO bid–qid (up to 1500 mg/day). *Sustained-release tablets:* 180–540 mg one to two times/day. **Pediatric:** 1–2 mg/kg PO q 3–4 hr. Individualize dosage. May give 1/30 PO dose IV/IM.
3. **Ileus:**
   a. Neostigmine: **Adult:** 0.25–1 mg IM/SQ q 4–6 hr.

4. **Tricyclic and anticholinergic poisoning:**
   a. Physostigmine: **Adult:** 0.5–2 mg IM/IV slowly. Individualize dosage, and repeat as necessary. **Pediatric:** 0.5 mg IV slowly; repeat q 5–10 min to max dose 2 mg.

Adverse Effects:

1. **Respiratory:** Bronchospasm, respiratory depression, increased secretions.
2. **Cardiovascular:** Arrhythmias, bradycardia (treat with atropine), hypotension, AV block, cardiac arrest.
3. **GI:** Nausea, vomiting, diarrhea, abdominal cramps, salivation, increased secretions, increased peristalsis.
4. **CNS:** Headache, dizziness, weakness, confusion, nervousness, sweating, seizures, hallucinations, muscle twitching, fasciculations, drowsiness.
5. **Dermatologic:** Rash.
6. **Other:** Miosis, blurred vision, conjunctivitis, lacrimation, diplopia, muscle cramps, urinary urgency, incontinence, vitreous hemorrhage, myopia, uveitis, iritis, cholinergic crisis.
7. **Use atropine** to blunt GI side effects or other muscarinic reactions.
8. **Overdosage** produces the clinical picture of increased parasympathetic action: GI stimulation, abdominal cramps, diarrhea, vomiting, salivation, pallor, sweating, urinary urgency, blurred vision, fasciculations, muscle weakness/paralysis, miosis, hypertension, bradycardia, anxiety.

Drug Interactions:

1. Cholinergic effect reversed by procainamide or quinidine.
2. Prolongs effect of succinylcholine.
3. Severe hypotension when used with ganglionic blockers.
4. Antagonized by magnesium.
5. Antagonized by corticosteroids.

Monitoring:

1. Blood pressure, heart rate.
2. Respiratory status.
3. Muscle strength.
4. Respiratory measurements; peripheral nerve stimulator.
5. Signs of cholinergic crisis.

BIBLIOGRAPHY

Miller RD (ed): *Anesthesia,* ed 4, New York, 1994, Churchill Livingstone.

Stoelting RK: *Pharmacology and Physiology in Anesthetic Practice,* ed 2, Philadelphia, JB Lippincott.

Denniston PL Jr (ed): *1995 Physicians GenRx,* Riverside, 1995, Denniston.

Physicians' Desk Reference, ed 49, Montvale, 1995, Medical Economics Data Production.

Gilman AG, Rall TW, Nies AS, Taylor P (eds): *Goodman and Gilman's The Pharmacological Basis of Therapeutics,* ed 8, New York, 1990, Macmillan.

ANTIDEPRESSANT MEDICATIONS

Antidepressants are rarely, if ever, prescribed in the Intensive Care Unit. Of greater concern to clinicians in Critical Care is the toxicity of this class of drugs. Therefore, the antidepressants will be discussed as a group, separated into the primary classifications of tricyclic and tetracyclic antidepressants (TCAs), monoamine oxidase (MAO) inhibitors, selective serotonin reuptake inhibitors (SSRIs), and other antidepressants. The primary mechanism of action of all these drugs is to increase the concentration of neurotransmitters in the CNS. The primary transmitters modulated by antidepressants are norepinephrine and serotonin. Virtually all the drugs listed below require many days to weeks of therapy before mood disturbances can be improved.

Tricyclic Antidepressants: The tricyclic antidepressants generally act through inhibition of neuronal reuptake of both norepinephrine and serotonin. The major adverse reactions that limit treatment with TCA drugs are the anticholinergic effects (dry mouth, constipation, urinary retention, blurred vision, flushing), orthostatic hypotension, sedation, and GI distress. TCA drugs also demonstrate an anti-/proarrhythmic effect on the myocardial conduction system that is similar to that of quinidine, and must be used with caution in patients with preexisting conduction disturbances or prior myocardial infarction. TCA drugs should be used with caution in combination with sedatives such as benzodi-azepines, and should not be combined with the MAO inhibitors. Although drug levels are available for most of the TCA drugs, the levels do not correlate with either the therapeutic effect or the tox-icity in cases of overdose.

The specific TCA drugs, recommended starting doses, and drug-specific side effects are listed in Table 4.

Monoamine Oxidase Inhibitors: Once the mainstay of the pharmacologic treatment of major depression, MAO inhibitors are generally reserved for use in patients who do not respond or who cannot tolerate either TCA or SSRI antidepressants. By inhibiting the primary metabolic pathway of CNS norepinephrine, epineph-rine, and serotonin, MAO inhibitors have effects similar to those of the other classes of antidepressant drugs in increasing the con-centrations of these neurotransmitters. MAO inhibitors interact with many other drugs and can cause a hypertensive crisis when combined with sympathomimetic medications, including over-the-counter cold preparations, levodopa, and pressor agents used in critical care. Spontaneous hypertensive urgencies have occurred with MAO inhibitors, and the drugs must be considered as an eti-ology for any hypertensive event (including headaches, blurred vision, delirium) in patients taking these medications. Extensive lists of foods that may induce a hypertensive crisis can be found in the PDR or other books. Because the effects may be potentiated, it is recommended that MAO inhibiting drugs should ***not*** be com-bined with other classes of antidepressants. The MAO inhibitors in common use are listed in Table 4.

Selective Serotonin Reuptake Inhibitors: The newest class of antidepressants is the SSRI drugs. While having a similar net effect in increasing CNS neurotransmitter concentrations, the SSRI antidepressants have a much more favorable side effect and toxicity profile. The lack of anticholinergic effects increases pa-tient compliance with these drugs, even though there may be a higher incidence of nausea, headache, nervousness, and insomnia with these drugs, especially early in the course of therapy. Most of the SSRI drugs have been reported to cause sexual dysfunction, including inability to achieve orgasm, but as a class the SSRI med-ications are very well tolerated. These agents are primarily metab-

TABLE 4.
Antidepressant medications

Name	Trade name	Usual starting dose	Specific side effects*
Amitriptyline	Elavil, Endep	25–75 mg per day	
Desipramine	Norpramin, Pertofrane	25–75 mg	
Doxepin	Adapin, Sinequan	25–75 mg per day	
Imipramine	Tofranil, Janimine, SK-Pramine	25–75 mg per day	
Nortriptyline	Pamelor, Aventyl	20–40 mg tid	
MAO Inhibitors			
Phenelzine	Nardil	15 mg tid	Postural hypotension
Tranylcypromine	Parnate	10 mg tid	Hypotension
SSRI Drugs			
Fluoxetine	Prozac, Lovan	20 mg per day	Akathisia, P-450 enzyme induction
Paroxetine	Paxil	20 mg once daily	May alter hepatic metabolism of other drugs
Sertraline	Zoloft	50 mg once daily	May potentiate effect of oral hypoglycemics; less drug interactions than other SSRI
Other Antidepressants			
Bupropion	Wellbutrin	100 mg bid	Seizures and CNS excitation
Maprotiline	Ludiomil	75 mg once daily	Seizures, proarrhythmic effect
Trazodone	Desyrel	50 mg bid–tid	Priapism (up to one third require surgery), sedation
Venlafaxine	Effexor	25 mg tid	Prolonged QT segment on ECG

*Side effects specific to the drug indicated. Does not include class-specific side effects discussed in the text.

olized by the liver, and fluoxetine does induce the P-450 microsomal enzyme system and may alter the metabolism of other drugs.

Other Antidepressants: Four additional drugs used for the treatment of depression do not fall into the above classification. The exact mechanisms have not been elucidated, but these agents also increase the CNS concentrations of norepinephrine and/or serotonin. Bupropion has been reported to cause seizures in up to 0.4% of patients and does induce hepatic enzymes, although the incidence of other significant side effects is relatively low. Maprotiline also has been reported to increase the incidence of seizures. Trazodone produces a high incidence of priapism and does cause increased sedation, and Venlafaxine has been associated with increased diastolic and systolic blood pressures.

ANTIDIARRHEALS

Trade Names:

Diphenoxylate and atropine: *Lomotil.*
Loperamide: *Imodium.*
Bismuth subsalicylate: *Pepto-Bismol.*
Attapulgite: *Diasorb.*
Kaolin, pectin, belladonna alkaloids: *Donnagel*; with opium, *Donnagel-PG.*
Kaolin and pectin: *Kaopectate.*
Paregoric, pectin, kaolin: *Parepectolin.*

Drug Action:

1. Diphenoxylate/atropine:
   a. Diphenoxylate acts locally and centrally to reduce GI motility.
   b. Atropine has antimuscarinic activity and reduces GI motility.
2. Loperamide: Reduces GI motility by direct effect on nerve endings and/or intramural ganglia within intestinal wall. May inhibit secretion or stimulate absorption.
3. Bismuth subsalicylate: Exact mechanism unknown. Does not have antiperistaltic activity, is not an antacid, and does not function as a mucosal protector. Decreases secretion.
4. Attapulgite: Physiologically inert clay that acts to absorb excess GI secretions. Can absorb 12 times its volume.

5. Kaolin: Absorbs bacteria and toxins, reduces water loss.
6. Pectins: Stimulate growth of intestine and colonic absorption.
7. Belladonna alkaloids (hyoscyamine, atropine, scopolamine): Decrease hypermotility and hypersecretion of GI tract via antimuscarinic activity.
8. Opium: Reduces GI motility, relieves tenesmus pain.
9. Paregoric: Reduces GI motility.

Indications:

1. Diphenoxylate/atropine and loperamide: Treatment of acute/chronic diarrhea.
2. Loperamide: Chronic diarrhea associated with inflammatory bowel disease; has been used to decrease ileostomy discharge.
3. Bismuth, attapulgite, kaolin, and pectin with additives: Only in acute setting for symptomatic relief of self-limited diarrheal illnesses.

Pharmacokinetics: *See* Table 5.

Drug Preparations:

Drug	Tabs/Caps	Syrup
Lomotil	2.5 mg diphenoxylate/ 25 μg atropine	2.5 mg/25μg/5 mL
Imodium	2 mg	1 mg/5 mL
Pepto-Bismol	262 mg	262 mg/5 mL
Diasorb	750 mg	750 mg/5 mL
Kaopectate	NA	Concentrated liquid: 290 mg kaolin/mL, 6.47 mg pectin/mL

Drug	Tabs/Caps	Syrup
Donnagel-PG	NA	6 gm kaolin/142 mg pectin, opium 24 mg/oz (2 tbsp)
Parepectolin	NA	5 gm kaolin/162 mg pectin, 15 mg opium, 3.7 mL paregoric/30 mL

None of the antidiarrheals are available in parenteral form.

TABLE 5.
Pharmacokinetics of Antidiarrheal Agents

Drug	Absorption	Metabolism	t½ (hr)	Duration (hr)	Excretion
Diphenoxylate	Not reported	Hepatic	2.5	3–4	Fecal/renal
Loperamide	Poor	—	10	9–14	Fecal/renal
Bismuth subsalicylate	Good	Hepatic	2–3	—	Fecal/renal
Attapulgite	Not absorbed	—	—	—	Fecal
Kaolin pectin	None	—	—	3–4	Fecal
Belladonna	—	Hepatic	—	3–4	Renal
Opium	Good	Hepatic	—	3–4	Hepatic/renal
Paregoric	Good	Hepatic	2–3	4–5	Hepatic/renal

Dosage (give PO):

1. *Lomotil:* 1–2 tabs or 1–2 tsp (5–10 mL) (2.5–5.0 mg diphen-oxylate/25–50 μg atropine) bid–tid.
2. *Imodium:*
   a. Short-term: 2 caps (4 mg), then 1 cap (2 mg) after each loose stool to a maximum of 8 caps (16 mg)/day.
   b. Long-term: 1 cap (2 mg) bid–qid.
3. *Pepto-Bismol:* 2 tsp or tabs q 1/2–1h, up to 8 doses/24 hr.
4. *Diasorb:* 4 tsp or tabs initially, then 2 tsp or tabs q 4–6 hr.
5. *Kaopectate:* 3–6 tbs (45–120 mL) after each loose bowel movement, up to 8 doses/24 hr.
6. *Donnagel-PG:* 2 tbs (30 mL) initially, then 1 tb q 3 hr.
7. *Parepectolin:* 1–2 tbs (15–30 mL) after each loose bowel movement, up to 8 doses/24 hr.

Adverse Effects:

1. Diphenoxylate/atropine: Bloating, abdominal pain (may indicate paralytic ileus or megacolon), drowsiness, respiratory depression, blurred vision, dry mouth, constipation, nausea/vomiting.
2. Loperamide: Bloating, abdominal pain (overdose can lead to toxic megacolon), drowsiness, dizziness, dry mouth, nausea/vomiting.
3. Bismuth subsalicylate: Salicylate toxicity (tinnitus, hyperthermia, hyperventilation, acidosis), epigastric upset/bleeding, dark stools mimicking melena (but Hemoccult negative).
4. Attapulgite: Constipation and impaction.
5. Kaolin and pectin: Constipation.
6. Kaolin, pectin, belladonna, opium: Belladonna alkaloids can suppress sweating and exacerbate hyperthermia. Constipation, abdominal cramping, anticholinergic symptoms (lightheadedness, dry mouth, flushing, confusion).
7. Kaolin, pectin, paregoric: Constipation, abdominal pain, drowsiness, confusion, allergic reactions (hives, pruritus).

Drug Interactions:

1. Diphenoxylate/atropine: Additive with other CNS depressants (alcohol, anxiolytics, anesthetics, tricyclic antidepressants); may predispose to pseudomembraneous colitis if used with antibiotics (cephalosporins, macrolides, penicillins, clindamycin).

2. Loperamide: May predispose to pseudomembranous colitis if used with antibiotics (cephalosporins, macrolides, penicillins, clindamycin).

3. Bismuth subsalicylate: Salicylates have many interactions: e.g., potentiate ototoxic medications (aminoglycosides, cisplatinum); potentiate bleeding in patients on anticoagulants; enhance effects of PO hypoglycemia medications; additive to platelet inhibitory medications.

4. Attapulgite: None reported.

5. Kaolin, pectin: Decrease absorption of digitalis, lincomycin, phenothiazines, xanthines.

6. Kaolin, pectin, belladonna, opium: Same as for kaolin, pectin. In addition, opium potentiates CNS depressants and is potentially addicting. Belladonna alkaloids antagonize metoclopramide and intensify antimuscarinic side effects of haloperidol. Ketoconazole absorption is decreased.

7. Kaolin, pectin, paregoric: Same as for kaolin, pectin. In addition, paregoric can potentiate other CNS depressants. May cause pseudomembranous colitis if given with antibiotics.

Comments and Recommendations: The textbook dictum is that suppressive agents should not be used to treat diarrhea. However, diarrhea is common and uncomfortable, and affected patients often seek medical attention promptly. Normal bowel patterns range from three movements per day to one every 3 days. Diarrhea is defined as increased volume (>250 mL/day) and frequency. Acute diarrhea is usually due to an infection or toxin, but a thorough history must consider other causes (e.g., inflammatory bowel disease, enzyme deficiencies [lactase or pancreatic insufficiency], irritable bowel, postgastrectomy, secretory diarrhea). Most US–acquired infectious diarrhea is caused by Norwalk or other viruses. These syndromes are characterized by watery diarrhea, usually with abdominal cramping, nausea, and vomiting, and occur in small epidemics. Patients are afebrile, with minimal or absent abdominal tenderness. There are no leukocytes or blood in the stool. The white blood cell count (WBC) is usually normal. In this setting, a short course (<3 days) of suppressive therapy often provides relief without exposing the patient to undue risk. We favor loperamide because it is non-narcotic and the absence of atropine limits troubling side effects and complications. In febrile patients with bloody diarrhea, leukocyte-positive stools, and elevation in WBC, infection (e.g., *Campylobacter, Shigella, Salmonella*) should be considered. Stool should be cultured for invasive pathogens, and antibiotics used when appropriate. In this setting, suppressive therapy is not indicated.

BIBLIOGRAPHY

AMA Drug Evaluations, ed 6, Philadelphia, 1986, WB Saunders.
Drug Information for the Health Care Provider, ed 6, 1986, US Pharmacopeial Convention.
Schiller L, Santa Ana C, Morawski S, et al: Mechanism of the antidiarrheal effect of loperamide, *Gastroenterology* 1984, 86:1475–1480.

ANTIEMETICS/ANTINAUSEANTS

Trade Names:

Promethazine (antihistamine, phenothiazine): *Phenergan.*
Meclizine (antihistamine): *Antivert, Bonine.*
Dimenhydrinate (antihistamine): *Dramamine.*
Hydroxyzine (antihistamine): *Vistaril.*
Prochlorperazine (phenothiazine): *Compazine.*
Trimethobenzamide (benzamide): *Tigan.*
Scopolamine: *Transderm Scop.*
Metoclopramide (benzamide): *Reglan.*
Ondansetron: *See* ondansetron.
Droperidol (butyrophenone): *See* droperidol.
Granisetron (Kytril): *See* granisetron.

Action:

1. Antihistamines (promethazine, meclizine, dimenhydrinate, hydroxyzine) have central antimuscarinic action. They also decrease vestibular stimulation and may act on the chemoreceptor trigger zone.
2. Prochlorperazine inhibits the medullary chemoreceptor trigger zone.
3. Trimethobenzamide inhibits the chemoreceptor trigger zone.

4. Scopolamine depresses conduction in the vestibular cerebellar pathway.
5. Metoclopramide at high doses raises the threshold of the chemoreceptor trigger zone.

Indications:

Nausea and vomiting.
Motion sickness (transdermal scopolamine, dimenhydrinate, meclizine).
Vertigo (meclizine).
Antiemetic for chemotherapy (ondansetron, promethazine, metoclopramide, droperidol, prochlorperazine).
Postoperative nausea: ondansetron, promethazine, metoclopramide, droperidol.

Pharmacokinetics: *See* Table 6.

Drug Preparations: *See* Table 7.

Dosage:

1. Promethazine: 12.5–50 mg PO/PR/IM q 4–6 hr; can titrate IV in 12.5 increments q15 min.
2. Hydroxyzine: 50–100 mg IM q 4–6 hr. Meclizine: 12.5–50 mg PO q d up to qid; max. dose 100 mg/day.
3. Dimenhydrinate: 50–100 mg PO/IM/IV q 4–6 hr to max. of 400 mg/day.
4. Scopolamine: one transdermal patch placed the day before departure; replace q 2 to 3 days.
5. Trimethobenzamide: 250 mg PO tid/qid or 200 mg PR/IM tid/qid.
6. Prochlorperazine: 5–10 mg PO/PR/IM/IV q 6–8 hr.
7. Metoclopramide: 1–2 mg/kg/IV prior to chemotherapy; can be repeated q 3–4 hr. 5–20 mg PO q 5–8 hr.

Adverse Effects:

1. Antihistamines.
   Anticholinergic effects include dry mouth, blurred vision, increased intraocular pressure, dilated pupils, constipation, urinary retention, and thick secretions. CNS effects include sedation, respiratory depression, confusion, restlessness, tremors, seizures, and dizziness. Extrapyramidal effects include

TABLE 6.
Pharmacokinetics

Drug	Absorption	Metabolism	t½ (hr)	Duration (hr)	Excretion
Antihistamines*	Good	Hepatic	6–12	4–8	Renal
Scopolamine	Good	Hepatic	8	Up to 72	Renal
Trimethobenzamide	Good	Hepatic	—	3–4	Renal
Prochlorperazine	Good	Hepatic	—	—	Renal
Metoclopramide	Good	Hepatic	4–6	1–2	Renal, 85%

*Promethazine, meclizine, dimenhydrinate, hydroxyzine.

TABLE 7.
Drug Preparations

Drug	Tablet	Liquid	Suppository	Parenteral
Antihistamines				
Promethazine	12.5, 25, 50 mg	6.25, 10, 25 mg/5mL	12.5, 25, 50 mg	25, 50 mg/mL
Hydroxyzine*	—	—	—	25 mg/mL
Meclizine	12.5, 25, 50 mg	—	—	—
Dimenhydrinate	50 mg	12.5 mg/4 mL	—	50 mg/mL
Scopolamine	0.5 mg cutaneous patch			
Trimethobenzamide	100, 250 mg	—	100, 200 mg	100 mg/mL
Prochlorperazine	5, 10, 25 mg	5 mg/5 mL	2.5, 5, 25 mg	5 mg/mL

*Hydroxyzine has antiemetic properties only when given parenterally.

parkinsonian syndrome, dystonia, dyskinesias, and akathisia. May cause tachycardia, bradycardia, hypotension, hypertension, or quinidine-like effects. Patients rarely develop leukopenia, agranulocytosis, or thrombocytopenia. GI effects include anorexia, constipation, and jaundice. Other effects include malignant neuroleptic syndrome, oral syndrome (red mucosa, cheiloses, loose teeth, vesicles, stomatitis), photosensitivity, and allergic reactions.

2. Trimethobenzamide can cause parksonian-like symptoms. Drowsiness, blurred vision, hypotension, diarrhea, hepatotoxicity, dizziness, headache, seizures, depression, coma, hypersensitivity reactions, and rare blood dyscrasias have been reported.

3. Prochlorperazine, a phenothiazine, can cause extrapyramidal side effects such as acute dystonic reactions and permanent tardive dyskinesia. (The treatment for acute dystonic reaction is diphenhydramine [Benadryl], 50 mg IM/IV.) Drowsiness, blurred vision, headache, agranulocytosis, cholestatic jaundice, and constipation have been reported.

4. Metoclopramide can cause extrapyramidal side effects such as acute dystonic reactions and permanent tardive dyskinesia. (The treatment for acute dystonic reaction is diphenhydramine [Benadryl], 50 mg IM/IV.) Drowsiness, dizziness, fatigue, and restlessness have been reported. Dopaminergic blockade can result in hyperprolactinemia, breast tenderness, galactorrhea, and menstrual irregularities.

5. Scopolamine is a belladonna alkaloid and should not be given to patients with glaucoma because of the drug's mydriatic effect. Dry mouth and drowsiness are frequent side effects.

6. Allergic reactions.

7. Hyperthermia: Phenothiazines (neuroleptic malignant syndrome).

Drug Interactions:

1. Antihistamines.
   Antihistamines potentiate other CNS depressants. MAO inhibitors potentiate effect. Additive sedative actions when combined with other CNS depressants, additive cardiotoxicity with quinidine, block α-adrenergic effect of epinephrine.

2. Trimethobenzamide potentiates other CNS depressants.

3. Prochlorperazine potentiates other CNS depressants. It also lowers the seizure threshold, particularly with metrizamide, a myelographic dye. It should not be given to patients taking antidepressants.
4. Scopolamine potentiates other CNS depressants and anticholinergic effects of other medications (antidepressants).
5. Metoclopramide potentiates other CNS depressants and accelerates gastric emptying of medications (long-acting preparations may not adequately dissolve.) Shortened transit time may decrease bioavailability.

Monitoring: Clinical response, blood pressure, heart rate.

Comments and Recommendations: Nausea with or without vomiting is common; generally it is of short duration and benign. However, prolonged severe nausea and vomiting can cause dehydration, electrolyte disturbances, alkalosis, and upper GI hemorrhage due to a gastroesophageal mucosal tear (Mallory-Weiss syndrome). Serious underlying causes such as closed head injury or bowel obstruction should be considered and excluded prior to institution of symptomatic therapy.

In treating nausea and vomiting, the route of administration is important. Rectal suppositories (in the absence of profuse diarrhea) and IV or IM routes are usually chosen initially to ensure adequate drug levels. Once the symptoms are controlled, PO medication can often be used.

Scopolamine given transdermally is effective prophylaxis against motion sickness. Dimenhydrinate and meclizine are less effective but cause less drowsiness.

Meclizine is useful in the short-term treatment of vertigo due to acute viral labyrinthitis.

BIBLIOGRAPHY

Triozzi PL, Laszlo J: Optimum management of nausea and vomiting in cancer chemotherapy, *Drugs* 1987, 34:136–149.

Sridhar KS, Donnelly E: Combination antiemetics for cisplatin chemotherapy, *Cancer* 1988, 61:1508–1517.

Ettinger DS: Preventing chemotherapy-induced nausea and vomiting: an update and review of emesis, *Semin Oncol* 1995, 22(4 suppl 10):6–18.

ANTITHROMBIN III (AT III)

Trade Name: *ATnativ, Thrombate III.*

Drug Actions: Inactivates thrombin, plasmin, and the activated forms of factors.

Indications: AT III is indicated for patients with AT III deficiency (hereditary or acquired) having surgical or obstetrical procedures, or when thromboembolism occurs.

Pharmacokinetics:

1. **Absorption:** Give IV.
2. **Onset of action:** Immediate.
3. **Half-life:** 3 days.
4. **Therapeutic level:** Goal of therapy is to raise AT III levels to 120% of normal.

Drug Preparations:

1. Produced from human plasma that has been heat sterilized for ≥ 10 hr. Powder for injection 500 units/10 mL.

Dosage:

$$\text{Units of AT III} = \frac{[\text{Desired level (\%)} - \text{baseline level (\%)}] \times \text{body wt (kg)}}{1.0\% \text{ (IU/kg)}}$$

This averages to 2000–4000 units per dose. Usually administered once every 24 hr.

Adverse Effects:

1. Generally minimal, although vasodilation and diuretic effects have been reported.
2. Chest pain, edema, shortness of breath.
3. Dizziness, fever, nausea, cramps.
4. Hypersensitivity reactions, hives.

Drug Interactions: Enhances anticoagulant effect of heparin.

Monitoring: Measuring AT III levels is the only way to adequately monitor the need for dosing.

BIBLIOGRAPHY

1. Ofosu FA: Mechanisms for the anticoagulant effects of synthetic antithrombins, *Adv Exp Med Biol* 1993, 340:213–226.
2. Menache D: Antithrombin III concentrates, *Hematol Oncol Clin North Am* 1992, 6:1115–1120.

APOMORPHINE

Generic Drug: *Apomorphine hydrochloride.*

Drug Action:

1. Dopaminergic agonist.
2. Induces vomiting by stimulating the chemoreceptor trigger zone in the brain.

Indications: Induction of vomiting in drug overdose and poisoning.

Pharmacokinetics:

1. **Absorption:** Give SQ.
2. **Metabolism:** Liver.
3. **Excretion:** Unknown.
4. **Onset of action:** Within 5–10 min in adults; 1–2 min in children.

Drug Preparations:

Tablets, soluble: 6 mg with lactose.

Dosage:

1. **Adult:** 5 mg SQ (range 2–10 mg).
2. **Pediatric:** 0.1 mg/kg SQ.

Adverse Effects:

1. Do not use in impending shock; corrosive poisoning; narcosis due to opiates, barbiturates, alcohol, or other CNS depressants.
2. **CNS:** Depression, confusion, drowsiness, restlessness, tremor, euphoria.
3. **Cardiovascular:** Hypotension, tachycardia, bradycardia, acute cardiovascular collapse.

4. **Respiratory:** Depression, shortness of breath.
5. **GI:** Nausea, vomiting.

Drug Interactions:

1. May be ineffective in narcotic poisoning because vomiting center is depressed.
2. Emetic effects blunted by antiemetics.
3. Antagonized by narcotic antagonists (e.g., naloxone).
4. Synergistic CNS depression when used in the presence of narcotics, barbiturates, alcohol, and other sedatives.

Monitoring:

1. Blood pressure, heart rate, respiratory rate.
2. Mental status.
3. Airway.

BIBLIOGRAPHY

Apomorphine. In *Drug Facts and Comparisons,* 1989, JB Lippincott, p 2183.

APROTININ

Trade Name: *Trasylol.*

Drug Actions: Aprotinin is a proteinase inhibitor with a multitude of effects on the coagulation system. It inhibits kallikrein and plasma, and inhibits the contact phase activation of the coagulation cascade, thus having the net effect to decrease fibrinolysis.

Indications: Aprotinin is used in conjunction with cardiopulmonary bypass surgery with extracorporeal circulation, to decrease intraoperative and postoperative bleeding. Available data suggest that aprotinin is more effective when given prior to initiation of extracorporeal circulation than when used after the bypass circuit is used.

Pharmacokinetics: Aprotinin is rapidly distributed into extracellular spaces after intravenous dosing, then the second phase of plasma elimination gives a plasma half life of approximately 150 min. The terminal elimination half life is approximately 10 hr.

Elimination: Approximately 20%–45% of aprotinin is excreted unchanged in the urine, with the remainder being degraded by lysosomal enzymes.

Drug Preparations:

10,000 units/mL in vials of 100 and 200 mL.

Dosage: A test dose of 1 mL (10,000 units) is followed by a loading dose of 200 mL (2 million units), which can also be given with the "pump priming" fluid. Continuous infusion of 50 mL/hr (500,000 units/hr) for 4–6 hr after completion of bypass surgery.

Adverse Effects: Hypersensitivity reactions have occurred, which is the reason for the initial test dose to determine allergic reactions. Studies to date have not been able to isolate side effects of aprotinin which can be distinguished from the effects of coronary artery bypass surgery (CABG). Initial concerns for coronary graft patency have been disputed, and there does not appear to be a reduction in graft patency.

Drug Interactions: Do not administer aprotinin with any other drugs in the intravenous line. There are not specific drug-drug interactions with aprotinin.

BIBLIOGRAPHY

Hardy JF, Belisle S: Natural and synthetic antifibrinolytics in adult cardiac surgery: efficacy, effectiveness and efficiency. *Can J Anaesth* 1994, 41:1104–1112.

ASPIRIN

Trade Names: *Bayer Aspirin, Anacin, Ecotrin, Empirin, Bufferin, Alka-Seltzer,* plus many others.

Drug Action:

1. The principal mechanism by which aspirin acts is via inhibition of prostaglandin synthesis. Specifically, the enzyme cyclooxygenase is irreversibly acetylated. The action of aspirin on pain and inflammation is primarily a peripheral effect in

which prostaglandin levels at peripheral nerve endings are decreased. This is in contrast to narcotics, which have no effect on prostaglandin levels and are central in action.

2. Aspirin probably exerts its antipyretic effect by also decreasing prostaglandin levels in the temperature-regulating hypothalamic nuclei, thus returning the temperature "set point" to normal. Aspirin is not effective in reducing body temperature when elevated as a consequence of exercise, thyrotoxicosis, defective heat loss mechanisms (e.g., heat stroke), or high environmental temperature.

3. Aspirin, by its effect on cyclooxygenase, causes reductions in thromboxane levels in platelets. Thus, inhibition of platelet aggregation occurs and lasts for the 7- to 10-day lifespan of platelets. 650 mg aspirin will double the bleeding time in normal subjects for approximately 7 days.

Indications:

1. **Analgesia:** Aspirin is often satisfactory for treatment of mild to moderate pain, e.g., from minor sprains, headaches, myalgias, neuralgias, dysmenorrhea, and some minor surgical procedures. Visceral pain is not well relieved with aspirin.

2. **Anti-inflammatory:** Aspirin is the drug of choice for initiation of therapy in rheumatoid and nonrheumatoid arthritis. The amount of drug required is frequently greater than that required for other types of pain.

3. **Antipyretic:** Aspirin is indicated in the treatment of fever induced by processes that alter the hypothalamic "set point," such as infections, collagen vascular disease, CNS lesions, toxins, blood transfusion reactions, and drug allergies.

4. **Inhibition of platelet aggregation:** Aspirin potentially reduces the nonfatal myocardial infarction rate in patients with previous infarctions or unstable angina and in patients with no history of myocardial infarction. It may also decrease the risk of cerebrovascular accident or transient ischemic attacks.

Pharmacokinetics:

1. **Absorption:** Orally administered aspirin is rapidly absorbed, primarily in the proximal small intestine and to a lesser extent in the stomach. Although there is little meaningful clinical dif-

ference in the absorption rates of buffered and nonbuffered products, the presence of food in the stomach significantly delays absorption. Rectal administration results in slower and less reliable absorption.

2. **Distribution:** Aspirin is distributed throughout most body tissues and fluids. Approximately 80% of salicylate is plasma protein bound, especially to albumin. Blood-brain barrier passage is slow because most of the drug is ionized at pH 7.40.

3. **Metabolism:** Aspirin is rapidly hydrolyzed into the pharmacologically active salicylic acid in the liver. Conjugation with glycine or glucuronide subsequently occurs.

4. **Excretion:** Metabolites, along with varying proportions of salicylic acid, are excreted mainly by the kidney. Alkalinization of urine increases the amount of free salicylic acid excreted.

5. **Half-life:** The half-life of aspirin is approximately 15 min; for salicylic acid, approximately 3 hr.

Drug Preparations:

Tablets, capsules, timed-release capsules: 80, 325, 500, 600 mg.
Suppositories: 60, 125, 200, 300, 600 mg.

Dosage:

Adult: for analgesia and antipyresis: 650 mg q 4 hr PO/PR. For arthritis: as much as 1000 mg q 4 hr.

Pediatric: Age ≥3 yr: 60 mg/kg/day in divided doses q 4–6 hr.

Adverse Effects: These are multiple and include various GI disorders such as dyspepsia, gastric irritation, ulceration, and bleeding; reversible hepatic injury; allergic reactions, which may be as minor as rashes or as major as anaphylaxis; bronchospasm; prolonged bleeding time; decreased urate excretion; renal dysfunction; hyperglycemia and glycosuria as well as depletion of glycogen stores with high-dose aspirin therapy; uncoupling of oxidative phosphorylation with subsequent increase in oxygen consumption and carbon dioxide production; and CNS stimulation of ventilation resulting in respiratory alkalosis.

Because of the possible association of salicylates with Reye's syndrome and viral illness, there should be a clear indication for using these agents in pediatric patients.

Drug Interactions:

1. **Anticoagulants:** Warfarin is easily displaced from protein-binding sites; platelet-coagulation cascade interactions.
2. **Probenecid:** Low to moderate doses of aspirin inhibit excretion of uric acid as well as the uricosuric action of probenecid.
3. **Dosage of protein-bound drugs** such as barbiturates, calcium channel blockers, propranolol, and phenytoin may need to be decreased. Oral hypoglycemic agents are also displaced from plasma protein-binding sites, and hypoglycemia may occur.
4. **Corticosteroids:** Bleeding from gastric ulcers may be increased as a result of inhibition of prostaglandin synthesis.

Monitoring: Therapeutic serum levels are 100–250 μg/mL but are seldom determined in the ICU.

BIBLIOGRAPHY

AMA Drug Evaluations, ed 6, Philadelphia, 1986, WB Saunders.
McEvoy GK (ed): *AHFS Drug Information 89,* Bethesda, 1989, American Society of Hospital Pharmacists.

ATOVAQUONE

Trade Name(s): *Mepron.*

Drug Actions: The mechanism of action against *Pneumocystis carinii* has not been elucidated, but in *Plasmodium* spp. the site of action appears to be the cytochrome bc$_1$ complex (Complex III). With blockade of the mitochondrial electron transport chain, inhibition of nucleic acid and ATP synthesis may ultimately occur.

Indications: Acute oral treatment of mild to moderate *P. carinii* pneumonia (PCP) in patients who are intolerant to trimethoprim/sulfamethoxazole (mild to moderate defined as A-a gradient ≤45 mm Hg or PaO$_2$ ≥60 mm Hg).

Pharmacokinetics:

1. **Absorption:** PO; is generally poor but better with new liquid suspension than the previously marketed tablets. Also, administration with food enhances absorption twofold.

2. **Metabolism:** Hepatic.
3. **Excretion:** 94% as unchanged atovaquone in feces. There is essentially no excretion in the urine (less than 0.6%).
4. **Half-life:** 67.0–77.6 hr.

Drug Preparations:

Suspension: 1 tsp (5 mL) contains 750 mg.

Dosage: 750 mg PO bid for 21 days (take with meals).

Adverse Effects:

1. Rash in 23%, but most cases were mild and did not require discontinuation of atovaquone.
2. Nausea (21%), diarrhea (19%), headache (16%), vomiting (14%), fever (14%), insomnia (10%), and others.
3. Laboratory abnormalities include elevated alkaline phosphatase (8%), elevated amylase (7%), hyponatremia (7%), anemia (6%), elevated ALT (6%), elevated AST (4%), and neutropenia (ANC <750/mm^3) in 3%.

Drug Interactions:

1. Concurrent rifampin administration decreases atovaquone plasma concentrations. (In a study of 13 HIV-infected patients receiving 600 mg of rifampin daily, atovaquone plasma concentrations decreased 52% and rifampin plasma concentrations increased 37%.)
2. Zidovudine (AZT) plasma concentrations increase mildly when taken with atovaquone, but this is not thought to be clinically significant.

BIBLIOGRAPHY

Physicians' Desk Reference, ed 50, Montvale, 1996, Medical Economics Co.

ATROPINE

Generic Drugs:

1. *Atropine sulfate:* Nonpolar; readily absorbed after inhalation; bronchodilator activity relatively low. Incidence of anticholinergic side effects high.

Drug Action:

1. Antagonizes actions of acetycholine (ACh) at its membrane-bound receptor site.
2. Blocks bronchoconstrictor effects of vagal efferent impulses within the airway.
3. Blocks ACh effects on SA and AV nodes, increasing nodal conduction and rate.
4. Decreases glandular secretion.

Indications:

1. Treatment of bronchospasm (by inhalation).
2. Bradycardia (IV).
3. Anticholinesterase insecticide poisoning (IV).
4. Diminishes secretions preoperatively (IV).

Pharmacokinetics:

1. **Metabolism:** Hepatic.
2. **Excretion:** Kidney, feces, bile.
3. **Absorption:** Atropine absorbed via trachea, IM/PO routes.
4. **Half-life:** Atropine: Biphasic: initial t½ hr; terminal t½ 12 hr.
5. **Onset of action:** 1–2 min for IV atropine.

Drug Preparations:

1. Atropine:
   Tablets: 0.4 mg.
   Injection: 0.05, 0.1, 0.3, 0.4, 0.5, 0.6, 0.8, 1, 1.2 mg/mL.

Dosage:

1. **For bronchospasm:**
   a. Atropine sulfate: 1.5–2.0 mg by updraft nebulizer q 6 hr.
2. **For Bradycardia:**
   a. **Adult:** 0.5–1 mg IV push; repeat q 5 min to max. of 3 mg.
   b. **Pediatric:** 0.01 mg/kg to max. of 0.4 mg IV.
3. **Preoperatively:**
   a. **Adult:** 0.4–0.6 mg IM 45–60 min before anesthesia.
   b. **Pediatric:** 0.01 mg/kg IM (max. 0.4 mg) 45–60 min before anesthesia.
4. **Anticholinesterase insecticide:** Atropine: 2 mg IM/IV repeated q 20–30 min until muscarinic symptoms disappear; up to 6 mg IM/IV q hr.

Adverse Effects (primarily with atropine):

1. **Cardiovascular:** Paradoxical slowing of heart rate (with doses <0.5 mg), dysrhythmias, tachycardia, myocardial ischemia, palpitations.
2. **CNS:** Headache, restlessness, ataxia, disorientation, delirium, coma, insomnia, dizziness, agitation, confusion.
3. **Urinary** retention.
4. **Other:** Increased intraocular pressure, rash, hyperpyrexia, mydriasis, photophobia, blurred vision, dry mouth, constipation, nausea, vomiting.

Drug Interactions: Additive with other anticholinergic drugs.

Drug Reversal: Overdose: Physostigmine reverses anticholinergic activity (cholinesterase inhibitor).

Monitoring:

1. Heart rate, ECG, blood pressure.
2. Respiratory rate, spirometry (for bronchospasm).

BIBLIOGRAPHY

Drugs used in the treatment of bronchial disorders. In *AMA Drug Evaluations,* ed 6, Philadelphia, 1986, WB Saunders, pp 393–418.
Respiratory drugs. In *Drug Facts and Comparisons,* New York, 1989, JB Lippincott, pp 755–756.

AZITHROMYCIN

Trade Name(s): *Zithromax.*

Drug Actions:

1. Inhibits bacterial protein synthesis by binding to the 50S ribosomal subunit.
2. Spectrum of activity includes gram-positive aerobes, *Haemophilus influenzae, Moraxella catarrhalis, Haemophilus Chlamydia trachomatis, Mycoplasma pneumoniae, pneumoniae Haemophilus ducreyi, Mycobacterium avium* complex (MAC), and others.

Indications:

1. Lower respiratory tract infections: acute bacterial exacerbations of chronic obstructive pulmonary disease or community-acquired pneumonia of mild severity.
2. Pharyngitis/tonsillitis due to *Streptococcus pyogenes* (alternative to penicillin, which should still be first-line therapy).
3. Uncomplicated skin and skin structure infections.
4. Nongonococcal urethritis and cervicitis (only agent offering a one dose treatment option).
5. Treatment of disseminated MAC disease. (Trials evaluating the effectiveness of azithromycin for prophylaxis of disseminated MAC disease in patients with AIDS are ongoing.)
6. Possible uses in toxoplasmosis, cryptosporidiosis, *Haemophilus ducreyi* (erythromycin-sensitive strains only), and Lyme disease.

Pharmacokinetics:

1. **Absorption:** PO. Azithromycin should not be taken with food, but rather at least 1 hour before or 2 hours after a meal. After oral administration, it is rapidly absorbed and widely distributed into tissues and cells, particularly phagocytes.
2. **Excretion:** Mostly biliary as unchanged drug (6% appears in urine, also as unchanged drug).
3. **Half-life:** 68 hr.

Drug Preparations:

Capsules: 250 mg.
Suspension (single-dose packet): 1 g.

Dosage: 500 mg PO as a single dose on day 1, followed by 250 mg PO qd on days 2–5. For treatment of nongonococcal urethritis/cervicitis, the dosage is 1 g PO once.

Adverse Effects: Azithromycin has a lower incidence of side effects than erythromycin. Most side effects are GI tract related: Diarrhea/loose stools (5%), nausea (3%), and abdominal pain (3%). Azithromycin is not recommended for use in patients under 16 years of age.

Drug Interactions:

1. Levels of digoxin, ergotamine or dihydroergotamine, triazolam, and drugs metabolized by the cytochrome P-450 system

(carbamazepine, cyclosporine, hexobarbital, phenytoin, and others) may be increased with azithromycin administration.
2. Macrolides in general have caused elevations in theophylline levels and prolongation of prothrombin times (in patients taking warfarin).

BIBLIOGRAPHY

Physicians' Desk Reference, ed 50, Montvale, 1996, Medical Economics Co.

AZLOCILLIN

Trade Name: *Azlin.*

Drug Action:
1. Interferes with cell wall synthesis.
2. Spectrum of activity includes gram-positive (but ***not*** penicillinase-producing staphylococci) and gram-negative (including extended coverage to *Pseudomonas aeruginosa, Proteus* spp., *Enterobacter* spp., *Klebsiella* spp., etc.) aerobes and anaerobes, including *Bacteroides fragilis.*

Indications:
1. Infections caused by susceptible organisms.
2. Most often used in combination with an aminoglycoside for synergy (especially against *P. aeruginosa*).

Pharmacokinetics:
1. **Absorption:** Give parenterally.
2. **Distribution:** Poor penetration into uninflamed meninges, bone, sputum.
3. **Metabolism:** Partial.
4. **Excretion:** Renal.
5. **Half-life:** Dose dependent, 55–70 min. Half-life prolonged in renal failure; removed by hemodialysis.

Drug Preparations:
Vials: 2, 3, 4 g for parenteral use.

Dosage:

1. **Normal renal function:** 200–350 mg/kg/day IV given in four to six divided doses; usual dose 3 g q 4 hr.
2. **Impaired renal function:**

Dose (g)	Creatinine Clearance	Interval (hr)
2–4	>80	4–6
	80–50	4–6
	50–10	8
	<10 (anuria)	12

Adverse Effects:

1. All the adverse effect potential as a penicillin class of antibiotics, such as hypersensitivity reactions, neurotoxicity. (*See* also Penicillin.)
2. **Sodium overload:** Monosodium salt with 2.17 mEq/g.
3. **Qualitative platelet defect** (binding to platelet adenosine diphosphate): Most common at high doses with uremia.
4. **Hypokalemia:** Large, nonreabsorbable anion load.
5. **Superinfection.**

Drug Interactions: Inactivated aminoglycosides if mixed in same delivery system. Tubular secretion blocked by probenecid. Inhibits renal excretion of methotrexate.

AZTREONAM

Trade Name: *Azactam.*

Drug Action:

1. Inhibits cell wall synthesis (monobactam antibiotic class).
2. Spectrum of activity specific for gram-negative aerobes (including *Pseudomonas aeruginosa*); *no* coverage against gram-positive aerobes or anaerobes.

Indications: Infections caused by gram-negative aerobes.

Pharmacokinetics:

1. **Absorption:** Give IM/IV.
2. **Distribution:** All body fluids, including CSF.
3. **Metabolism:** Partial.
4. **Excretion:** Renal, feces.
5. **Serum half-life:** 1.7 hr. Removed by hemodialysis and peritoneal dialysis.

Drug Preparations:

Vials: 500 mg, 1, 2 g for injection.

Dosage:

1. **Normal renal function:** 0.5–2 g q 6–12 hr parenterally (IV/IM).
2. **Impaired renal function:**

Dose (g)	Creatinine Clearance	Interval (hr)
0.5–2	>80	6–12
	80–50	8–12
	50–10	12–24
	<10 (anuria)	24–36

Adverse Effects:

1. Similar to other β-lactams, e.g., hypersensitivity, elevation of serum transaminase levels.
2. Poor cross-allergenicity with other β-lactams; no anaphylaxis after use in patients with positive skin tests to penicillin.

β-ADRENERGIC AGONIST BRONCHODILATOR THERAPY

Trade Names:

1. Nonselective β-agonists: Both β_1 and β_2 receptor activity:
   Isoproterenol: *Isuprel:* Pure β-agonist.
   Epinephrine: *Adrenaline:* Both α- and β-agonist activity.

2. Selective β-agonists: Predominantly β_2-receptor activity:
   Metaproterenol: *Alupent, Metaprel:* Not very β_2 selective.
   Isoetharine: *Bronkosol:* Relatively short duration of action.
   Bitolterol: *Tornalate:* Available only as metered dose inhaler.
   Terbutaline: *Brethaire, Bricanyl.*
   Albuterol: *Proventil, Ventolin.*
   Pirbuterol: *Maxair:* Available only as metered-dose inhaler
   Salmeterol: *Serevent* (long-acting β-agonist)

Drug Action:

1. β_2:
   a. Bronchial smooth muscle relaxation, thereby reducing air flow resistance.
   b. Increased mucociliary clearance.
   c. Decreased bronchopulmonary secretion.
   d. Increased hepatic glycogenolysis/gluconeogenesis (causes hyperglycemia).
   e. Increased uterine relaxation.
   f. Increased pancreatic β-cell secretion.
   g. Increased renin secretion.
   h. Increased skeletal muscle tremor.
   i. Peripheral vasodilation.
   j. CNS stimulation.
   k. Intracellular potassium shift.
2. β_1: Positive chronotropic and inotropic cardiac effects: increased heart rate and contractility.
3. **Epinephrine:** Inhibits antigen-induced release of histamine and leukotrienes (possibly also true of isoproterenol, metaproterenol, isoetharine, ephedrine). Antagonizes histamine-induced bronchiolar constriction, vasodilation, edema.

Indications:

1. Bronchospasm.
2. Treatment of anaphylactic and anaphylactoid reactions (**epinephrine** only).
3. Premature labor (IV β_2 agonists).
4. Mild hyperkalemia.

Dosage and Pharmacokinetics: *See* also Table 8:

1. **Metabolism:** Hepatic; also lungs and other tissues for epinephrine, isoproterenol, isoetharine.
2. **Excretion:** Renal, both unchanged and as metabolites.

Adverse Effects:

1. **Cardiovascular:** Palpitations, tachycardia, hypertension, arrhythmias, angina pectoris. Use with caution in patients with coronary artery disease, congestive heart failure, hyperthyroidism, diabetes.
2. **CNS:** Tremor, anxiety, excitability, insomnia, disorientation, seizures, headache, dizziness, weakness, tinnitus, diaphoresis.
3. **GI:** Nausea, vomiting, reflux.
4. **Other:** Muscle cramps, hyperglycemia, hypersensitivity reactions (to drug and sulfite preservatives), paradoxical bronchoconstriction, urinary retention, hypokalemia.
5. **Warning:** do not exceed recommended doses since fatalities have been reported in association with excessive use of inhaled sympathomimetic drugs.

Drug Interactions:

1. Potentiates other cardiovascular agents: general anesthetics (e.g., halothane, cyclopropane), theophylline derivatives, digitalis, levodopa, thyroid hormones, monoamine oxidase inhibitors, tricyclic antidepressants, ergot alkaloids.
2. Additive side effects with other sympathomimetics.
3. Antagonized by β-adrenergic blockers.

Monitoring:

1. Heart rate, blood pressure, ECG.
2. Forced expiratory flow in 1 sec (FEV_1), expiratory flow rates (spirometry).

BIBLIOGRAPHY

Drugs used in bronchial disorders. In *AMA Drug Evaluations,* ed 6, Philadelphia, 1986, WB Saunders, pp 393–418.

Respiratory drugs. In *Drug Facts and Comparisons,* New York, 1989, JB Lippincott, pp 716–729.

Firemen P: β$_2$ agonists and their safety in the treatment of asthma. *Allergy Proc* 1995, 16:235–239.

TABLE 8.
Beta Agonist Agents and Pharmacokinetics

Drug	Drug Form	Dosing Route	Dose*	Onset of Action (min)	Duration of Action (hr)
Albuterol (β_2)	90 µg/spray	MDI	2–3 inhalations (0.18–0.27 mg)	5–10	3–6
	2 mg/5 mL	Nebulizer	2 mg in 2–3 mL saline solution	5–10	3–6
	2, 4 mg tab	PO	2–4 mg	30–45	≥8
Bitolterol (β_2)	370 µg/spray	MDI	2–3 inhalations (0.74–1.11 mg)	5	4–7
Epinephrine (α, β_1, β_2)	160, 200, 250 µg/spray	MDI	2 inhalations (0.4–0.5 mg)	5	1–2
	1%, 1.25%, 2.25%	Nebulizer	5 mg (5 mL 0.1% solution)	5	1–2
	1 mg/mL (1:1,000)	SC	0.2–0.5 mg	5–10	0.75–3
Isoetharine (β_2)	340 µg/spray	MDI	2–3 inhalations (0.68–1.02 mg)	5	2–4
	0.062%–1% solution	Nebulizer	5 mg (0.5 mL 1% solution in 3 mL saline solution)	5	2–4
Isoproterenol (β_1, β_2)	120, 131 µg/spray	MDI	2–3 inhalations (0.16–0.26 mg)	5	0.5–2
	0.25%, 0.5%, 1%	Nebulizer	2.5 mg in saline solution	5	0.5–2
	200 µg/mL	IV (rarely)	0.01–0.02 mg	1–5	<1
Metaproterenol (β_2, β_1)	0.65 mg/spray	MDI	2–3 inhalations (1.3–1.95 mg)	5	3–5
	0.6%, 5% solution	Nebulizer	15 mg (0.3 mL 5% solution in 3 mL saline solution)	5	3–5
Pirbuterol (β_2)	10, 20 mg tab	PO	20 mg	30–45	4
	0.2 mg/spray	MDI	2–3 inhalations	5–10	4–6
Salmeterol (β_2)	21 µg/spray	MDI	2 inhalations	10–20	10–12
Terbutaline (β_2)	200 µg/spray	MDI	2–3 inhalations (0.4–0.6 mg)	5	3–6
	1 mg/mL	Nebulizer	2 mg (2 mL parenteral solution)	5	3–6
	2.5, 5 mg tab	PO	2.5–5 mg	45–60	6–8
	1 mg/mL	SC	0.25 mg	5–10	2–3

*No adjustment in dose for renal/hepatic disease.
MDI, metered dose inhaler.

β-ADRENERGIC RECEPTOR ANTAGONISTS

Trade Names:

Nonselective (β_1 and β_2 antagonism):
  Propranolol: *Inderal.*
  Timolol: *Blocadren.*
  Nadolol: *Corgard.*
Cardioselective (β_1 antagonism predominates):
  Esmolol: *Brevibloc.*
  Metoprolol: *Lopressor.*
  Atenolol: *Tenormin.*
  Acebutolol: *Sectral.*
Intrinsic sympathomimetic activity (ISA):
  Pindolol: *Visken.*
Combined α- and β-antagonist:
  Labetolol (See Labetolol).

Drug Action: Competitive binding to β-receptors results in blockade of adenyl cyclase activation, which prevents increases in intracellular levels of cyclic adenosine monophosphate (cAMP), blunting the second messenger β-response. Drugs with ISA have both agonist and antagonist properties (pindolol). Cardioselectivity results in minimal binding to β-receptors at low drug levels, but with greater binding as the levels increase. Propranolol and pindolol have membrane stabilizing activity, which reduces the excitability of depolarizing cells.

1. β_1 blocking effects:
   a. **Cardiac:** Reduced chronotropy, inotropy, excitability.
   b. **Noncardiac:** Reduced renin release and aqueous humor production.
2. β_2 blocking effects:
   a. **Cardiac:** Reduced chronotropy, inotropy.
   b. **Metabolic:** Decreased insulin secretion, gluconeogenesis, glycogenolysis, lipolysis.
   c. Peripheral vasoconstriction.
   d. Bronchoconstriction.
   e. Increased uterine tone.
   f. Prevents decrease in serum potassium caused by β_2 stimulation.

Indications:

1. Myocardial ischemia.
2. Hypertension.
3. Cardiac arrhythmias.
4. Post myocardial infarction.
5. Hypertrophic obstructive cardiomyopathy.
6. Mitral valve prolapse.
7. Hyperthyroidism.
8. Migraine.
9. Essential tremor.

Pharmacokinetics: IV drugs only:

1. Propranolol (Inderal):
   a. **Metabolism:** Hepatic.
   b. **Excretion:** Renal.
   c. **Protein binding:** 90%–95%.
   d. **Onset of action:** Almost immediate (after IV administration).
   e. **Plasma half-life:** IV: 2.5 hr; PO: 3–6 hr.
2. Metoprolol (Lopressor):
   a. **Metabolism:** Hepatic.
   b. **Excretion:** Renal.
   c. **Protein binding:** 10%.
   d. **Onset of action:** Almost immediate (after IV administration).
   e. **Plasma half-life:** 3–7 hr.
3. Esmolol (Brevibloc):
   a. **Metabolism:** Red blood cell esterase.
   b. **Excretion:** Renal.
   c. **Protein binding:** 55%.
   d. **Onset of action:** Immediate.
   e. **Plasma half-life:** 9 min.

Drug Preparations:

1. Propranolol (Inderal):
   Vials: 1 mg/mL.
   Extended release capsules: 80, 120, 160 mg.
   Tablets: 10, 20, 40, 60, 80, 90 mg.
2. Metoprolol (Lopressor):
   Vials: 5 mg/5 mL.
   Tablets: 50, 100 mg.
3. Esmolol: *Vials:* 2.5 g/10 mL, 100 mg/10 mL.

4. Atenolol: *Tablets:* 50, 100 mg.
5. Nadolol: *Tablets:* 20, 40, 80, 120, 160 mg.
6. Pindolol: *Tablets:* 5, 10 mg.
7. Timolol: *Tablets:* 5, 10, 20 mg.

Dosage:

1. Propranolol (Inderal):
   a. *IV:* If serum levels of β-blockers present, 0.5–1 mg IV, titrated to effect. If no serum levels, up to 0.1 mg/kg IV may be given to achieve full β-antagonism.
   b. *PO:* 10–80 mg bid–qid; 80–160 mg/day of extended-release capsules.
2. Metoprolol (Lopressor):
   a. *IV:* If serum levels present, 1–2 mg IV, titrated to effect. If no serum levels, up to 0.2 mg/kg may be necessary.
   b. *PO:* 100–450 mg/day in single or divided doses.
3. Esmolol (Brevibloc): 0.5–1 mg/kg loading dose, with 50 µg/kg/min continuous infusion. Continuous infusion may be increased by 50 µg/kg/min, preceded by a loading dose up to 300 µg/kg/min. Titrate to effect.
4. Atenolol: 50–100 mg PO once/day.
5. Nadolol: 40–320 mg PO once/day.
6. Pindolol: 5–30 mg PO bid.
7. Timolol: 10–30 mg PO bid.

Adverse Effects:

1. **Bradycardia;** less with pindolol (ISA).
2. Worsening **congestive heart failure;** less with pindolol (ISA).
3. **Bronchospasm;** less with cardioselective β-antagonists. Pindolol (ISA) may provide even more protection against bronchospasm.
4. Signs of **tachycardia** and **diaphoresis** with hypoglycemia may be masked. Also, $β_2$-blocking effects of decreased insulin secretion, gluconeogenesis, and glycogenolysis may make hypoglycemia worse or more likely (propranolol).
5. **Peripheral vasoconstriction** with $β_2$-blockade may worsen peripheral vascular disease (propranolol).
6. **Hypotension;** worse with cardioselective drugs by allowing $β_2$-stimulation (decreased systemic resistance) while decreasing cardiac output.

7. Worsening preexisting **cardiac conduction disturbances.**
   Asystole and heart block reported with simultaneous IV β- and
   calcium channel antagonists.
8. Sudden β-antagonist withdrawal may precipitate tachycardia,
   hypertension, myocardial ischemia, myocardial infarction, and
   death.

Monitoring:

1. Hemodynamic signs, heart rate, blood pressure, etc.
2. Drug levels (propranolol) available depending on hospital laboratory.

Drug Reversal: β-agonists reverse competitively β-antagonism
(isoproterenol, dobutamine, dopamine, epinephrine).

BIBLIOGRAPHY

Slogoff S: Beta adrenergic blockers. In Kaplan J (ed): *Cardiac
   Anesthesia,* vol 2, *Cardiovascular Pharmacology,* New York,
   1983, Grune & Stratton, pp 181–208.
Weiner N: Drugs that inhibit adrenergic nerves and block adrenergic receptors. In Gilman AG, Goodman LS, Gilman A (eds):
   The Pharmacological Basis of Therapeutics, ed 6, New York,
   1980, Macmillan, pp 176–210.

BRETYLIUM

Trade Names: *Bretylol, Bretylium Tosylate.*

Drug Action:

1. Initially causes release of norepinephrine, then prevents norepinephrine release.
2. Electrophysiologic effects may cause chemical defibrillation.
   Prolongs refractoriness in atria and ventricles.
3. Increases significantly ventricular fibrillation threshold.
4. Reduces disparity between action potential duration and refractory period in regions of normal and ischemic myocardium, thus decreasing reentry arrhythmias.
5. No myocardial depression.
6. May produce hypotension by α-blocking properties.

Indications:

1. Drug-resistant ventricular arrhythmias.
2. Treatment and prophylaxis of ventricular fibrillation in cardiopulmonary resuscitation.

Pharmacokinetics:

1. **Absorption:** Give IV/IM.
2. **Metabolism:** None.
3. **Excretion:** Intact in urine.
4. **Plasma half-life:** 7–8 hr.
5. **Onset of action:** Ventricular; fibrillation: rapid. For suppression of ventricular tachycardia, onset may be 20 min–2 hr.

Drug Preparations:

Vials: 500 mg/10 mL, 1 g/20 mL.

Dosage: Bolus: 5–10 mg/kg over 10–20 min IV, followed by continuous infusion 1–5 mg/min.

Adverse Effects:

1. Hypotension.
2. Transient hypertension.
3. CNS effects.
4. Bradycardia.
5. Early increased frequency of premature ventricular contractions.
6. Nausea/vomiting.

Drug Interactions:

1. Hypersensitivity to dopamine, epinephrine, norepinephrine.
2. Questionable efficacy when combined with procainamide or quinidine.
3. May exacerbate ventricular arrhythmias associated with digitalis intoxication.

Monitoring: Blood pressure is a limiting factor; ECG.

BIBLIOGRAPHY

Bigger JT Jr, Hoffman BF: Antiarrhythmic drugs. In Gilman AG, Goodman LS, Gilman A (eds): *The Pharmacological Basis of Therapeutics,* ed 6, New York, 1980, Macmillan, pp 761–792.

Zipes DP: Management of cardiac arrhythmias: pharmacological, electrical, and surgical techniques. In Braunwald E (ed): *Heart Disease: A Textbook of Cardiovascular Medicine,* Philadelphia, 1988, WB Saunders, pp 621–657.

BUMETANIDE

Trade Name: *Bumex.*

Drug Action:

1. Inhibits absorption of sodium and chloride in the ascending limb of the loop of Henle by blocking the chloride site of the $Na-K_2-Cl$ cotransport system.
2. May inhibit sodium and chloride reabsorption in the proximal convoluted tubules.

Indications:

1. **Acute oliguria:** Possible adjunct to therapy for oliguria when attempting to prevent acute renal failure. Other measures must also be taken to ensure adequate circulating blood volume and renal perfusion.
2. **Edematous states:** Indicated for treatment of edema associated with congestive heart failure, liver failure, renal disease (including nephrotic syndrome).
3. **Pulmonary edema:** Indicated as adjunctive therapy in treatment of acute pulmonary edema.
4. **Hypertension:** May be useful in acute management of hypertension or as an adjunct in management of mild to moderate hypertension. Not considered the drug of choice in treatment of chronic essential hypertension.
5. **Hypercalcemia:** Can be used in treatment of severe hypercalcemia by promoting diuresis and calcium wasting.

Pharmacokinetics:

1. **Metabolism:** Limited, and produces inactive metabolites.
2. **Excretion:** 81% renal (45% unchanged), 2% biliary.
3. **Volume of distribution:** 0.1 L/kg.
4. **Protein binding:** 94%–96%.

5. **Plasma half-life:** 60–90 min; prolonged in renal disease.
6. **Absorption:** 72%–76% of PO dose.

Drug Preparations:

Tablets: 0.5, 1, 2 mg.
Solution: 0.025% for dilution and IV administration.

Dosage:

1. **Adult:**
   a. Diuretic:
      (1) **IV:** 0.5–1.0 mg, repeated in 2–3 hr if necessary. Usual prescribing limit 10 mg/day.
      (2) **PO:** 0.5–2.0 mg/day in single dose; can be increased by adding a second or third daily dose at 4–5 hr intervals. Usual prescribing limit 10 mg/day.
2. **Pediatric:**
   a. Diuretic: IV/PO not established.

Adverse Effects:

1. Common: Hypokalemia, hyponatremia, dizziness, glucose intolerance, hypomagnesemia, hypovolemia, hyperuricemia, prerenal azotemia, hypotension.
2. Uncommon: Ototoxicity (usually reversible and associated with rapid infusion of excessively large doses), syncope, hyperosmolality, thromboembolic complications, encephalopathy in preexisting liver disease.

Drug Interactions:

1. **Increased hypokalemia:**
   a. Adrenocorticoids.
   b. Antihypertensives.
   c. Amphotericin B.
2. **Increased effects:**
   a. Anticoagulants.
   b. Oral hypoglycemics, insulin.
   c. Nondepolarizing neuromuscular blocking agents.
   d. Lithium.
3. **Decreased effects:**
   a. Allopurinol.
4. **Nephrotoxicity increased:**
   a. Aminoglycosides.

5. **Ototoxicity increased:**
   a. Aminoglycosides.
   b. Cisplatin.
6. **Digoxin toxicity** (secondary to hypokalemia).

Monitoring:

1. Follow urinary output and taper to desired effect.
2. Monitor for adverse effects:
   a. Blood pressure.
   b. Serum electrolyte determinations.
   c. BUN, creatinine, serum uric acid.
   d. Hearing examinations.
   e. Hepatic function.
   f. Renal function.

BIBLIOGRAPHY

Diuretics and cardiovasculars. In *Drug Facts and Comparisons,* New York, 1995, JB Lippincott, pp 607–614.

Diuretics, loop (systemic). In *Drug Information for the Health Care Provider,* ed 15, Rockville, 1995, US Pharmacopeial Convention, pp 1144–1151.

Weiner IM, Mudge GH: Diuretics and other agents employed in the mobilization of edema fluid. In Gilman A, Goodman L, Rall T, et al (eds): *Goodman and Gilman's The Pharmacologic Basis of Therapeutics,* ed 7, New York, 1985, Macmillan, pp 896–900.

BUPRENORPHINE

Trade Name: *Buprenex.*

Drug Actions:

1. Buprenorphine is a partial μ-opioid agonist. 0.4 mg of buprenorphine is equivalent to 10 mg of morphine for pain relief.
2. Buprenorphine and morphine have similar respiratory depressant activity when administered at comparable analgesic doses. Peak respiratory depression may not occur for 3 hr. A ceiling effect for respiratory depression is likely but has not been

clearly demonstrated, and clinically significant respiratory depression has occurred.
3. Because it is a partial agonist and dissociates slowly from the μ-opioid receptor, buprenorphine can antagonize the analgesic effects of other opioids such as morphine. It may also have κ-opioid antagonist effects.

Indications:

1. For the relief of moderate to severe pain and as an adjunct to local regional or general anesthesia.

Pharmacokinetics:

1. Absorption: Well absorbed by the sublingual and intramuscular routes.
2. Onset of actions: Slower onset than morphine, pharmacologic effects after IM injection occur in 15 min, peak effects at 1 hr and duration of action is 6 hr or longer. Faster onset after IV use. Peak blood concentrations occur in 2 hr after sublingual administration.
3. Metabolism: Metabolized by the liver, and clearance is related to hepatic blood flow.
4. Excretion: Majority is excreted unchanged in the feces. Small amount of N-dealkylated and conjugated metabolites excreted in the urine.
5. Half-life: Elimination half-lifes have ranged from 1.2 to 7.2 hr. The consensus value is approximately 3 hr.
6. Therapeutic level:

Drug Preparations:

Ampules: 0.3 mg/mL

Dosage: IM: 0.3 mg; IV: 0.03–0.3 mg slowly over 2 min; SL: 0.4–0.8 mg q 4–6 hr in a 70-kg adult.

Adverse Effects:

1. Similar to morphine: Sedation, respiratory depression, decrease in blood pressure or pulse rate, increase in intracranial pressure, nausea, dizziness, and vertigo.
2. Opioid antagonists such as naloxone may not be effective in reversing the respiratory depression produced by buprenorphine.
3. Buprenorphine can precipitate withdrawal symptoms in narcotic addicts.

4. After prolonged administration a withdrawal syndrome can develop, which is delayed in onset for up to 15 days and is typically less severe than observed during withdrawal from morphine.

Drug Interactions:

1. Sedation is additive with other CNS depressants (e.g., phenothiazines, hypnotics, and tranquilizers). However, buprenorphine has been used to reverse narcotic-induced respiratory depression following surgery in which significant doses of narcotics were used as part of the surgery. This effect is the result of the partial agonist activity at the μ-opioid receptor. Buprenorphine is probably not a good choice for antagonism of respiratory depression, since antagonism of buprenorphine induced respiratory depression is unpredictable and pure antagonists such as naloxone are readily available.
2. Coadministration with diazepam has been reported to result in respiratory and cardiovascular collapse.
3. Interaction with MAO inhibitors is unknown and caution is advised.

Monitoring: Respiratory rate, blood pressure, heart rate, mental status.

BIBLIOGRAPHY

Wallenstein SL, Kaiko RF, Rogers AG, Houde RW: Crossover trials in clinical analgesic assays: studies of buprenorphine and morphine, *Pharmacotherapy* 1986, 6:228–235.
Boysen K, Hertel S, Chraemmer-Jorgensen B, et al. Buprenorphine antagonism of ventilatory depression following fentanyl anesthesia, *Acta Anaesthesiol Scand* 1988, 32:490–492.

BUSPIRONE

Trade Name: *Buspar.*

Drug Actions: Antianxiety drug unrelated to benzodiazepines, barbiturates, or other sedative-hypnotic drugs. Does not have anticonvulsant or muscle relaxant effects. Selective antagonist at 5-HT_{1A} receptors.

Indications: For treatment of anxiety disorders or temporary relief of symptoms of anxiety.

Pharmacokinetics:

1. **Absorption:** Rapidly absorbed with extensive first-pass metabolism.
2. **Onset of action:** 40–90 min.
3. **Metabolism:** Hepatic. 95% of drug is protein bound.
4. **Excretion:** Two thirds renal, one third fecal.
5. **Half-life:** About 2–3 hr.
6. **Therapeutic level:** None.

Drug Preparations:

 Tablets: 5 mg, 10 mg.

Dosage: Initial dose of 15 mg/day in three doses can be increased to maximum of 60 mg/day.

Adverse Effects: May increase liver enzyme levels. Dizziness, drowsiness, and GI distress all reported, although to a lesser extent than with the benzodiazepines.

Drug Interactions: May displace protein-bound drugs, including digoxin. Hypertension is reported with the combination of Buspar and MAO inhibitors—the combination use is not recommended.

Monitoring: Level of sedation.

BIBLIOGRAPHY

Eison AS, Eison MS: Serotonergic mechanisms in anxiety. *Prog Neuropsychopharmacol Biol Psychiatry* 1994, 18:47–62.

Barrett JE, Vanover KE: 5-HT receptors as targets for the development of novel anxiolytic drugs—models, mechanisms and future directions, *Psychopharmacology* 1993, 112:1–12.

BUTORPHANOL

Trade Name: *Stadol.*

Drug Action:

1. Butorphanol is an opiate receptor agonist-antagonist. Unlike morphine and related compounds, butorphanol has little if any

activity at the μ-receptor, which mediates analgesia and respiratory depression. There appears to be moderate affinity at the κ-receptor, which also mediates analgesia, and low affinity at the σ-receptor, which mediates dysphoria.

2. Dose of 2 mg IM approximates 10 mg intramuscular morphine sulfate. Unlike morphine, respiratory depression in healthy adults plateaus after 3–4 mg IV butorphanol, and increasing the dose usually results in no further respiratory depression. There is also a plateau with respect to its analgesic properties.

Indications: Butorphanol can be used to treat moderate to severe pain, as a preoperative sedative, and as part of a general anesthetic.

Pharmacokinetics:

1. **Absorption:** IM administration results in onset of action of about 10–20 min, compared with 1 min when given IV. Both IV and IM administration results in 3–4 hr duration of action. Although it is well absorbed from the GI tract, the PO route is limited because more than 80% of butorphanol undergoes first-pass metabolism in the liver.
2. **Metabolism:** Hydroxylation, dealkylation, and glucuronide conjugation in liver.
3. **Excretion:** Primarily in urine.
4. **Half-life:** 3–4 hr.

Drug Preparations:

Vial: 1, 2 mg/mL.

Dosage:

1. **IM:** 2 mg q 3–4 hr, but dose may vary from 1–4 mg, depending on patient requirements.
2. **IV:** 1 mg q 3–4 hr. Dose may range from 0.5–2 mg q 3–4 hr. Dosage should be decreased in severe liver disease.

Adverse Effects:

1. May precipitate a withdrawal syndrome in narcotic addicts because of its agonist-antagonist properties.
2. Sedation, dysphoria, nausea and vomiting, confusion, lethargy.
3. Use with caution in patients at risk for increased intracranial pressure.

4. Administer carefully in patients with myocardial ischemia, because drug may increase pulmonary artery and left ventricular filling pressure, as well as systemic blood pressure.

Drug Interactions: As with morphine, butorphanol is additive to other CNS depressants.

Monitoring:

1. Mental status.
2. Heart rate, blood pressure.
3. Respiratory rate.

BIBLIOGRAPHY

McEvoy GK (ed): *AHFS Drug Information 89,* Bethesda, 1989, American Society of Hospital Pharmacists.

Gilman AG, Goodman LS, Rall TW, et al (eds): *Goodman and Gilman's The Pharmacological Basis of Therapeutics,* ed 7, New York, 1985, Macmillan.

Physicians' Desk Reference, ed 42, Oradell, 1988, Medical Economics Co.

CALCITONIN

Trade Names:

Salmon origin: *Osteocalcin, Miacalcin.*
Human: *Calcimar, Cibacalcin.*

Drug Action: Hypocalcemic agent. Inhibits bone resorption of calcium; inhibits renal tubular calcium resorption. Increases urinary excretion of calcium, phosphorus, and sodium. Also inhibits secretion of pancreatic enzymes and gastric secretion.

Indications:

1. Hypercalcemia.
2. Paget's disease of bone.

Pharmacokinetics:

1. **Absorption:** Must be given parenterally.
2. **Metabolism:** Kidney and peripheral tissues.

3. **Excretion:** Urine as inactive metabolites.
4. **Half-life:** 1–2 hr.
5. **Duration:** 8–24 hr after SC/IM dose; 0.5–12 hr after IV injection. Max. effect 2–4 hr.

Drug Preparations:

Salmon: 200 IU/mL (2 mL vials).
Human: 0.5 mg/syringe.

Dosage:

1. **Hypercalcemia:** (salmon calcitonin) 4–8 IU/kg IM/SQ q 12 hr; may increase to 8 IU/kg q 6 hr. Effectiveness may decrease after several days of use. 0.5 mg human calcitonin q 6–8 hr.
2. **Paget's disease of bone:**
   a. Salmon: 50–100 IU SQ/IM per day.
   b. Human: 0.5 mg SQ/IM per day (Cibacalcin).
3. **Postmenopausal osteoporosis:** 100 IU SQ per day.

Adverse Effects:

1. **CNS:** Headache, dizziness, tingling, weakness.
2. **Cardiovascular:** Flushing.
3. **GI:** Nausea/vomiting, diarrhea, anorexia, epigastric discomfort, abdominal pain.
4. **GU:** Diuresis, increased urination.
5. **Hyperglycemia, hypocalcemia, tetany.**
6. **Rash, pain, and swelling** at injection site.
7. **Urticaria, anaphylaxis, allergic reaction.**

Drug Interactions: Hypocalcemic action antagonized by calcium and vitamin D.

Monitoring:

1. Serum calcium, phosphate.
2. Alkaline phosphatase, urine hydroxyproline (Paget's disease).

BIBLIOGRAPHY

Zaloga GP, Chernow B: Divalent ions: calcium, magnesium, and phosphorus. In Chernow B (ed): *The Pharmacologic Approach to the Critically Ill Patient,* ed 3, Baltimore, 1994, Williams & Wilkins, pp 777–804.

Warrell RP, Israel R, Frisone M, et al: Gallium nitrate for acute treatment of cancer related hypercalcemia. A randomized, double-blind comparison to calcitonin, *Ann Intern Med* 1988, 108:669–674.

Ralston SH, GArdner MD, Dryburgh FJ, et al: Comparison of amino-hydroxypropylidine diphosphonate, mithramycin, and corticosteroids/calcitonin in treatment of cancer associated hypercalcemia, *Lancet* 1985, 2:907–909.

Avioli LV: Calcitonin therapy in osteoporotic syndromes, *Rheum Dis Clin North Am* 1994, 20:777–785.

CALCIUM SALTS

Trade Names:

Calcium carbonate: *Alka-2, Alka-Mints, Amitone, Cal Carb-HD, Calcilac, Calglycine, Caltrate 600, Chooz, Dicarbosil, Equilet, Mallamint, Os-Cal, Titracid, Titralac, Tums, Tums Liquid Extra-Strength,* and others.

Calcium chloride: *Cal Plus.*

Calcium glubionate: *Neo-Calglucon.*

Calcium gluceptate.

Calcium gluconate.

Calcium lactate.

Calcium phosphate: Dibasic calcium phosphate.

Calcium citrate: *Citracal.*

Calcium acetate: *Phos-Ex, PhosLo.*

Drug Action:

1. Calcium is required for function of all cells in the body. It is essential for excitation-contraction coupling, stimulus-secretion coupling, enzyme activity, cardiac action potential, cell division, and many other metabolic activities. It is a major cell messenger and is important for membrane and bone structure.
2. Calcium binds phosphorus in the GI tract, decreasing its absorption.

Indications:

1. Ionized hypocalcemia.
2. Vasopressor action (hypotension).
3. Osteoporosis.
4. Hyperkalemia, hypermagnesemia, hyperphosphatemia.
5. Calcium channel blocker overdose.
6. Antacid (carbonate).
7. Cardiac arrest due to hypocalcemia, hyperkalemia, hypermagnesemia, calcium channel blocker toxicity.

Pharmacokinetics:

1. **Absorption:** Small bowel; increased by vitamin D; 30% absorbed; absorbed in soluble ionized form; solubility (except calcium lactate) increased by acid pH; calcium carbonate absorption impaired in achlorhydria.
2. **Distribution:** Primarily extracellular space and bone.
3. **Metabolism:** None.
4. **Excretion:** Urine, stool.
5. **Half-life:** 30–60 min with normal renal function.

Drug Preparations: (Ca = elemental calcium):

1. Calcium chloride (27.2% Ca): 10% solution (100 mg/mL) in 10 mL containing 1 g = 272 mg Ca. May be given IV.
2. Calcium gluceptate (8.2% Ca): 1.1 g in 5-mL ampules (90 mg Ca) or 50-mL vials. May be given IV.
3. Calcium gluconate (9% Ca): 10% solution in 10-mL ampules (1 g = 90 mg Ca) may be given IV; 500 (45 mg Ca), 650, 975, 1000-mg tablets.
4. Calcium carbonate (40% Ca): 350, 420, 500, 650, 750, 850, 1250-, 1500-mg Ca tablets; 1250 mg/5 mL suspension (400 mg Ca/gm); liquid (Tums Extra-Strength) 1000 mg/5 mL; powder (Cal Carb-HD) 6.5 g/packet.
5. Calcium citrate (21% Ca): 950-mg tablets (211 mg Ca/g).
6. Calcium glubionate syrup (6.5% Ca): 1.8 g/5 mL (65 mg Ca/g).
7. Calcium lactate (13% Ca): 325, 650-mg tablets (130 mg Ca/g).
8. Calcium phosphate, dibasic (23% Ca): 468-mg tablets (230 mg Ca/g).
9. Calcium acetate (25% Ca): 500 mg capsules; 250–1000 mg tablets.

Dosage:

1. **Ionized hypocalcemia:**
   a. Initial dose 90 mg Ca IV by slow push, then 0.5–2.0 mg/kg/hr Ca by IV infusion. Taper to ionized calcium level.
   b. **PO:** Give 1–1.5 g Ca three to four times/day.
   c. Calcium gluceptate may be given IM.
2. **Antacid:** Calcium carbonate: 1–2 tabs (500 mg) q 4–6 hr.
3. **Hyperkalemia, hypermagnesemia, calcium blocker overdose:** 90–180 mg Ca by slow IV push; repeat if necessary. Begin definitive therapy at same time.
4. **Osteoporosis:** 1–1.5 g Ca/day PO.
5. **Hyperphosphatemia:** Calcium acetate 500 mg with each meal or calcium carbonate 250–500 mg with each meal; increase dose to bring serum phosphate to <6 mg/dL.
6. **RDA:** 800–1000 mg Ca/day (adults).

Adverse Effects:

1. Hypercalcemia, hypophosphatemia.
2. Milk-alkali syndrome with calcium carbonate.
3. **CNS:** Depressed sensorium, headache, confusion, lethargy, coma, flushing, weakness.
4. **GI:** Anorexia, nausea/vomiting, constipation, abdominal pain, pancreatitis, hepatic injury.
5. **GU:** Polyuria, renal stones, nephrocalcinosis, renal failure.
6. **Cardiovascular:** Hypertension, arrhythmias, bradycardia, AV block.
7. Cellular damage during ischemic and shock states.
8. Ectopic calcification, pruritus, erythema, conjunctivitis, dry mouth.
9. Necrosis after IM/SQ injection or IV infiltration.

Drug Interactions:

1. Potentiates digitalis; may precipitate toxicity.
2. Binds with tetracycline in gut and decreases its absorption.
3. Blunts action of epinephrine.
4. Antagonizes decreased contractile effects of calcium channel blockers.
5. Oxalic acid (rhubarb, spinach), phytic acid (bran, whole-grain cereals), phosphorus may interfere with gut absorption.
6. Thiazides decrease renal excretion of calcium.

7. Corticosteroids decrease gut calcium absorption.
8. Calcium decreases phenytoin absorption.
9. Calcium carbonate increases urinary pH and may decrease excretion of quinidine.

Monitoring:

1. Serum calcium (ionized calcium is best).
2. Urine calcium.
3. Serum phosphate.
4. ECG (during IV administration), blood pressure.

BIBLIOGRAPHY

Zaloga GP, Chernow B: Divalent ions—calcium, magnesium, and phosphorus. In Chernow B (ed): *The Pharmacologic Approach to the Critically Ill Patient,* ed 3, Baltimore, 1994, Williams & Wilkins, pp 777–804.

Haynes RC: Agents affecting calcification—calcium, parathyroid hormone, calcitonin, vitamin D, and other compounds. In Gilman AG, et al (eds): *The Pharmacological Basis of Therapeutics,* ed 8, New York, 1993, McGraw-Hill, pp 1496–1522.

CARBAMAZEPINE

Trade Name: *Tegretol*; generics.

Drug Action: The pharmacologic actions of carbamazepine are similar to those of the hydantoins. These medications limit seizure propagation by reduction of post-tetanic potentiation of the synaptic transmission. The drug has also demonstrated sedative, anticholinergic, antidepressant, muscle relaxant, antiarrhythmic, antidiuretic, and neuromuscular transmission inhibiting actions. Carbamazepine has only slight analgesic properties.

Indications:

1. **Seizures:** Carbamazepine is used in the treatment of complex partial (e.g., psychomotor or temporal lobe) seizures. It may also be of benefit in generalized tonic-clonic seizures and partial seizures with complex symptoms. As with nearly all anticonvulsants, patient response, according to seizure type, is

variable. Carbamazepine is not effective in the management of absence seizures, myoclonic seizures, or akinetic seizures.

2. **Trigeminal neuralgia:** Tegretol is effective in the treatment of pain associated with trigeminal neuralgia. It has not been found effective in other causes of facial pain, except that in some patients glossopharyngeal neuralgia may respond to carbamazepine.

3. **Pain:** Carbamazepine has been used in the control of neuropathic pain such as in tabes dorsalis, acute polyneuritis, posttraumatic pain, diabetic neuropathy, and postherpetic pain.

4. **Other:** Carbamazepine has been used in the treatment of postconcussion syndromes, hemifacial spasm, and dystonia in children and has been used for its antidiuretic effects in the management of diabetes insipidus.

Pharmacokinetics:

1. **Metabolism:** 90% of carbamazepine is biologically available after PO dosing. Carbamazepine's major metabolic pathway appears to be oxidation by the liver microsomal enzymes system to the 1,11-epoxide. This is then almost completely metabolized to the trans-10,11-dihydroxy form and is excreted in the urine. Carbamazepine induces liver enzymes, and may speed its own metabolism and metabolism of other similarly metabolized drugs.

2. **Excretion:** Only 1%–3% of the drug is excreted unchanged in the urine.

3. **Volume of distribution:** 75%–90% of carbamazepine is bound to plasma proteins; 15% of the plasma concentration is found in the cerebrospinal fluid.

4. **Clearance:** 1.4 ± 0.4 mL/min/kg.

5. **Plasma half-life:** 6.1 ± 0.7 hr; in some cases may extend for as long as 25–65 hr.

Dosage: 10–20 mg/kg/day is suggested, depending on therapeutic response and steady-state blood levels. Therapy must be started at low levels and increased slowly (200 mg/day at weekly intervals is suggested). More rapid or slower increases must be made as tolerated.

1. **Adult:** Usual dose 800–1200 mg/day in divided doses q 6–8 hr PO. Some patients may require 1600–2400 mg/day, depending on other drug exposure and metabolic rates.

2. Pediatric:
>12 yr: Usual dose 800–1200 mg/day in two to four divided doses PO.
<12 yr: 400–800 mg/day in two to four divided doses PO is common.

Drug Preparations:

Tablets: 200 mg.
Chewable tablets: 100 mg.
PO suspension: 100 mg/5 mL.
No parenteral preparations are available at present.

Adverse Reactions:

1. Carbamazepine can result in an allergic reaction to the medication, necessitating prompt discontinuance of its use.
2. Carbamazepine may induce the stimulation of antidiuretic hormone, resulting in hyponatremia and water intoxication.
3. Carbamazepine is associated with a long list of potential adverse reactions. Many of the side effects are associated with too rapid increase in dosage. More frequently encountered side effects include blurred or double vision, confusion or behavioral changes, headache, nausea/vomiting, drowsiness, and weakness. For a complete list of potential side effects or adverse effects, the reader is directed to the references cited.

Drug Interactions: Multiple drug interactions are potential in patients receiving carbamazepine with other therapeutic agents. Carbamazepine is a powerful, microsomal enzyme inducer, and may stimulate its own metabolism and the metabolism of other therapeutic agents. The following are believed to be of enough significant clinical importance to be included:

1. Carbamazepine may decrease the therapeutic effect of adrenocorticoid therapy, requiring increased adrenocorticoid dosing.
2. Carbamazepine may increase the risk of hepatotoxicity in patients taking large amounts of acetaminophen.
3. Carbamazepine increases the metabolism of anticoagulant agents, requiring dosage adjustment based on results of coagulation studies.
4. Concomitant use of carbamazepine with other anticonvulsants, such as phenytoin, barbiturates, benzodiazepines, and valproic acid, may increase the metabolism of both agents, requiring

careful blood concentration monitoring and appropriate dosage modifications.

5. Cimetidine, erythromycin, and some calcium channel blockers may inhibit the metabolism of carbamazepine, resulting in toxic levels of the agent.
6. Carbamazepine may induce the metabolism of isoniazide, resulting in increased levels of toxic metabolites and resultant hepatic toxicity.
7. Concurrent use of carbamazepine and monoamine oxidase inhibitors may result in a hypertensive, hyperpyretic crisis; convulsions; and death.
8. Numerous other drug interactions of equal or lesser clinical significance can occur. Again, the reader's attention is directed to the more encyclopedic pharmacologic text.

Monitoring: Therapeutic plasma concentrations range from 4–12 μg/mL. Reliable drug level testing is available in most hospitals and reference laboratories.

NOTE: A rare but serious drug effect that may be associated with carbamazepine is leukopenia, and more rarely aplastic anemia. Before starting carbamazepine therapy, baseline complete blood cell count and differential should be determined. Follow-up hematologic profiles should be obtained at monthly intervals during the first 6 months of therapy and at 6-month intervals thereafter, if no major hematologic derangements are encountered. The drug should be discontinued if the white blood cell (WBC) count falls below the normal range. In this author's experience, minimal decrease in WBC count is encountered frequently, but this rarely falls below the normal range, and likewise rarely requires discontinuance of the drug or modification of dosage.

Owing to carbamazepine's short half-life in monitoring of blood levels, the assay should be determined at an appropriate trough, usually drawn in the morning, before the morning dose.

BIBLIOGRAPHY

Cohen, S, Armstrong M: *Drug Interactions: A Handbook for Clinical Use,* Baltimore, 1974, Williams & Wilkins.

Drug Information for the Health Care Professional, ed 8, Rockville, 1988, US Pharmacopeial Convention.

Evans WE, Oellerich M: *Therapeutic Drug Monitoring Clinical Guide,* ed 2, Irving, 1984, Abbott Laboratories Publications.

Gilman A, Goodman L, Rall T, et al (eds): *The Pharmacological Basis of Therapeutics,* ed 7, New York, 1985, Macmillan.

Johnson G: *Blue Book of Pharmacologic Therapeutics,* Philadelphia, 1985, WB Saunders.

McEvoy GK: *Drug Information 88,* Bethesda, 1988, American Society of Hospital Pharmacists.

CARBENICILLIN

Trade Names: *Geopen, Geocillin.*

Drug Action:

1. Inhibits cell wall synthesis (penicillin).
2. Spectrum of activity includes non-β-lactamase-producing gram-positive aerobes (streptococci but not staphylococci), most gram-negative aerobes (including *Pseudomonas aeruginosa* but **not** *Klebsiella* species), and anaerobes (including *Bacteroides fragilis*).

Indications: Infections caused by susceptible organisms (often combined with aminoglycosides for synergy).

Pharmacokinetics:

1. **Absorption:** Poor after PO administration. Must give IM/IV.
2. **Distribution:** Minimal penetration into uninflamed meninges; slight penetration into bone and sputum.
3. **Metabolism:** Partial.
4. **Excretion:** Renal.
5. **Plasma half-life:** 72 min. Removed by hemodialysis but not by peritoneal dialysis.

Drug Preparations:

    Vials: 2, 5 g for IV/IM.
    Tablets: Equivalent to 0.382 g carbenicillin.

Dosage:

1. **Normal renal function:** 5–6.5 g q 4–6 hr IV/IM
2. **Impaired renal function** (IV/IM):

Dose (g)	Creatinine Clearance	Interval (hr)
5–6.5	>80	4–6
	80–50	6
2–3	50–10	6–8
2	<10 (anuria)	12

3. **Hemodialysis:** Supplement anuric dosage schedule with 2 g after each dialysis. Daily dose during peritoneal dialysis is 2 g q 6 hr.
4. Oral drug used only for urinary tract infections: 1–2 tablets q 6 hr.

Adverse Effects:

1. **Sodium overload:** 108 mg or 4.7 mEq sodium/g.
2. **Convulsions,** especially with high doses and renal insufficiency.
3. **Qualitative platelet defect** secondary to binding to platelet ADP, especially when high dose used in renal insufficiency.
4. **Hypokalemia:** Large nonreabsorbable anion load.
5. **Hypersensitivity reactions** (e.g., rash), GI effects (e.g., nausea) and other side effects shared with penicillins.

Drug Interactions: Inactivation of aminoglycosides if mixed together in same IV solution.

Monitoring: Serial electrolytes and bleeding times (with bleeding problems).

CARBICARB

Trade Name: Carbicarb is a registered trade name for an equimolar solution of 50% sodium bicarbonate ($NaHCO_3$) and 50% sodium carbonate (Na_2CO_3).

Drug Action: Systemic alkalinization: Raises blood pH by increasing plasma bicarbonate levels and buffering excess hydrogen ions in the blood in a manner similar to that of sodium bicarbonate alone but without changing $PaCO_2$ levels.

Indications:

1. **Metabolic acidosis:** May be useful in acute treatment of circulatory insufficiency or cardiac arrest.
2. **Respiratory acidosis:** May be a useful adjunct in the treatment of acute respiratory acidosis with severe acidemia. Since Carbicarb appears to buffer blood pH without increasing $PaCO_2$, it may be useful in the treatment of acute respiratory acidosis while other definitive therapy is being initiated.

Pharmacokinetics:

1. **Metabolism:** None.
2. **Excretion:** CO_2 formed as HCO_3^- reacts with H^+ to form H_2CO_3; is excreted by the lungs.
3. **Volume of distribution:** Extracellular fluid (0.2 L/kg).
4. **Basal circulating levels:** 24 mEq/L.
5. **Plasma half-life:** Indeterminate.

Drug Preparations: *Parenteral:* Carbicarb is an equimolar solution of sodium bicarbonate ($NaHCO_3$) and sodium carbonate (Na_2CO_3).

Dosage:

1. **Adult/Pediatric:**
   a. **Systemic alkalinization:**
      (1) For severe acidosis, initial dose 1.0 mEq/kg IV, followed by 0.5 mEq/kg body weight; adjust dose as indicated by clinical condition and blood pH measurements.
      (2) For less urgent therapy, may be given as a continuous IV infusion, 2–5 mEq/kg over 4–8 hr.

Adverse Effects:

1. With excessive administration, severe metabolic alkalosis can occur.
2. Irregular heartbeat, muscle cramps or pain, peripheral edema, mood or mental changes, nervousness, nausea, vomiting all occur uncommonly.

Drug Interactions: Because Carbicarb contains sodium bicarbonate, the same drug interactions that occur with parenterally administered sodium bicarbonate can also occur with parenteral administration of Carbicarb. These include but are not necessarily limited to:

1. Decreased pharmacologic effects: Benzodiazepines, ketoconazole, lithium, salicylates, sulfonylureas, tetracyclines, phenobarbital.
2. Increased pharmacologic effects: Quinidine, amphetamines, flecainide, sympathomimetics.
3. Hypokalemia enhanced: Glucocorticoids, diuretics, mineralocorticoids.

Monitoring:

1. Arterial blood pH determinations.
2. Serum bicarbonate determinations.
3. Urinary pH determinations.

BIBLIOGRAPHY

Bersin RM, Arieff AI: Improved hemodynamic function during hypoxia with Carbicarb, a new agent for the management of acidosis, *Circulation* 1988, 77:227–233.

Filley GF, Kindig NB: Carbicarb, an alkalizing ion-generating agent of possible clinical usefulness, *Trans Am Clin Climatol Assoc* 1984, 96:141–152.

Gastrointestinal drugs. In *Drug Facts and Comparisons,* Philadelphia, 1989, JB Lippincott, pp 1275–1280.

CEFACLOR

Trade Name: *Ceclor.*

Drug Action:

1. Inhibits cell wall synthesis (cephalosporin).
2. Spectrum of activity includes gram-positive aerobes (including β-lactamase producers such as *Staphylococcus aureus*) and common gram-negative aerobes (including β-lactamase-positive and -negative *Haemophilus influenzae*).

Indications: Infections caused by susceptible organisms.

1. Commonly used in upper respiratory tract infections (otitis media, sinusitis).

Pharmacokinetics:

1. **Absorption:** Well absorbed after PO administration with or without food.
2. **Distribution:** Poor CSF penetration.
3. **Excretion:** 60%–85% excreted unchanged in urine within 8 hr.
4. **Serum half-life:** 0.6–0.9 hr. Removed by hemodialysis.

Drug Preparations:

Capsules: 250, 500 mg.
Suspension: 125, 250 mg/5 mL in 75, 150 mL size.

Dosage:

1. **Normal renal function:**
   a. **Adult:** 250–500 mg q 8 hr PO.
   b. **Pediatric:** 6.6–13.3 mg/kg q 8 hr PO.
2. **Impaired renal function: Adult:**

Dose (mg)	Creatinine Clearance	Interval (hr)
250–500	>80	8
	80–50	8
	50–10	8
	<10 (anuria)	8

3. **Hemodialysis:** Repeat dose after each dialysis.

Adverse Effects:

1. Hypersensitivity and GI effects similar to other cephalo-sporins.
2. Serum sickness–like reaction.
   a. Arthralgias, fever, rashes such as erythema multiforme or purpura occur in 1%–2% of patients and last 3–4 days after drug discontinuation.
   b. More common in children after a second course (hypersensitivity reaction).
   c. Antihistamines and corticosteroids enhance resolution.
3. Dizziness, headache, seizures, somnolence, rash, nausea/vomiting, diarrhea, anorexia, pseudomembranous colitis, dyspepsia, nephrotoxicity, leukopenia, anemia.

CEFAZOLIN

Trade Names: *Ancef, Kefzol.*

Drug Action:

1. Inhibits cell wall synthesis (first-generation cephalosporin).
2. Spectrum of activity includes common gram-positive (including β-lactamase-producing staphylococci but **not** enterococci, *S. pneumoniae,* streptococci) and gram-negative aerobes (e.g., *Pseudomonas aeruginosa, Serratia,* indole-positive *Proteus, E. coli, H. influenzae, Klebsiella,* Enterobacteriaceae).

Indications:

1. Infections caused by susceptible organisms.
   a. Wide spectrum of infections, including respiratory tract, urinary tract, skin structure, biliary tract, bone and joint, blood-borne (including endocarditis).
2. Perioperative prophylaxis:
   a. Short course, primarily in contaminated or potentially contaminated cases (e.g., vaginal hysterectomy, cholecystectomy) in high risk patients (including age >70 yr, acute cholecystitis, obstructive jaundice, common duct bile stones).
   b. In surgical patients in whom infection at operative site would present serious risk (e.g., open-heart surgery or prosthetic arthroplasty).

Pharmacokinetics:

1. **Absorption:** Give IV/IM.
2. **Distribution:** Poor CSF penetration.
3. **Excretion:** Unchanged in urine.
4. **Serum half-life:** 1.8 hr IV, 2 hr IM. Removed by hemodialysis and peritoneal dialysis.
5. **Bile level** in patients *without* obstruction up to five times serum level.

Drug Preparations:

Vials: 0.25, 0.5, 1, 5, 10 g.

Dosage:

1. **Normal renal function:** 0.5–1.5 g q 6–8 hr IV/IM.
2. **Impaired renal function:**

Dose (g)	Creatinine Clearance	Interval (hr)
0.5–1.5	>80	6–8
	80–50	8
0.5–1	50–10	8–12
0.5–1	<10 (anuria)	24

3. **Hemodialysis:** Supplement 0.25–0.5 g to anuric dose after each dialysis.

Adverse Effects: Shares side effects in common with other β-lactams:

1. Elevation in alkaline phosphatase level common.
2. Positive Coombs test.
3. To avoid false-positive reactions for glucose, use enzyme-based tests (e.g., Clinistic, Tes-Tape).
4. Dizziness, headache, seizures, rash, nausea/vomiting, diarrhea, dyspepsia, abdominal cramps, pseudomembranous colitis, leukopenia, anemia, hypersensitivity reactions, nephrotoxicity.

Drug Interactions: Probenecid decreases renal tubular secretion, resulting in increased and more prolonged serum levels. Bacteriostatic agents may interfere with bactericidal activity.

CEFIXIME

Trade Name: *Suprax.*

Drug Actions:

1. Inhibits bacterial cell wall synthesis (is highly stable in the presence of β-lactamase enzymes); is an oral third-generation cephalosporin.

2. Spectrum of activity: *Streptococcus pyogenes, S. pneumoniae,* and gram-negative aerobes (including *H. influenzae, Moraxella catarrhalis,* and *Neisseria gonorrhoeae*). Cefixime does not have good activity against staphylococci, enterococci, *Pseudomonas* spp., *Enterobacter* spp., *Bacteroides fragilis,* and *Clostridia* spp. (Of the cephalosporins, cefixime is among the poorest in antistaphylococcal activity and should *not* be used for treatment of staphylococcal infections.)

Indications:

1. Uncomplicated urinary tract infections due to *E. coli* and *Proteus mirabilis.*
2. Otitis media.
3. Pharyngitis/tonsillitis (but penicillin is drug of choice).
4. Acute bronchitis.
5. Acute exacerbations of chronic bronchitis.
6. Gonorrhea (cefixime offers an effective one-dose PO therapy).

Pharmacokinetics:

1. **Absorption:** PO.
2. **Excretion:** 50% unchanged in urine; >10% in bile.
3. **Half-life:** 3–4 hr (up to 9 hr in some healthy patients).

Drug Preparations:

Tablets: 200, 400 mg.
Oral suspension: 100 mg/5 mL.

Dosage:

400 mg PO q day or 200 mg PO bid.
For gonococcal cerviciti/urethritis: 400 mg PO once.

Adverse Effects:

1. Approximately 30% of patients experience GI side effects: diarrhea (16%), nausea (7%), loose or frequent stools (6%), flatulence (4%), abdominal pain (3%), dyspepsia (3%).
2. Other adverse effects characteristic of cephalosporins (e.g., hypersensitivity reactions, cytopenias, hepatic dysfunction, eosinophilia, superinfection).

Drug Interactions: None reported.

BIBLIOGRAPHY

Physicians' Desk Reference, ed 50, Montvale, 1996, Medical Economics Co.

CEFOPERAZONE

Trade Name: *Cefobid.*

Drug Action:

1. Inhibits cell wall synthesis (advanced cephalosporin).
2. Spectrum of activity includes gram-positive and gram-negative aerobes (including *Pseudomonas aeruginosa*) and anaerobes (but generally **not** *Bacteroides* group).

Indications: Infections caused by susceptible organisms, especially when *P. aeruginosa* is potential or known pathogen.

Pharmacokinetics:

1. **Absorption:** Give IV/IM.
2. **Serum half-life:** 2 hr (allowing q 8–12 hr dosing in some settings). Prolonged in patients with biliary obstruction or cirrhosis.
3. **Excretion:** Mainly biliary.

Drug Preparations:

Sterile powder in vials or piggyback: 1, 2 g units.

Dosage:

1. **Normal renal function:** 1–4 g q 6–12 hr IV/IM.
2. **Impaired renal function:**

Dose (g)	Creatinine Clearance	Interval (hr)
1–4	>80	6–12
	80–50	6–12
	50–10	6–12
	<10 (anuria)	6–12

3. **Hemodialysis:** Because of biliary excretion, no supplemental dose needed.

Adverse Effects:

1. Similar to other cephalosporins (e.g., hypersensitivity reactions, GI effects).
2. Contains MTT side chain (along with cefamandole, cefotetan, moxalactam) with potential for unique side effects:
   a. **Hypoprothrombinemia:** Prevent or treat with vitamin K; more common in patients with vitamin K depletion (e.g., poor nutritional status, alcoholism).
   b. **Disulfiram-like reaction:** Flushing, sweating, tachycardia, headache if alcohol ingested within 72 hr after cefoperazone administration.

Drug Interactions: Disulfiram-like reaction with alcohol.

Monitoring: Serial PT and PTT determinations in patients with potential for vitamin K depletion.

CEFOTAXIME

Trade Name: *Claforan.*

Drug Action:

1. Inhibits cell wall synthesis (advanced cephalosporin).
2. Spectrum of activity includes gram-positive (but **not** enterococci or MRSA) and gram-negative (including many resistant Enterobacteriaceae and β-lactamase-producing *H. influenzae* but **not** *P. aeruginosa*) aerobes, with only variable antianaerobic activity.

Indications: Infections caused by susceptible organisms:

1. Empiric coverage providing broad spectrum when *P. aeruginosa* not a major pathogen.
2. Special indication for CNS infections (meningitis and ventriculitis) caused by common pathogens (meningococci, pneumococci, *H. influenzae*) and less common pathogens (especially gram-negative bacilli such as *E. coli* and *Klebsiella*).

Pharmacokinetics:

1. **Absorption:** Give IV/IM.
2. **Distribution:** Good CSF penetration.
3. **Metabolism:** 15%–25% into desacetyl derivative, which contributes to bactericidal activity, and 20%–25% into two other metabolites.
4. **Excretion:** Renal.
5. **Penetration into CNS** allows use in CNS infections.
6. **Elimination half-life:** 1–2 hr; prolonged in renal failure.

Drug Preparations:

Vials: 1, 2 g for parenteral use.

Dosage:

1. **Normal renal function:** 1–2 g q 4–6 hr IV/IM.
2. **Impaired renal function:**

Dose (g)	Creatinine Clearance	Interval (hr)
1–2	>80	4–6
	80–50	4–6
	50–10	6–12
	<10 (anuria)	12

3. **Hemodialysis:** 50% maintenance dose as supplement after each dialysis.

Adverse Effects: Similar to other cephalosporins (e.g., hypersensitivity, GI effects, phlebitis).

CEFOTETAN

Trade Name: *Cefotan.*

Drug Action:

1. Inhibits cell wall synthesis (cephamycin drug).
2. Spectrum of activity includes gram-positive (but **not** enterococci or MRSA) and common gram-negative (but **not**

P. aeruginosa) and anaerobes (including *B. fragilis* but **not** some others e.g., *B. distasonis, B. ovatus*).

Indications: Infections caused by susceptible organisms:

1. Used where mixed aerobic/anaerobic infections suspected (intraabdominal or pelvic):
   a. **Therapeutically** (e.g., intraabdominal infection not involving resistant organisms, such as *P. aeruginosa*).
   b. **Prophylactically** (e.g., intraabdominal or pelvic surgery).

Pharmacokinetics:

1. **Absorption:** Give IV/IM.
2. **Distribution:** Poor CSF penetration; good biliary penetration.
3. **Excretion:** Renal.
4. **Serum half-life:** 3–4.6 hr (allowing q 12 hr dosing).

Drug Preparations:

Vials: 1, 2, 10 g.

Dosage:

1. **Normal renal function:** 1–2 g q 12 hr IV/IM.
2. **Impaired renal function:**

Dose (g)	Creatinine Clearance	Interval (hr)
1–2	>30	12
	30–10	24
	<10 (anuria)	48

3. **Hemodialysis:** One fourth usual recommended dose q24 hr on days between dialysis, and one half usual recommended dose on day of dialysis.

Adverse Effects:

1. Similar to other β-lactams (e.g., hypersensitivity reactions, GI problems, phlebitis, hematologic laboratory abnormalities).
2. Contains MTT side chain (along with moxalactam, cefoperazone, and cefamandole) with potential for:
   a. **Hypoprothrombinemia:** Prevent or treat with vitamin K.
   b. **Disulfiram-like reaction** with alcohol.

Drug Interactions: Disulfiram-like reaction when alcohol ingested within 72 hr of cefotetan.

Monitoring: Serial PT and PTT in patients predisposed to vitamin K depletion.

CEFOXITIN

Trade Name: *Mefoxin.*

Drug Action:

1. Inhibits cell wall synthesis (cephamycin).
2. Spectrum of activity includes gram-positive (but **not** enterococci or MRSA) and gram-negative (but **not** *P. aeruginosa*) aerobes and anaerobes including *Bacteroides* family.

Indications: Infections caused by susceptible organisms:

1. Used where mixed aerobic-anaerobic infections suspected (intraabdominal or pelvic areas):
   a. **Therapeutically** (e.g., intraabdominal infections where *P. aeruginosa* not present).
   b. **Prophylactically** (e.g., pelvic surgery).

Pharmacokinetics:

1. **Absorption:** Give IV/IM.
2. **Distribution:** Poor CSF penetration.
3. **Excretion:** Renal.
4. **Serum half-life:** 1 hr. Removed by hemodialysis but not by peritoneal dialysis.

Drug Preparations:

   Vials: 1, 2, 10 g.

Dosage:

1. **Normal renal function:** 1–2 g q 4–6 hr or 3 g q 8 hr IV/IM.
2. **Impaired renal function:**

Dose (g)	Creatinine Clearance	Interval (hr)
1–3	>80	4–6
1–3	80–50	8
1–2	50–10	12
0.5–1	<10 (anuria)	12–24

3. Supplement 1–2 g after each dialysis.

Adverse Effects:

1. Similar to other β-lactams (e.g., rash, pain of IM injection, phlebitis, cytopenias, elevation of liver enzymes).
2. Powerful inducer of β-lactamase in some organisms (e.g., *Enterobacter*).

CEFPODOXIME PROXETIL

Trade Name: *Vantin.*

Drug Actions:

1. Inhibits bacterial cell wall synthesis (is highly stable in the presence of β-lactamase enzymes); is an oral third-generation cephalosporin.
2. Spectrum of activity: staphylococci (not MRSA), *Streptococcus pyogenes, S. pneumoniae,* gram-negative aerobes including *Haemophilus influenzae, Moraxella catarrhalis,* and *Neisseria gonorrhoeae* (not *Pseudomonas* spp. or *Enterobacter* spp.). Cefpodoxime proxetil, like other cephalosporins, is inactive against most enterococci.

Indications:

1. Acute, community-acquired pneumonia.
2. Acute bacterial exacerbation of chronic bronchitis.
3. Gonococcal cervicitis/urethritis. Additionally, anorectal infections in women can be treated with cefpodoxime proxetil (efficacy in anorectal infections in men is not established).
4. Skin and skin structure infections.
5. Acute otitis media.

6. Pharyngitis/tonsillitis (but penicillin remains drug of choice).
7. Uncomplicated urinary tract infections due to *E. coli, Klebsiella pneumoniae, Proteus mirabilis,* and *Staphylococcus saprophyticus.*

Pharmacokinetics:

1. **Absorption:** PO.
2. **Metabolism:** Cefpodoxime proxetil is a prodrug that is deesterified to the active metabolite cefpodoxime.
3. **Half-life:** 2.09–2.84 hr (increased in renal impairment).

Drug Preparations:

Tablets: 100, 200 mg.
Oral suspension: 50 mg/5 mL, 100 mg/5 mL.

Dosage:

1. Pharyngitis/tonsillitis, urinary tract infections: 100 mg PO q 12 hr.
2. Pneumonia, chronic bronchitis exacerbations: 200 mg PO q 12 hr.
3. Skin and skin structure infections: 400 mg PO q 12 hr.
4. Uncomplicated gonorrhea (men and women) and anorectal gonococcal infections (women): 200 mg PO once.
5. For children (5 mo–12 yr): Acute otitis media: 10 mg/kg PO q 24 hr or 5 mg/kg PO q12 hr. Pharyngitis/tonsillitis: 5 mg/kg q 12 hr.

Adverse Effects:

1. Diarrhea (7.2%) and nausea (3.8%) are the most common side effects.
2. Other adverse effects associated with cephalosporins may occur (e.g., hypersensitivity reactions, cytopenias, hepatic dysfunction, eosinophilia, superinfection).

Drug Interactions: High doses of antacids or H_2 blockers reduce absorption and peak plasma levels.

BIBLIOGRAPHY

Physicians' Desk Reference, ed 50, Montvale, 1996, Medical Economics Co.

CEFPROZIL

Trade Name: *Cefzil.*

Drug Actions:

1. Inhibits bacterial cell wall synthesis; is an oral second-generation cephalosporin.
2. Spectrum of activity: *Staphylococcus aureus* (including penicillinase-producing strains but not MRSA), *Streptococcus pyogenes, S. pneumoniae, Haemophilus influenzae,* (including β-lactamase–positive strains), *Moraxella catarrhalis,* and others.

Indications:

1. Pharyngitis/tonsillitis (but penicillin is drug of choice).
2. Otitis media. (Cefprozil has somewhat lower bacterial eradication rates for β-lactamase–producing organisms than agents containing a specific β-lactamase inhibitor).
3. Secondary bacterial infection of acute bronchitis.
4. Acute bacterial exacerbation of chronic bronchitis.
5. Uncomplicated skin and skin structure infections.

Pharmacokinetics:

1. **Absorption:** PO; 95% absorbed.
2. **Onset of action:** Peak plasma concentrations within 1 hr.
3. **Excretion:** Approximately 60% of administered dose is recovered in the urine.
4. **Half-life:** 1.2 hr.

Drug Preparations:

Tablets: 250, 500 mg.
Oral Suspension: 125 mg/5 mL, 250 mg/5 mL.

Dosage:

1. Pharyngitis/tonsillitis: 500 mg PO q 24 hr.
2. Otitis media, secondary bacterial infection of acute bronchitis, acute bacterial exacerbation of chronic bronchitis: 500 mg PO q 12 hr.
3. Uncomplicated skin and skin structure infections: 250 mg PO q 12 hr, 500 mg PO q 24 hr, or 500 mg PO q 12 hr.

4. For children (2–12 yr): Pharyngitis/tonsillitis: 7.5 mg/kg PO q 12 hr.
5. For infants and children (6 mo–12 yr): Otitis media: 15 mg/kg PO q 12 hr.

Adverse Effects:

1. Nausea (3.5%) and diarrhea (2.9%).
2. Other adverse effects associated with cephalosporins may occur (e.g., hypersensitivity reactions, cytopenias, hepatic dysfunction, eosinophilia, superinfection).

Drug Interactions: None specifically. (Nephrotoxicity has been reported following concomitant administration of aminoglycosides and cephalosporins.)

BIBLIOGRAPHY

Physicians' Desk Reference, ed 50, Montvale, 1996, Medical Economics Co.
Sanford JP, Gilbert DN, Sande MA (eds): *The Sanford Guide to Antimicrobial Therapy,* ed 26, Dallas, 1996, Antimicrobial Therapy.

CEFTAZIDIME

Trade Names: *Fortaz, Tazicef, Tazidime.*

Drug Action:

1. Inhibits cell wall synthesis (advanced cephalosporin).
2. Spectrum of activity includes gram-positive (but not enterococci or methicillin-resistant *S. aureus* [MRSA]) and gram-negative (especially *Pseudomonas aeruginosa*) aerobes and anaerobes (but not *Bacteroides* family).

Indications: Infections caused by susceptible organisms, especially when *P. aeruginosa* proven or suspected.

Pharmacokinetics:

1. **Absorption:** Give IV/IM.
2. **Distribution:** Good CSF penetration.
3. **Metabolism:** None.

4. **Excretion:** Renal.
5. **Serum half-life:** 1.9 hr.

Dosage:

1. **Normal renal function:** 0.5–2 g q 8–12 hr IV/IM.
2. **Impaired renal function:**

Dose (g)	Creatinine Clearance	Interval (hr)
0.5–2	>80	8–12
	80–50	8–12
1	50–10	12–24
0.5	<10 (anuria)	24–48

3. **Hemodialysis:** 1 g IV after each hemodialysis.

Drug Preparations:

Vials: 0.5, 1, 2 g for IV/IM.

Adverse Effects: Similar to other cephalosporins, including rash, GI problems, mild hepatic dysfunction, cytopenias, eosinophilia, phlebitis.

CEFTIBUTEN

Trade Name: *Cedax.*

Drug Actions:

1. Inhibits bacterial cell wall synthesis; is an oral second-generation cephalosporin.
2. Spectrum of activity: *Streptococcus pyogenes, Neisseria gonorrhoeae, N. meningitidis,* and *Haemophilus influenzae* (including β-lactamase–producing strains). Ceftibuten is moderately active against *Moraxella catarrhalis,* weakly active against *Streptococcus pneumoniae* (pneumococci) and has *no* activity against staphylococci (similar to cefixime in this respect). It has the broadest gram-negative spectrum of any oral cephalosporin, with activity against most strains of *E. coli, Salmonella* spp., *Shigella* spp., and *Yersinia* spp. Enterococci,

Pseudomonas spp., and gram-negative anaerobes are usually resistant to ceftibuten.

Indications:

1. Acute bacterial exacerbations of chronic bronchitis (but if *M. catarrhalis* is isolated, ceftibuten is less effective).
2. Acute bacterial otitis media (not when due to *S. pneumoniae*).
3. Pharyngitis/tonsillitis (but penicillin is drug of choice).

Pharmacokinetics:

1. **Absorption:** PO. Food delays the time to peak serum concentration, lowers the peak concentration, and decreases the amount of drug absorbed.
2. **Onset of action:** 2–3 hr.
3. **Excretion:** In urine.
4. **Half-life:** Approximately 2 hr.

Drug Preparations:

Capsules: 400 mg.
Oral suspension: 90 mg/5 mL, 180 mg/5 mL.

Dosage:

1. Adults: 400 mg PO q day.
2. Children: 9 mg/kg PO q day (and give the suspension at least 2 hr before or 1 hr after a meal).

Adverse Effects:

1. Diarrhea is the most common side effect.
2. Other adverse effects associated with cephalosporins may occur (e.g., hypersensitivity reactions, cytopenias, hepatic dysfunction, eosinophilia, superinfection).

Drug Interactions: None reported.

BIBLIOGRAPHY

The Medical Letter on Drugs and Therapeutics 1996, 38: 23–24.
Sanford JP, Gilbert DN, Sande MA (eds): *The Sanford Guide to Antimicrobial Therapy,* ed 26, Dallas, 1996, Antimicrobial Therapy.

CEFTIZOXIME

Trade Name: *Cefizox.*

Drug Action:

1. Inhibits cell wall synthesis (advanced cephalosporin).
2. Spectrum of activity includes gram-positive (but **not** entero-cocci or MRSA) and gram-negative (including many resistant and β-lactamase–producing strains but **not** *Pseudomonas aeruginosa*) aerobes and anaerobes (including many *Bacteroides* species).

Indications: Infections caused by susceptible organisms not involving *P. aeruginosa.*

1. Because of CNS penetration, may be used in gram-negative bacillary meningitis.
2. Various nosocomial infections at multiple sites.

Pharmacokinetics:

1. **Absorption:** Give IV/IM.
2. **Metabolism:** None.
3. **Excretion:** Renal.
4. **Serum half-life:** 1.7 hr.
5. **Good penetration** into most tissues, including CNS.

Drug Preparations:

Vials: 1, 2 g IV/IM.

Dosage:

1. **Normal renal function:** 1–4 g q 8–12 hr IV/IM.
2. **Impaired renal function:**

Dose (g)	Creatinine Clearance	Interval (hr)
1–4	>80	8–12
0.15–1.5	80–50	8
0.25–1	50–10	12
0.25–1	<10 (anuria)	24–28

3. **Hemodialysis:** Give scheduled dose after each dialysis as supplement.

Adverse Effects: Similar to other cephalosporins (e.g., rash, GI problems, phlebitis, cytopenias, superinfection, eosinophilia).

CEFTRIAXONE

Trade Name: *Rocephin.*

Drug Action:

1. Inhibits cell wall synthesis (cephalosporin).
2. Spectrum of activity includes gram-positive (but not enterococci or MRSA) and gram-negative (including resistant and β-lactamase producers but **not** *Pseudomonas aeruginosa*) aerobes and anaerobes (but **not** most *Bacteroides* species).

Indications: Infections caused by susceptible organisms not involving *P. aeruginosa.*

1. Nosocomial infections at multiple sites.
2. CNS infections (meningitis and ventriculitis caused by meningococci, pneumococci, *Haemophilus influenzae,* and gram-negative bacilli).
3. Lyme borreliosis.

Pharmacokinetics:

1. **Absorption:** Give IV/IM.
2. **Metabolism:** Partial.
3. **Excretion:** Renal and biliary tract.
4. **Serum half-life:** 6+hr (allows q 12–24 hr dosing). Not removed by dialysis.
5. **Penetration** into most tissues, including CNS.

Drug Preparations:

Vials: 0.25, 0.5, 1, 2 g for IV/IM.

Dosage:

1. **Normal renal function:** 0.5–1 g q 12–24 hr IV/IM.
2. **Impaired renal function:**

Dose (g)	Creatinine Clearance	Interval (hr)
0.5–1	>80	12–24
	80–50	12–24
	50–10	12–24
	<10 (anuria)	12–24

3. **Hemodialysis:** No supplemental dose needed.

Adverse Effects: Similar to other cephalosporins (e.g., phlebitis, rash, cytopenias, fever, GI problems).

CEFUROXIME

Trade Names:

Cefuroxime sodium: *Kefurox, Zinacef.*
Cefuroxime axetil: *Ceftin.*

Drug Action:

1. Inhibits cell wall synthesis (cephalosporin).
2. Spectrum of activity includes gram-positive (but **not** enterococci or MRSA) and many gram-negative (including β-lactamase–producing *Haemophilus influenzae* but **not** *Pseudomonas aeruginosa* or resistant nosocomial pathogens) aerobes and some anaerobes (but **not** *Bacteroides* species).

Indications: Community-acquired infections caused by susceptible organisms.

1. Useful in multiple sites, including upper and lower respiratory tract, skin and skin structures, bone and joint, and meninges (most prefer advanced cephalosporins).

Pharmacokinetics:

1. **Absorption:** Cefuroxime sodium: Give IV/IM. Cefuroxime axetil: well absorbed from GI tract.
2. **Metabolism:** None.
3. **Excretion:** Renal.
4. **Serum half-life:** 80 min.
5. **Good penetration** into most tissues, including CNS.

Drug Preparations:

1. Cefuroxime sodium: *Vials:* 0.75, 1.5 g for IV/IM.
2. Cefuroxime axetil: *Tablets:* 125, 250, 500 mg.

Dosage:

1. **Normal renal function:**
   a. **Parenteral:** 0.75–1.5 g q 8 hr IV/IM.
   b. **PO:** 125–500 mg q 8 hr.
2. **Impaired renal function:**

Dose (g)	Creatinine Clearance	Interval (hr)
0.75–1.5 IV/IM	>80	8
	80–50	8
	50–10	12
	<10	24

3. **Hemodialysis:** Add supplemental dose after each dialysis.

Adverse Effects:

1. Similar to other cephalosporins (e.g., rash, fever, cytopenias, GI problems, phlebitis).
2. Bitter taste of tablets decreases acceptance to children.

CEPHALEXIN

Trade Names: *Cephalexin, Keflet, Keflex, Keftab.*

Drug Action:

1. Inhibits cell wall synthesis (cephalosporin).
2. Spectrum of activity includes gram-positive (but **not** enterococci or MRSA) and common gram-negative (but **not** resistant nosocomial pathogens or *Pseudomonas aeruginosa*) aerobes and some anaerobes (but **not** *Bacteroides* family).

Indications: Community-acquired infections caused by susceptible organisms.

1. Useful in multiple sites, including respiratory tract, urinary tract, skin and skin structures, bone and joint.

Pharmacokinetics:

1. **Absorption:** PO.
2. **Distribution:** Most tissues; poor CSF penetration.
3. **Metabolism:** None.
4. **Excretion:** Renal.
5. **Half-life:** 30–60 min; prolonged in renal failure. Removed by dialysis.

Dosage:

1. **Normal renal function:** 0.25–1 g q 6 hr PO.
2. **Impaired renal function:**

Dose (g)	Creatinine Clearance	Interval (hr)
0.25–1 PO	>80	6
	80–50	6
	50–10	8–12
	<10 (anuria)	24–48

3. **Hemodialysis:** 0.25–1 g supplemental dose after each dialysis.

Drug Preparations:

Tablets/capsules: 250, 500 mg.
Suspension: 125, 250 mg/5 mL.

Adverse Effects: Similar to other cephalosporins, including hypersensitivity reactions (e.g., rash, fever), GI problems (e.g., nausea, diarrhea), cytopenias, increase in liver function tests.

CEPHRADINE

Trade Names:

1. Parenteral: *Velocef.*
2. PO: Anspor, *Cephradine, Velocef.*

Drug Action:

1. Inhibits cell wall synthesis (first-generation cephalosporin).
2. Spectrum of activity includes gram-positive (including penicillinase-producing staphylococci but **not** enterococci or MRSA)

and common community-acquired gram-negative (but **not** *Pseudomonas aeruginosa*) aerobes and some anaerobes (but **not** *Bacteroides* family).

Indications: Community-acquired infections caused by susceptible organisms.

Pharmacokinetics:

1. **Absorption:** PO/IV/IM.
2. **Distribution:** Most tissues; poor CSF penetration.
3. **Metabolism:** None.
4. **Excretion:** Renal.
5. **Half-life:** 30–120 min; prolonged in renal failure. Removed by dialysis.

Drug Preparations:

Capsules: 250, 500 mg
Suspension: 125, 250 mg/5 mL.
Vials: 0.25, 0.5, 1 g

Dosage:

1. **Normal renal function:**
   a. **PO:** 0.25–1 g q 6 hr.
   b. **Parenteral:** 1–2 g q 6 hr.
2. **Impaired renal function:**

Dose (g)	Creatinine Clearance	Interval (hr)
1–2	>80	6
	80–50	6
	50–10	8
	<10 (anuria)	12–24

3. **Hemodialysis:** 1–2 g supplemental dose after each hemodialysis.

Adverse Effects: Similar to other cephalosporins, including hypersensitivity reactions (e.g., rash, fever, eosinophilia), GI problems (e.g., nausea, diarrhea), cytopenias.

CHLORAL HYDRATE

Trade Names: *SK-Chloral Hydrate, Aquachloral.*

Drug Action: CNS depressant (primary site of action: Reticular activating system).

Indications: Sedation, sleep.

Pharmacokinetics:

1. **Absorption:** Oral, rectal.
2. **Metabolism:** Liver, erythrocytes, kidney; metabolized to active metabolite trichloroethanol.
3. **Excretion:** Urine, bile.
4. **Plasma half-life:** 8–10 hr.
5. **Onset of sleep:** 30–60 min after 0.5–1 g dose (adults).

Drug Preparations:

> *Capsules:* 250, 500 mg.
> *Syrup:* 250, 500 mg/5 mL.
> *Suppositories:* 325, 500, 650 mg.

Dosage:

1. **Sedation:**
   a. **Adult:** 250 mg PO/PR tid.
   b. **Pediatric:** 8 mg/kg PO tid (max. dose 500 mg tid).
2. **Sleep:**
   a. **Adult:** 500–1000 mg PO/PR 15–30 min before bedtime.
   b. **Pediatric:** 50 mg/kg PO/PR (max. dose 1000 mg).

Adverse Effects:

1. **GI:** Nausea, vomiting, diarrhea, flatulence, gastric irritation, altered taste.
2. **Dermatologic:** Rash, urticaria, dermatitis.
3. **Hematologic:** Leukopenia, eosinophilia.
4. **CNS:** Drowsiness, headache, hangover, ataxia, hallucinations, confusion, disorientation, nightmares, paranoia, excitement.
5. May precipitate **acute intermittent porphyria.**
6. **Dependence** may develop; withdrawal can occur with discontinuation.
7. **Overdose** may cause hypotension, ventilatory depression, arrhythmias, myocardial depression, coma.

Drug Interactions:

1. Increased sedation when used with other sedatives (e.g., alcohol, narcotics, antihistamines, barbiturates).
2. Displaces thyroid hormone and warfarin from binding proteins (potentiates effects of these agents).
3. Increases metabolism of coumarin anticoagulants, reducing their effectiveness (monitor PT/PTT).
4. Administration of chloral hydrate after Iv furosemide may result in a hypermetabolic state due to displacement of thyroid hormone.

Monitoring: Mental status.

BIBLIOGRAPHY

Chloral hydrate. In *Drug Facts and Comparisons,* Philadelphia, 1989, JB Lippincott, p 1127.
Chloral hydrate. In *AMA Drug Evaluations,* ed 6, Philadelphia, 1986, WB Saunders, p 106.

CHLORAMPHENICOL

Trade Name: *Chloromycetin.*

Drug Action:

1. Binds reversibly with bacterial 50S ribosomal subunits and inhibits protein synthesis.
2. Spectrum of activity includes most gram-positive and gram-negative (but **not** *Pseudomonas aeruginosa*) aerobes and essentially all anaerobes plus the rickettsiae and chlamydiae.

Indications:

1. Severe salmonellosis. A drug of choice in typhoid fever but should not be used to treat carriers.
2. Rickettsial infections, including Rocky Mountain spotted fever, when tetracyclines contraindicated (e.g., pregnancy, renal failure, allergy to tetracycline, ?children)
3. CNS and parameningeal infections:
   a. Pneumococcal or meningococcal meningitis in penicillin-allergic patients.

b. Should **not** be used to treat gram-negative bacillary meningitis, because of poor clinical experience.
c. *Haemophilus influenzae* meningitis with significant penicillin allergy.
d. Anaerobic brain abscesses, especially due to *Bacteroides* species.

Pharmacokinetics:

1. **Absorption:** PO.
2. **Excretion:** 90% inactivated in the liver by glucuronidation and excreted in urine.
3. **Penetration excellent** into all tissues, including CNS.
4. **Plasma half-life:** 1.5–4.5 hr; prolonged in hepatic/renal failure.

Drug Preparations:

1. Chlormycetin sodium succinate: *Parenteral prep:* 100 mg/mL.
2. *Kapseals:* 250 mg capsules.
3. *Skin cream* (1%), *ophthalmic ointment/solution* (1%), *otic solution.*

Dosage:

1. **Normal/impaired renal function:** 12.5–25 mg/kg q 6 hr PO/IV.
2. **With dialysis:** No change in dose.
3. Excess accumulation possible with hepatic dysfunction, with increased toxicity.

Adverse Effects:

1. Reversible interference with protein synthesis (common, dose related), resulting in inhibition of mitochondrial protein synthesis.
   a. Reversible anemia, leukopenia, thrombocytopenia (revert in 1–2 wk).
2. Irreversible blood dyscrasia (**aplastic anemia,** other).
   a. Often after cessation of therapy (up to 6+ mo).
   b. Idiosyncratic reaction (not dose related).
   c. More common after multiple courses and after PO use.
   d. Incidence 1:20,000–1:40,000.
3. **Gray syndrome:**
   a. Premature and neonatal infants with high serum concentrations of unconjugated drug secondary to immature hepatic (inactivation) and renal (excretion) function.

    (1) Usually within first 48 hr of life.
    (2) Symptoms appear 3–4 days after continuous use of high doses and include abdominal distention, vomiting, diarrhea, hypotonia, progressive ashen-gray cyanosis, vasomotor collapse.
    (3) High mortality (40% within a few hours).
4. Hemolysis in glucose-6-phosphate dehydrogenase–deficient patients.
5. Hypersensitivity reactions.
6. Herxheimer reaction with syphilis, typhoid fever, brucellosis.
7. Optic or peripheral neuritis, headache, confusion.
8. **GI:** Nausea/vomiting, diarrhea, jaundice, stomatitis, colitis.

Drug Interactions:

1. **Acetaminophen:** Possible increased chloramphenicol toxicity secondary to decreased metabolism.
2. **Alcohol:** Minor disulfiram reactions.
3. **Barbiturates:** Increased barbiturate effect, decreased chloramphenicol effect (increased antibiotic metabolism).
4. **Cimetidine:** Aplastic anemia.
5. **Dicumarol:** Increased anticoagulant effect.
6. **Hypoglycemics, sulfonylurea:** Increased hypoglycemic effect.
7. **Iron salts:** Hematologic response to iron may be decreased.
8. **Phenytoin:** Increased phenytoin toxicity (decreased metabolism), decreased chloramphenicol effect (increased metabolism).

Monitoring: Follow up with white blood cell counts, hemoglobin, platelet counts, and reticulocyte counts at onset of therapy, after 1 wk, and q 3 days thereafter.

CHLORDIAZEPOXIDE

Trade Name: *Librium.*

Drug Action: Anxiety reduction, sedation, anticonvulsant activity, muscle relaxation, amnesia.

Indications: Anxiety, alcohol withdrawal, anesthetic agent pre-medication.

Pharmacokinetics:

1. **Metabolism:** Hepatic oxidation.
2. **Half-life:** 9.9 hr (mean); may be ≥24 hr in some patients.
   a. Desmethylchlordiazepoxide 24–96 hr.
3. **Excretion:** Renal excretion of inactive metabolites.
4. **Dialyzable?:** Limited.
5. **Renal failure:** Monitor for sedation.
6. **Hepatic failure:** Reduce dose, use with extreme caution, be-cause of greatly prolonged half-life.

Drug Preparations:

   Tablets: 5, 10, 25 mg.
   Capsules: 5, 10, 25 mg.
   Injection: 100 mg/ampule.

Dosage: For anxiety: 5–25 mg q 6–8 hr. May be given PO/IM/IV. Reduce dose to 10 mg/day initially in elderly.

Adverse Effects: Sedation, psychomotor impairment, depres-sion, amnesia, confusion, impaired concentration, weakness, im-paired sexual function, paradoxical agitation.

Drug Interactions:

1. Additive effect with other CNS depressants.
2. Induces liver enzymes.

Monitoring: Excess sedation vs. therapeutic effect.

BIBLIOGRAPHY

Drugs used for anxiety and sleep disorders. In *AMA Drug Evalua-tions*, ed 6, Philadelphia, 1986, WB Saunders, pp 81–110.
Sussman N: The benzodiazepines: selection and use in treating anxiety, insomnia, and other disorders, *Hosp Formul* 1985, 20:298–305.

CHLORPROMAZINE

Trade Name: *Thorazine.*

Drug Action: Antipsychotic effect thought to be caused by blockade of dopamine receptors in forebrain and basal ganglia.

Indications: Treatment of psychotic symptoms and/or agitation resulting from a variety of psychiatric or medical illnesses. Reduces nausea/vomiting, hiccups.

Pharmacokinetics:

1. **Absorption:** PO/PR/IM.
2. **Metabolism:** Hepatic, with several active metabolites.
3. **Half-life:** Approximately 30 hr, although metabolites may be excreted in urine for months.
4. **Excretion:** Both hepatic and renal. Less than 1% of drug is excreted unchanged by the kidneys.
5. **Dialyzable(?):** Minimal.
6. **Renal failure:** Reduce dosage.
7. **Hepatic failure:** Use with extreme caution, at greatly reduced dosage.

Drug Preparations:

Tablets: 10, 25, 50, 100, 200 mg.
Ampules: 25 mg/mL (1, 2 mL).
Suppositories: 25, 100 mg.
Multidose vials: 25 mg/mL (10 mL).
Concentrate: 30 mg/mL (4 oz), 100 mg/mL (8 oz).

Dosage:

1. **Adult:**
   a. **Severe psychosis:** Initial dose 200–600 mg/day PO in 2–4 divided doses.
   b. **Psychosis with agitation:** 25–100 mg IM q 1–4 hr until control is achieved.
   c. **Elderly patients** usually require one third to one half adult dose.
   d. **Nausea/vomiting:** 25–200 mg PO/IM q 4–6 hr; 50–100 mg PR q 6–8 hr.
   e. **Hiccup:** 25–50 mg PO/IM q 4–6 hr.

Adverse Effects:

1. Sedation, extrapyramidal reactions (e.g., dystonias, akathisia, parkinsonism), anticholinergic effects (e.g., dry mouth, blurred vision, urinary retention, constipation), orthostatic hypotension.
2. Rare allergic, hematologic, neuroendocrine, respiratory, GI, and cardiac effects.
3. Neuroleptic malignant syndrome.
4. Tardive dyskinesia.

Drug Interactions:

1. Enhances effects of other CNS depressants.
2. Additive effect with other anticholinergic drugs.
3. Antagonizes antihypertensive effect of guanethidine.

Monitoring: Blood levels for routine therapeutic monitoring are currently unavailable.

BIBLIOGRAPHY

Antipsychotic drugs. In *AMA Drug Evaluations,* ed 6, Philadelphia, 1986, WB Saunders, pp 111–130.
Schatzberg A, Cole J (eds): Antipsychotic drugs. In *Manual of Clinical Psychopharmacology,* Washington, 1986, American Psychiatric Press, pp 67–106.

CIPROFLOXACIN

Trade Name: *Cipro.*

Drug Action:

1. Rapidly bactericidal (replicating and stationary bacteria) by inhibiting DNA gyrase (topoisomerase II).
2. Spectrum of activity includes staphylococci (plus MRSA) and most gram-negative aerobes (*Pseudomonas aeruginosa* but **not** other *Pseudomonas* species); moderately active against streptococci; inactive against anaerobes.
   a. Also active against a number of other pathogens, including *Acinetobacter, Aeromonas, Brucella, Branhamella, Campylobacter, Pasteurella, Vibrios, Yersinia,* and *Plesiomonas.*

Indications:

1. **Urinary tract infections:** Active against most uropathogens associated with cystitis, pyelonephritis, prostatitis.
   a. Reserved for complicated urinary tract infections or resistant pathogens.
2. **Gastrointestinal infections:** Active against most GI pathogens, including *Escherichia coli, Salmonella, Shigella, Yersinia, Vibrios, Campylobacter.*
   a. Not active against *Clostridium difficile.*
3. **Sexually transmitted diseases:** Effective for gonorrhea at all sites and against resistant organisms.
   a. Not useful against chlamydial infections as single dose.
4. **Osteomyelitis:** Active against staphylococci and gram-negative organisms, such as *P. aeruginosa.*
5. **Skin and soft tissue infections, medical prophylaxis** (e.g., granulocytopenia and bacterial gastroenteritis).

Pharmacokinetics:

1. **Absorption:** Well absorbed orally (70% bioavailability).
2. **Excretion:** Renal.
3. **Serum half-life:** 4 hr.
4. **Penetrates well** into most tissues (CNS only 10% of peak serum level).

Drug Preparations:

Tablets: 250, 500, 750 mg.
Vials: 200, 400 mg IV.

Dosage:

1. **Normal renal function:** 250–750 mg q 12 hr.
2. **Impaired renal function:**

Dose (g)	Creatinine Clearance	Interval (hr)
0.25–0.75	>50	12
0.25–0.5	50–30	12
0.25–0.5	29–5	18

3. **Hemodialysis/peritoneal dialysis:** 250–500 mg q 24 hr after each dialysis.

Adverse Effects:

1. Generally well tolerated, adverse reactions occur in 5%, including GI problems (e.g., nausea, diarrhea, vomiting), CNS problems (e.g., headache, restlessness), rash.
2. Cartilage damage in experimental animals. **Not approved** in patients <18 yr or in pregnant or nursing women.

Drug Interactions:

1. **Antacids** containing magnesium or aluminum: Interferes with bioavailability if concurrently administered.
2. **Theophylline:** Prolongation of serum elimination, with high theophylline levels, increasing risk for CNS problems, including seizure activity.

CISAPRIDE

Trade Name: *Propulsid.*

Drug Actions: Gastrointestinal prokinetic agent increases gastric emptying, enhances release of acetylcholine by myenteric plexus, serotonin (5-HT4) receptor agonist, increases lower esophageal sphincter pressure.

Indications: Gastroesophageal reflux disease, increased gastric emptying during enteral nutrition.

Pharmacokinetics:

1. **Absorption:** Give PO; bioavailability 35%–40%, rapidly absorbed, peak levels 1–1.5 hr.
2. **Onset of action:** 20–60 min after PO administration.
3. **Metabolism:** Hepatic.
4. **Excretion:** Urine, feces.
5. **Half-life:** Terminal t½ 6–12 hr.

Drug Preparations:

Tablets, 10 mg.

Dosage: 10 mg PO qid (can be increased to 20 mg qid).

Adverse Effects: Do not administer to patients in whom an increase in GI motility may be harmful (i.e., GI obstruction or perforation). May cause headache, diarrhea, abdominal pain, urinary frequency, abnormal vision. Rare cases of cardiac arrhythmias (ventricular, torsades de pointe) have been reported in patients taking cisapride with ketoconazole, itraconazole, meconazole, erythromycin, clarithromycin, or fluconazole.

Drug Interactions: Absorption decreased by reduced gastric acidity (i.e., H_2 blockers). May increase sedative effects of benzodiazepines and alcohol. Anticholinergic compounds decrease effect. May alter absorption of other drugs owing to GI effects. May increase effects of anticoagulants. Drugs that inhibit hepatic metabolism such as ketoconazole, meconazole, clarithromycin, erythromycin, fluconazole, or troleandomycin can lead to elevated cisapride blood levels.

Monitoring: Reflux symptoms, gastric emptying (i.e., check residuals), ECG for arrhythmias or QT prolongation.

BIBLIOGRAPHY

Washabau RJ, Hall JA: Cisapride, *J Am Vet Med Assoc* 1995, 207:1285–1288.

Duan LP, Braden B, Caspary WF, Lembcke B: Influence of cisapride on gastric emptying of solids and liquids monitored by 13_c breath tests. *Dig Dis Sci* 1995, 40:2200–2206.

CLARITHROMYCIN

Trade Name: *Biaxin.*

Drug Actions:

1. Inhibits bacterial protein synthesis by binding to the 50S ribosomal subunit.
2. Spectrum of activity includes gram-positive aerobes, *Haemophilus influenza, Mycoplasma pneumoniae, Moraxella catarrhalis, Mycobacterium avium* complex (MAC), and others.

Indications:

1. Pharyngitis/tonsillitis due to *Streptococcus pyogenes* (alternative to penicillin).
2. Acute maxillary sinusitis.
3. Lower respiratory tract infections: Acute bacterial exacerbation of chronic bronchitis or pneumonia (due to *S. pneumoniae, H. influenzae,* or *M. catarrhalis*).
4. Uncomplicated skin and skin structure infections.
5. Treatment of disseminated MAC infections, and prophylaxis of disseminated MAC disease in patients with AIDS.

Pharmacokinetics:

1. **Absorption:** PO; rapidly absorbed after PO administration and may be given with or without food.
2. **Onset of action:** Peak serum concentrations are attained within 2 hr of dosing.
3. **Metabolism:** Has active 14-OH metabolite.
4. **Excretion:** Liver and kidney (20%–40% in urine).
5. **Half-life:** 3–4 hr with 250 mg PO q 12 hr; 5–7 hr with 500 mg PO q 12 hr.

Drug Preparations:

Tablets: 250, 500 mg.
Suspension: 125 mg/5 mL, 250 mg/5 mL.

Dosage: 250–500 mg PO q 12 hr. For MAC prophylaxis in HIV-infected patients, 500 mg PO bid is recommended.

Adverse Effects: Clarithromycin has a lower incidence of side effects than erythromycin. GI intolerance (3%) and abnormal, unpleasant taste (3%) are reported among others. Clarithromycin should not be used in pregnancy.

Drug Interactions:

1. Increased: Theophylline, digoxin, triazolam, and active metabolite of terfenadine.
2. Drugs metabolized by the cytochrome P-450 system may also be increased (carbamazepine, cyclosporine, phenytoin, and others).
3. Effects of oral anticoagulants may be potentiated.
4. Zidovudine concentrations are decreased (OK to give clarithromycin 2–4 hr prior to zidovudine).

BIBLIOGRAPHY

Physicians' Desk Reference, ed 50, Montvale, 1996, Medical Economics Co.

CLINDAMYCIN

Trade Name: *Cleocin.*

Drug Action:

1. Suppression of protein synthesis by binding to 50S ribosomal subunit.
2. Spectrum of activity includes gram-negative aerobes (but **not** enterococci or MRSA) and most anaerobes (including *Bacteroides fragilis* but **not** *Clostridium difficile*).
   a. **Not** active against aerobic and facultative gram-negative organisms.
   b. Resistance increasing among staphylococci and *Bacteroides* group.

Indications: Infections caused by susceptible organisms (primarily gram-positive aerobes and anaerobes).

1. Anaerobic lung abscess.
2. Intraabdominal and pelvic infections (generally with another drug with gram-negative aerobic activity, such as an aminoglycoside).
3. Topically for acne.
4. Alternative (used with primaquine) to trimethoprim/sulfamethoxazole for treatment of *Pneumocystis carinii* pneumonia.

Pharmacokinetics:

1. **Absorption:** PO/IV/IM.
2. **Distribution:** Most tissues; poor CSF penetration.
3. **Metabolism:** Hepatic.
4. **Excretion:** Renal as metabolites. Not removed by dialysis.
5. **Penetration good** except in CSF, even with inflamed meninges (may concentrate in brain abscess).
6. **Serum half-life:** 3 hr in adults.

Drug Preparations:

> *Capsules:* 75, 150, 300 mg.
> *Topical solution/gel:* 10 mg/mL.
> *Clindamycin phosphate:* 150 mg/mL IV/IM.

Dosage:

1. **Normal renal function:** 150–900 mg q 6 hr PO/IM/IV.
2. **Renal dysfunction or dialysis:** No dosage change necessary.
3. **Severe hepatic dysfunction:** Dosage modification.

Adverse Effects:

1. **GI:** Diarrhea 7%, pseudomembranous colitis (1 : 7500), metallic taste, nausea/vomiting, abdominal pain, diarrhea, anorexia, elevated hepatic enzymes.
2. **Hypersensitivity reactions:** Rash, eosinophilia.
3. **Neuromuscular blockage** (with apnea).
4. **Hematologic:** Leukopenia, eosinophilia, thrombocytopenia.

Drug Interactions:

1. **Chloramphenicol and erythromycin:** Act at same site, with potential for antagonism.
2. **Neuromuscular blocking agents:** Additive effect.

CLOFAZIMINE

Trade Name: *Lamprene.*

Drug Actions:

1. Binds preferentially to mycobacterial DNA, but precise mechanisms of antimycobacterial action are not known.
2. Exerts slow bactericidal effect on *Mycobacterium leprae,* and also inhibits *Mycobacterium avium* complex (MAC) and *M. bovis.*
3. Clofazimine is thought to have anti-inflammatory properties (controls erythema nodosum leprosum reactions).

Indications:

1. Lepromatous leprosy.
2. MAC disease (in HIV-negative and AIDS patients).

Pharmacokinetics:

1. **Absorption:** PO; should be taken with meals.
2. **Excretion:** Small amounts in feces, sputum, sebum, sweat, and urine (negligible).
3. **Half-life:** 70 days.

Drug Preparations:

Capsules: 50, 100 mg.

Dosage: 100–200 mg PO q day.

Adverse Effects:

1. Red-brownish black skin discoloration in 75%–100% (may reverse after discontinuation of clofazimine, but takes several months to years). Discoloration of conjunctivae, lacrimal fluid, sweat, sputum, urine, and feces may also occur.
2. Abdominal pain: (50%)—rarely severe.
3. Dryness (20%).
4. Pruritus (5%).

Drug Interactions: None proven.

BIBLIOGRAPHY

Physicians' Desk Reference, ed 50, Montvale, 1996, Medical Economics Co.

CLONAZEPAM

Trade Names: *Klonopin* (formerly Clonopin).

Drug Action: As with all benzodiazepines, clonazepam is thought to exert its pharmacologic action by enhancing GABA-mediated chloride conductance across the neural membrane.

Indications:

1. Second-line drug to ethosuximide or valproate for treatment of absence seizures and akinetic seizures.
2. Treatment of myoclonic seizures and status epilepticus, and as adjunctive treatment for focal motor seizures.

   NOTE: 30% of patients lose efficacy over 3 mo.

Pharmacokinetics:

1. **Metabolism:** 98% ± 31% of the drug is bioavailable after PO dosing. Readily metabolized by reduction of nitro group to produce inactive 7-amino derivatives.
2. **Excretion:** Less than 1% of clonazepam is excreted unchanged in the urine; five major metabolites are renally excreted.
3. **Volume of distribution:** 3.2 ± 1.1 L/kg.
4. **Clearance:** 1.55 ± 0.28 mL/min/kg.
5. **Effective concentrations:** 5–70 ng/mL; 86% ± 0.5% of clonazepam bound to plasma protein.
6. **Plasma half-life:** 23 ± 5 hr; may be as long as 50 hr.

Drug Preparations:

Tablets: 0.5, 1, 2 mg.
Parenteral forms not available in the United States at this time.

Dosage: All doses must be individualized on basis of response and clinical requirements. Doses should be divided in equal amounts or with the largest dose given at bedtime.

1. **Adult:** Initial dose should not exceed 1.5 mg/day divided in 3 doses PO. Dosage should not be increased more than 0.5–1 mg every third day. Adult maintenance dose should not exceed 20 mg/day.
2. **Pediatric** (infants/children ≤10 yr or 30 kg): Usual doses 0.01–0.03 mg/kg/day. Initial dose should not exceed 0.05 mg/kg/day given in two to three divided doses. Dosage may be increased by 0.5 mg every third day. Pediatric maintenance dose should not exceed 0.2 mg/kg/day.

Adverse Reactions:

1. Behavioral effects characterized by irritability, aggression, hyperactivity, disobedience, and antisocial activities have been reported.
2. Sedation, decreased alertness, and drowsiness are common.
3. Increased salivation and hypersecretion in upper airway may occur and can pose problems in the very young or in patients who have difficulty in maintaining airway patency.
4. Transient elevation in alkaline phosphatase assays may occur.
5. Dysuria, enuresis, nocturia, and urinary retention have been reported.

6. Anemia, leukopenia, thrombocytopenia, eosinophilia may be noted.
7. Dermatologic manifestations may include rash, hair loss, facial edema.
8. Contraindicated in patients with angle-closure glaucoma or hepatic disease.
9. May increase serum levels of phenytoin.
10. Additive effect with other CNS depressants.
11. Physical and/or psychological dependence may occur.
12. Acute toxicity manifested by somnolence, confusion, ataxia, hyporeflexia, coma.
13. May increase incidence of generalized tonic-clonic (grand mal) seizures.

Monitoring: Quantitative levels of clonazepam are available through most hospital and reference laboratories.

BIBLIOGRAPHY

Cohen S, Armstrong M: *Drug Interactions: A Handbook for Clinical Use,* Baltimore, 1974, Williams & Wilkins.

Drug Information for the Health Care Professional, ed 8, Rockville, 1988, US Pharmacopeial Convention.

Evans WE, Oellerich M: *Therapeutic Drug Monitoring Clinical Guide,* ed 2, Irving, 1984, Abbott Laboratories Publications.

Gilman A, Goodman L, Rall T, et al: *The Pharmacological Basis of Therapeutics,* ed 7, New York, 1985, Macmillan.

Johnson G: *Blue Book of Pharmacologic Therapeutics,* Philadelphia, 1985, WB Saunders.

McEvoy GK: *Drug Information 88,* Bethesda, 1988, American Society of Hospital Pharmacists.

CLONIDINE

Trade Names: *Catapres, Catapres-TTS.*

Drug Action:

1. Stimulates central α_2-adrenergic receptors, decreasing sympathetic outflow.
2. Reduces peripheral vascular resistance.

3. Inhibits renin release, catecholamine secretion, aldosterone secretion.

Indications:

1. Hypertension.
2. Withdrawal (e.g., opiates, nicotine, alcohol).
3. Prophylaxis against vascular headache.

Pharmacokinetics:

1. **Absorption:** GI and cutaneous.
2. **Metabolism:** Liver (50%).
3. **Excretion:** Urine (50% unchanged), feces.
4. **Plasma half-life:** 12–16 hr.
   a. **Renal failure:** 25–40 hr.
5. **Onset:** 30–60 min after PO administration (max. effect at 2–4 hr, duration 8 hr).
   a. Therapeutic levels achieved 2–3 days after transdermal application.

Drug Preparations:

Tablets: 0.1, 0.2, 0.3 mg.

Transdermal: TTS-1 (0.1 mg/24 hr), TTS-2 (0.2 mg/24 hr), TTS-3 (0.3 mg/24 hr).

Dosage:

Adult:

1. **Hypertension:**
   a. PO: 0.1 mg bid; increase by 0.1–0.2 mg/day until desired response achieved. Usual dose 0.2–1.2 mg/day in divided doses; max. dose 2.4 mg/day.
      (1) **Hypertensive emergencies:** 0.2 mg, then 0.1 mg/hr to 0.7 mg or blood pressure controlled.
   b. **Transdermal:** Apply once q7 days. Start with 0.1 mg, and increase weekly by 0.1 mg (peak effect occurs 2–3 days after increasing dose).
2. **Withdrawal:** 5–17 µg/kg PO in divided doses.

Adverse Effects:

1. **Cardiovascular:** Hypotension, bradycardia, rebound hypertension and tachycardia when suddenly stopped.
2. **GI:** Constipation, anorexia, nausea/vomiting.

3. **GU:** Urinary retention, impotence.
4. **Dermatologic:** Rash, pruritus, urticaria.
5. **CNS:** Dizziness, drowsiness, nervousness, headache, fatigue, sedation, insomnia, delirium, depression, coma, seizures.
6. **Other:** Dry mouth, glucose intolerance, weakness, hypothermia.

Drug Interactions:

1. Increased sedation when used with other depressants (e.g., alcohol, barbiturates).
2. Antihypertensive effects diminished by tricyclic antidepressants, monoamine oxidase inhibitors, tolazoline.
3. Paradoxical hypertension when used with β-adrenergic blockers.

Monitoring: Blood pressure, heart rate.

BIBLIOGRAPHY

Clonidine. In *Drug Facts and Comparisons,* New York, 1989, JB Lippincott, p 622.
Clonidine. In *AMA Drug Evaluations,* ed 6, Philadelphia, 1986, WB Saunders, p 516.

CLORAZEPATE

Trade Name: *Tranxene.*

Drug Action: A benzodiazepine. Anxiety reduction, sedation, anticonvulsant activity, muscle relaxation, amnesia.

Indications: Anxiety, seizure disorders, alcohol withdrawal.

Pharmacokinetics:

1. **Absorption:** PO.
2. **Metabolism:** Hepatic oxidation.
3. **Half-life:** 50–100 hr (mean).
4. **Excretion:** Renal excretion of inactive metabolites.
5. **Dialyzable(?):** Limited.
6. **Renal failure:** Monitor for sedation.

7. **Hepatic failure:** Reduce dosage, use with caution because of prolonged half-life.

Drug Preparations:

Tablets: 3.75, 7.5, 11.25, 15, 22.5 mg.
Capsules: 3.75, 7.5, 15 mg.

Dosage:

1. **Anxiety:** 15–60 mg/day in two to four divided doses.

Adverse Effects: Sedation, psychomotor impairment, depression, amnesia, impaired concentration, weakness, impaired sexual function, paradoxical agitation, respiratory depression, hypotension.

Drug Interactions:

1. Additive effect with other CNS depressants.
2. Induces liver enzymes.

Monitoring: Excess sedation vs. therapeutic effect.

BIBLIOGRAPHY

Drugs used for anxiety and sleep disorders. In *AMA Drug Evaluations,* ed 6, Philadelphia, 1986, WB Saunders, pp 81–110.
Sussman N: The benzodiazepines: selection and use in treating anxiety, insomnia, and other disorders, *Hosp Formul* 1985, 20:298–305.

CODEINE

Trade Names: Various companies make codeine phosphate or codeine sulfate either as single-drug formulations or in combination with other agents:

With aspirin: *Empirin With Codeine.*
With acetaminophen: *Tylenol With Codeine.*

Drug Action: Codeine has a low affinity for the μ and κ opioid receptors. The analgesic effect of codeine may be secondary to 10% demethylation to morphine in vivo. Codeine 100 mg IM is approximately equianalgesic to morphine sulfate 10 mg IM or aspirin 1000 mg.

Indications:

1. Mild to moderate pain.
2. Antitussive.
3. Antidiarrheal (not commonly used).

Pharmacokinetics:

1. **Absorption:** Rapid after PO administration.
2. **Onset of action:**
   a. **PO:** 15–20 min, with analgesic effects lasting 4–6 hr.
   b. **IM:** More rapid onset, and similar duration.
3. **Metabolism:** 10% demethylated to morphine in the liver.
   a. Other routes of demethylation and glucuronide conjugation result in inactive metabolites.
4. **Excretion:** Metabolites and small portions of unchanged drug excreted primarily in urine.
5. **Half-life:**
   a. **PO:** 2.5 hr.
   b. **IM:** 3.5 hr.

Drug Preparations:

1. Codeine sulfate: *Tablets:* 15, 30, 60 mg.
2. Codeine phosphate:
   a. Variety of PO combinations with other drugs, including aspirin and acetaminophen.
   b. 15, 30, 60 mg/mL SQ/IM.

Dosage:

1. **Mild to moderate pain:**
   a. **Adult:** 15–60 mg PO/SQ/IM q 4 hr.
   b. **Pediatric:** 0.5 mg/kg PO/SQ/IM q 4 hr.
2. **Antitussive:** Similar doses can be used.

Adverse Effects:

1. With equianalgesic doses, respiratory depression is similar to that with morphine. This may be of great significance in patients with elevated intracranial pressure.
2. Drowsiness, dysphoria, nausea/vomiting, constipation.

Drug Interactions:

1. Combinations of codeine with aspirin or acetaminophen are additive in analgesic effect.

2. If used in combination with sedatives, antihistamines, alcohol, or other similar drugs, significant sedation may occur.

Monitoring: Respiratory rate, blood pressure, heart rate, mental status.

BIBLIOGRAPHY

McEvoy GK (ed): *AHFS Drug Information 89,* Bethesda, 1989, American Society of Hospital Pharmacists.

AMA Drug Evaluations, ed 6, Philadelphia, 1986, WB Saunders.

Gilman AG, Goodman LS, Rall TW, et al (eds): *Goodman and Gilman's The Pharmacological Basis of Therapeutics,* ed 7, New York, 1985, Macmillan.

CYCLOSPORINE

Trade Name: *Sandimmune.*

Drug Action:

1. Immunosuppressive; inhibits production and release of inter-leukin 2 and inhibits interleukin 2–induced activation of T cells.
2. Inhibits T helper cells.

Indications: Immunosuppressant: Prevention of organ rejection after transplantations, autoimmune disease.

Pharmacokinetics:

1. **Absorption:** 30% from GI tract (highly variable).
2. **Metabolism:** Liver. Clearance decreased in patients with liver disease.
3. **Excretion:** Primarily bile; 6% in urine; present in breast milk.
4. **Peak levels after PO administration:** 3.5 hr.
5. **Plasma half-life:** Biphasic, with terminal half-life of 19 hr.

Drug Preparations:

Oral solution: 100 mg/mL (may mix with milk, orange juice).

Capsules: 25, 50, 100 mg

Injection: 50 mg/mL (mix each 50 mg in 20–100 mL saline or D_5W solution and give over 2–6 hr).

Dosage:

1. **PO:** 15 mg/kg/day, beginning 4–12 hr before transplantation. Continue this dose for 1–2 wk after transplantation, then reduce by 5%/wk to a maintenance dose of 5–10 mg/kg/day.
2. **IV:** 5–6 mg/kg/day over 2–24 hr, beginning 4–12 hr before transplantation. Switch to oral drug for long-term therapy. IV dose is administered at one third the oral dose.

Adverse Effects:

1. **Cardiovascular:** Chest pain, hypertension, tachycardia
2. **GI:** Nausea/vomiting, abdominal pain, diarrhea, constipation, anorexia, difficulty swallowing, hepatotoxicity, pancreatitis.
3. **GU:** Nephrotoxicity, renal failure.
4. **Dermatologic:** Acne, brittle nails, hirsutism, oily skin.
5. **Oronasopharynx:** Gum hyperplasia, oral thrush, mouth ulcers, sore throat.
6. **Hematologic:** Leukopenia, anemia, thrombocytopenia.
7. **CNS:** Seizures, tremor, headache, ataxia, paresthesia, depression, mania, encephalopathy, hallucinations.
8. **Other:** Infection, anaphylaxis (IV), flushing, leg cramps, visual disturbances, night sweats, gynecomastia, hypomagnesemia, hyperuricemia, hyperkalemia, second malignancy, (e.g., lymphoma), myositis, respiratory distress.

Drug Interactions:

1. **Increased nephrotoxicity** when used with amphotericin B, aminoglycosides, sulfamethoxazole, trimethoprim, nonsteroidal anti-inflammatory agents.
2. Increased risk of **second malignancy** when used with other immunosuppressive agents.
3. **Increased cyclosporin plasma levels (increased effect):** Erythromycin, fluconazole, ketoconazole, diltiazem, verpamil, corticosteroids, danazol, methyltestosterone, oral contraceptives, imipenem-cilastatin, metoclopramide.
4. **Lower cyclosporin plasma levels (decreased effect):** Phenytoin, rifampin, phenobarbital, co-trimoxazole, carbamazepine, isoniazid.
5. **Hyperkalemia** with potassium-sparing diuretics.
6. **Increased risk of seizures** with glucocorticoids.

Monitoring:

1. Plasma and blood levels (obtain 12–18 hr after dose or just before next dose): trough levels: 100–400 ng/mL for whole blood (depends on organ transplanted).
2. Blood cell counts.
3. BUN, creatinine.
4. Liver function tests.
5. Magnesium, potassium.
6. Blood pressure, heart rate.

BIBLIOGRAPHY

Cyclosporine. In *Drug Facts and Comparisons,* New York, 1989, JB Lippincott, p 2241.

Matl I, Jirka J, Petrasek R, Vitko S: Triple therapy with cyclosporin A in kidney transplant patients, *Transplant Proc* 1995, 28:2573.

Hoyer PE: Complications of cyclosporin therapy, *Contrib Nephrol* 1995, 114:111–123.

Galla F, Marzocchi V, Croattino L, et al: Oral and intravenous disposition of cyclosporin in psoriatic patients, *Ther Drug Monit* 1995, 17:302–304.

DANTROLENE

Trade Name: *Dantrium.*

Drug Action:

1. Decreases excitation-contraction coupling in skeletal muscle by apparently reducing the amount of calcium released from sarcoplasmic reticulum without affecting reuptake.
2. Does not alter contraction in cardiac or smooth muscle.

Indications:

1. Drug of choice in treatment of malignant hyperthermia, a rare syndrome in which certain anesthetics trigger a fulminant, frequently fatal episode characterized by a hypermetabolic state. Body temperature can reach 41.5°–42°C (107°–108°F), and severe metabolic disturbances may occur.

2. Possibly efficacious in treatment of neuroleptic malignant syndrome.
3. Used PO to treat chronic spasticity.
4. Prophylaxis of malignant hyperthermia.

Pharmacokinetics:

1. **Absorption:** PO administration results in slow (several hr and incomplete uptake. IV administration results in rapid onset of action.
2. **Metabolism:** Hepatic, resulting in hydroxyamino and acetylamino metabolites.
3. **Excretion:** Urinary and biliary.
4. **Half-life:** 4–8 hr after IV administration.

Drug Preparations:

Capsules: 25, 50, 100 mg (for use in treatment of spasticity).

Vials: 20 mg. (Dantrolene must be reconstituted with *sterile water for injection USP*). Each vial contains 3 g mannitol, and significant diuresis may occur.

Dosage:

1. **Malignant hyperthermia:**
   a. **Initial dose:** 1–2 mg/kg IV via rapid infusion. This dose may be given repeatedly to a total of 10 mg/kg if needed.
   b. **Subsequent therapy** after initial event, not clearly defined. We recommend 2–5 mg/kg q4 hr for 24 hr, with careful monitoring in the ICU.
   c. PO administration, 1–2 mg/kg qid, may be necessary for 1–3 days to prevent recurrence of the event.
   d. In patients potentially susceptible to malignant hyperthermia, prophylactic dantrolene can be administered, 2.5 mg/kg IV 1.5 hr before surgery.
2. **Spasticity:**
   a. Initial dose 25 mg PO once/day. Increase to 25 mg PO qid. Gradually increase by 25 mg q 4–7 days to max. daily dose of 400 mg given in four divided doses.

Adverse Effects: Both IV and PO administration of dantrolene can result in weakness, dizziness, lethargy, and malaise. Consult appropriate text for a complete description of adverse effects following long-term PO administration.

Drug Interactions:

1. When used in treatment of malignant hyperthermia, few significant interactions of clinical importance. There may be an additive effect with nondepolarizing neuromuscular blocking agents.
2. In experimental studies, marked myocardial depression has occurred when verapamil and dantrolene were coadministered.

Monitoring: Muscle rigidity, temperature, improvement in acid-base status.

BIBLIOGRAPHY

Gilman AG, Rall TW, Nies AS, Taylor P (eds): *Goodman and Gilman's The Pharmacological Basis of Therapeutics,* ed 8, New York, 1990, Macmillan.

Denniston PL Jr (ed): 1995 *Physicians GenRx,* Riverside, 1995, Denniston Publishing.

Physicians' Desk Reference, ed 49, Montvale, 1995, Medical Economics Data Production.

Miller RD (ed): *Anesthesia,* ed 4, New York, 1994, Churchill Livingstone.

Stoelting RK: *Pharmacology and Physiology in Anesthetic Practice,* ed 2, Philadelphia, 1991, JB Lippincott.

DAPSONE

Trade Name: *Dapsone.*

Drug Actions:

1. Inhibits microbial folic acid synthesis.
2. Spectrum of activity: *Mycobacterium leprae* and *Pneumocystis carinii.*

Indications:

1. Leprosy.
2. Alternative to trimethoprim/sulfamethoxazole for prophylaxis of *P. carinii* pneumonia in patients with AIDS or other conditions of immunodeficiency.

3. Treatment of *P. carinii* pneumonia (used with trimethoprim) in patients allergic/intolerant to trimethoprim/sulfamethoxazole.
4. Dermatitis herpetiformis.

Pharmacokinetics:

1. **Absorption:** PO.
2. **Metabolism:** Rapidly and almost completely absorbed. Peak concentrations are reached in 4–8 hr. Dapsone is acetylated in the liver.
3. **Excretion:** 85% of daily dose is recoverable from urine in the form of water-soluble metabolites.
4. **Half-life:** 10–50 hr with an average of 28 hr.

Drug Preparations:

Tablets: 25, 100 mg.

Dosage: 100 mg PO q day. (50–300 mg/day or higher is used in treatment of dermatitis herpetiformis.)

Adverse Effects:

1. Hemolysis, particularly in patients with G6PD or methemoglobin deficiencies, or hemoglobin M (patients should be screened for G6PD deficiency prior to dapsone initiation). In patients without G6PD deficiency, significant hemolysis occurs with dosages 200 mg/day. Interrelated changes of a loss of 1–2 g of hemoglobin, reticulocytosis (2%–12%), shortened red blood cell life span, and a rise in methemoglobin occur in nearly all patients receiving dapsone. Methemoglobinemia, when clinically significant (cyanosis generally occurs at or around 15 g/L), can be treated with 1 mg/kg IV methylene blue.
2. Hyperbilirubinemia—more common in G6PD patients.
3. Toxic hepatitis.
4. Cholestatic jaundice.
5. Agranulocytosis, aplastic anemia, and other blood dyscrasias—rare.
6. Severe dermatologic reactions (e.g., erythema multiforme, toxic epidermal necrolysis, and others)—rare.
7. Nausea, vomiting, abdominal pains, pancreatitis, vertigo, blurred vision, tinnitus, paresthesias, reversible peripheral neuropathy, insomnia, fever, headache, psychosis, phototoxicity, pulmonary eosinophilia, tachycardia, albuminuria, nephrotic syndrome, hypoalbuminemia without proteinuria, renal papil-

lary necrosis, male infertility, drug-induced lupus erythematosus, and mononucleosis-like syndrome have all been reported.
(The mononucleosis-like blood picture with fever and exfoliative dermatitis has been termed the dapsone syndrome.)
8. In general, dapsone is continued when leprosy reactional states
occur.

Drug Interactions:

1. Use of dapsone with other folic acid antagonists may increase
the likelihood of hematologic reactions.
2. Rifampin lowers dapsone levels seven- to tenfold.

Monitoring: Serial complete blood counts.

BIBLIOGRAPHY

Alford RH, Wallace RJ Jr: Antimycobacterial agents. In Mandell
GL, Bennett JE, Dolin R (eds): *Mandell, Douglas and Bennett's
Principles and Practice of Infectious Diseases,* ed 4, New York,
1995, Churchill Livingstone, pp 389–400.
Bunn HF: Disorders of hemoglobin. In Wilson JD, Braunwald E,
Isselbacher KJ, et al (eds): *Harrison's Principles of Internal
Medicine,* ed 12, New York, 1991, McGraw-Hill, pp
1543–1552.
Physicians' Desk Reference, ed 50, Montvale, 1996, Medical Eco-
nomics Co.
Sanford JP, Gilbert DN, Sande MA (eds): *The Sanford Guide to
Antimicrobial Therapy,* ed 26, Dallas, 1996, Antimicrobial
Therapy.

dDAVP (DESMOPRESSIN)

Trade Name: *DdAVP.*

Drug Action:

1. Antidiuretic; decreases free water excretion.
2. Hemostatic; increases factor VIII levels (i.e., in patients with
hemophilia and von Willebrand's disease type I) and improves
platelet function.

Indications:

1. **Neurogenic (central) diabetes insipidus.**
2. **Bleeding:** Hemophilia A with factor VIII levels >5%, von Willebrand disease (type I), uremia, bleeding after cardiac surgery.

Pharmacokinetics:

1. **Absorption:** Destroyed by GI tract; 10%–20% absorbed from nasal mucosa.
2. **Peak effect:** Intranasal 1–5 hr, IV 1.5–3 hr.
3. **Metabolism:** Tissues.
4. **Serum half-life:** Fast phase 8 min; slow phase 75 min.
5. **Duration of antidiuretic effect:** Intranasal 8–20 hr; IV 12–24 hr.

Drug Preparations:

Nasal spray: 5 mL bottles, 10 mg/dose.
Rhinal tube: 2.5 mL vial, 0.1 mg/mL.
Injection (IV/SQ): 1 and 10 mL vials, 4 μg/mL.

Dosage:

1. **Neurogenic diabetes insipidus:**
   a. **Intranasal:**
      (1) **Adult:** 0.1–0.4 mL (10–40 μg) or 1-4 sprays one to two times/day.
      (2) **Pediatric:** 0.05–0.1 mL (5–10 μg) or 1 spray one to three times/day.
   b. **Parenteral:** Adults 0.5–1 mL (2–4 μg) IV/SC bid. (Use IV form; IV preparation 10 times more potent as intranasal preparation.)
2. **Hemostasis:**
   a. Adult and pediatric dose: 0.3–0.4 μg/kg IV in saline solution over 15–30 min; may be repeated. Effect decreases with repeated injections.

Adverse Effects:

1. **CNS:** Headache, seizures, confusion, dizziness, drowsiness, coma (water intoxication).
2. **Cardiovascular:** Hypotension with rapid IV injection, hypertension with very large doses, flushing.
3. **GI:** Nausea/vomiting, abdominal cramps.
4. Nasal congestion, rhinitis.

5. Oliguria.
6. Local pain, flushing, hypersensitivity reactions.
7. Weight gain.
8. Water intoxication, hyponatremia, hypoosmolality.
9. Platelet aggregation may be induced in patients with von Willebrand disease type IIb, rare thrombus formation.

Drug Interactions:

1. **Potentiate antidiuretic action:** Carbamazepine, chlorpropamide, clofibrate, fludrocortisone.
2. **Decrease antidiuretic action:** Demeclocycline, lithium, epinephrine, norepinephrine, heparin, alcohol.

Monitoring:

1. Serum sodium.
2. Urine and plasma osmolality.
3. Urine output.
4. Fluid balance.
5. Body weight.
6. Signs of water intoxication.
7. Blood pressure and heart rate (during IV infusion).
8. When used for hemostasis: Factor VIII antigen levels, PTT, bleeding time.

BIBLIOGRAPHY

Hayes RM: Agents affecting the renal conservation of water. In Gilman AG, et al (eds): *The Pharmacological Basis of Therapeutics,* 8th ed, New York, 1993, McGraw-Hill, pp 732–742.
Robertson GL: Diabetes insipidus, *Endocrinol Metab Clin North Am* 1995, 24:549–572.
Cobb WE, Spare S, Reichlin S: Neurogenic diabetes insipidus: management with dDAVP (l-desamino-8-D-arginine vasopressin), *Ann Intern Med* 1978, 88:183–188.
Mannucci PM: Desmopressin: a nontransfusional form of treatment for congenital and acquired bleeding disorders, *Blood* 1988, 72:1449–1455.
Zaloga GP: Hormones—vasopressin, growth hormone, glucagon, somatostatin, prolactin, G-CSF, GM-CSF. In Chernow B (ed): *The Pharmacologic Approach to the Critically Ill Patient,* ed 3, Baltimore, 1994, Williams & Wilkins, pp 700–714.

DEMECLOCYCLINE

Trade Names: *Declomycin, Ledermycin.*

Drug Action:

1. **Antibiotic** (tetracycline; bacteriostatic, inhibits protein synthesis): Effective against gram-negative and gram-positive organisms, *Mycoplasma, Rickettsia, Chlamydia,* spirochetes, agents of psittacosis and ornithosis, lymphogranuloma venereum.
2. **Inhibits antidiuretic hormone** action on renal tubules.

Indications:

1. Infection with susceptible organisms.
2. Syndrome of inappropriate antidiuretic hormone secretion (SIADH).

Pharmacokinetics:

1. **Absorption:** 60%–80% absorbed from GI tract; peak 3–4 hr. Absorption reduced by food or milk.
2. **Distribution:** Body tissues and fluids; crosses placenta; concentrated in bile; present in breast milk.
3. **Metabolism:** None.
4. **Excretion:** Unchanged in urine. Adjust dose in renal failure. Excreted in feces.
5. **Plasma half-life:** 10–17 hr in normal renal function.

Drug Preparations:

Tablets: 150, 300 mg.

Dosage:

1. **Infection:** Adults: 150 mg q 6 hr or 300 mg q 12 hr; children >8 yr: 3–6 mg/lb/day divided into two to four doses. Reduce dose for renal impairment.
2. **SIADH:** 600–1200 mg/day in divided doses (1 hr before or 2 hr after meals).

Adverse Reactions:

1. Photosensitivity reactions, rashes, dermatitis, urticaria, anaphylaxis.

2. Lightheadedness, vertigo, pseudotumor cerebri, headache, blurred vision, tinnitus.
3. Discolored nails and teeth, enamel hypoplasia, impaired bone growth.
4. Anorexia, nausea/vomiting, diarrhea, glossitis, stomatitis, dysphagia, anogenital inflammation, enterocolitis, pancreatitis, esophagitis.
5. Pericarditis, exacerbation of systemic lupus erythematosus.
6. Nephrotoxicity, hepatotoxicity.
7. Elevated BUN (increased catabolism), neutropenia, eosinophilia, hemolytic anemia, thrombocytopenia.
8. Nephrogenic diabetes insipidus.

Drug Interactions:

1. Chelated (absorption decreased) by antacids, iron, dairy products, food, laxatives, sodium bicarbonate.
2. Binds to calcium ions.
3. Antagonizes bactericidal effects of penicillins.
4. Increased nephrotoxicity with methoxyflurane.
5. Enhances effects of PO anticoagulants.
6. Increases digoxin bioavailability.
7. False test for glucose (glucose oxidase method) in urine.
8. False elevation for catecholamines in urine (fluorometric test).
9. Oral contraceptives less effective.

Monitoring:

1. Serum sodium, osmolality.
2. Urine output.
3. BUN, creatinine.
4. Liver function tests, blood counts.

BIBLIOGRAPHY

Forrest JN Jr, Cox M, Hong C, et al: Superiority of demeclocycline over lithium in treatment of chronic syndrome of inappropriate secretion of antidiuretic hormone, *N Engl J Med* 1978, 298:173–177.

Sande MA, Mandell GL: Antimicrobial agents. In Gilman AG, et al (eds): *The Pharmacologic Basis of Therapeutics,* ed 8, New York, 1993, McGraw-Hill, pp 1117–1125.

DEXTRAN

Trade Name:

Dextran 40 (low molecular weight):

Rheomacrodex (10% dextran in 5% dextrose or 0.9% sodium chloride solution), *Dextran 40, Gentran-40, 10% LMD*.

Dextran 70 (high molecular weight):

Macrodex (6% dextran solution in 0.9% sodium chloride), *Dextran 70, Hyskon Hysteroscopy Fluid* (32% dextran solution in 10% dextrose).

Dextran 75 (high molecular weight):

Dextran 75, Gentran 75.

Drug Action:

1. Volume expansion:
   a. Colloid volume expander.
2. Prevention of thromboembolism:
   a. Direct anticoagulant effects:
      (1) Increased antithrombin III activity.
      (2) Reduced activation of factor V (proaccelerin) to accelerin by thrombin.
      (3) Decreased serum fibrinogen levels.

   Hemostatic defects are related to molecular weight (the larger mol wt dextrans possessing increased anticoagulant effect) and the amount of dextran administered (increased affect at >120 mL/kg/day).

   b. Antiplatelet effects:
      (1) Coating of platelet surfaces.
      (2) Decreased platelet adhesiveness, resulting in incrased bleeding time.
3. Promotion of peripheral blood flow:
   a. Inhibits erythrocyte aggregation.
   b. Coats endothelial cell surfaces, which inhibits sludging and cellular aggregation in microcirculation.

Pharmacokinetics:

1. **Absorption:** Give IV.
2. **Metabolism:** Larger molecules slowly taken up by reticuloendothelial system (mostly liver) and eventually oxidized to carbon dioxide and water.

3. **Excretion:** Renal. Smaller particles (mol wt <15,000) are very rapidly filtered and excreted by kidneys. Renal threshold for filtration occurs at mol wt about 55,000.
4. **Onset of action:** Concurrent with administration. However, time lag of 3–12 hr has been observed between end of dextran infusion and max. anticoagulant effect.
5. **Plasma half-life:** Dependent on molecular size: only minutes for molecules <15,000 mol wt. In general, two thirds of dextran 40 and one third of dextran 70 is eliminated in first 12 hr after infusion.

Drug Preparations: Dextran is a biosynthetic sucrose product of the bacterium *Leuconostoc*. Partial hydrolysis and fractionation determine average mol wt of the commercial end product.

Dosage:

1. **Hypovolemia, shock:** 10 mL/kg high mol wt dextran as rapid IV infusion, with total dose not to exceed 20 mL/kg in first 24 hr. If therapy is continued longer than 24 hr, subsequent total daily dose should not exceed 10 mL/kg. Therapy should be limited to no more than 5 days.
   May use Dextran 40 also. Taper to hemodynamic effect.
2. **Prophylaxis of thromboembolism, or antiplatelet effect:** Give continuous IV infusion of dextran 40 (Rheomacrodex) at 30–50 mL/hr. Monitor urine specific gravity and urine output (*see* Adverse Effects, below). Continue infusion for 2–3 days from time of surgery; thereafter may administer 500 mL every 2–3 days for up to 2 wk.

Adverse Effects:

1. **Anticoagulant effect:** When used primarily as a volume expander, anticoagulant actions may cause bleeding problems, especially at higher doses.
2. **Antigenicity:** Dextran is a potent antigen, cross-reacting with a number of bacterial polysaccharides. Severe anaphylaxis may occur, usually within the first 30 min after infusion is initiated. Less severe hypersensitivity reactions manifested by rash, hives, and pruritus are also possible.
3. **Renal failure:** Filtered dextran markedly increases urine viscosity and may contribute to acute tubular obstruction in states of low urine output and avid water reabsorption by renal tubules.

4. **Laboratory abnormalities:** Dextran may interfere with cross-matching of blood.

Drug Interactions: Anticoagulant effect of dextran will clinically potentiate anticoagulant effects of heparin, warfarin, or other antiplatelet agents. Excess bleeding may result.

Monitoring:

1. Urine osmolality, urine volume.
2. Daily BUN, creatinine.
3. Coagulation studies not routinely monitored.

BIBLIOGRAPHY

Plasma expanders. In *Drug Facts and Comparisons,* Philadelphia, 1996, JB Lippincott, pp 384–391.

Blood, blood components, and blood substitutes. In *AMA Drug Evaluations,* ed 6, Philadelphia, 1986, WB Saunders, pp 637–638.

Gruber UF, Saldeen T, Brokop T, et al: Incidences of fatal postoperative pulmonary embolism after prophylaxis with dextran 70 and low-dose heparin: an international multicentre study, *Br Med J* 1980, 280:69–72.

Manger D, Gerson JI, Constantine RM, et al: Pulmonary edema and coagulopathy due to Hyskon (32% dextran-70) administration, *Anesth Analg* 1989, 68:686–687.

Mudge GH: Agents affecting volume and composition of body fluids. In Gilman AG, Goodman LS, Rall TW, et al (eds): *The Pharmacologic Basis of Therapeutics,* ed 7, New York, 1985, Macmillan, pp 846–878.

Rainey TG, English JF: Pharmacology of colloids and crystalloids. In Chernow B (ed): *The Pharmacologic Approach to the Critically Ill Patient,* Baltimore, 1988, Williams & Wilkins, pp 219–240.

DIAZEPAM

Trade Name: *Valium.*

Drug Action: Anxiety reduction, sedation, anticonvulsant activity, muscle relaxation, amnesia, anesthesia induction.

Indications: Anxiety, preanesthetic, anesthetic induction, skeletal muscle relaxation, seizure disorder, alcohol withdrawal, tetanus and stiff-man syndrome.

Pharmacokinetics:

1. **Absorption:** PO, parenteral.
2. **Onset of action:** 30–60 min after PO administration; 15–30 min after IM use; 1–5 min after IV injection.
3. **Metabolism:** Hepatic oxidation.
4. **Half-life:** 10–100 hr; prolonged in elderly or patients with renal/hepatic disease.
5. **Excretion:** Renal excretion of inactive metabolites.
6. **Dialyzable(?):** Limited.
7. **Renal failure:** Monitor for sedation.
8. **Hepatic failure:** Reduce dose, use with caution.

Drug Preparations:

Tablets: 2, 5, 10 mg.
PO solution: 5 mg/5 mL.
Injection: 5 mg/mL; compounded with 40% propylene glycol and 10% ethyl alcohol.

Dosage:

1. **Anxiety:** 4–40 mg/day in two to four divided doses PO, IV, IM.
2. **Status epilepticus:** 5–10 mg IV (1–2 mg/min).
3. Dosage highly variable for other indications.

Adverse Effects: Sedation, psychomotor impairment, depression, amnesia, impaired concentration, weakness, impaired sexual function, paradoxical agitation, hypotension, dysrhythmias (IV), hypersensitivity.

Drug Interactions:

1. Additive effect with other CNS depressants.
2. Induces liver enzymes.
3. Prolonged effect with agents that diminish hepatic metabolism (e.g., cimetidine, disulfiram, PO contraceptives).
4. Decreased digoxin clearance.

Monitoring: Excess sedation vs. therapeutic effect.

BIBLIOGRAPHY

Drugs used for anxiety and sleep disorders. In *AMA Drug Evaluations,* ed 6, Philadelphia, 1986, WB Saunders, pp 81–110.

Sussman N: The benzodiazepines: selection and use in treating anxiety, insomnia, and other disorders, *Hosp Formul* 1985, 20:298–305.

DIAZOXIDE

Trade Names: *Hyperstat IV Injection, Proglycem.*

Drug Action:

1. Vasodilator.
2. Elevates blood glucose (inhibits insulin secretion).

Indications:

1. Hypertensive crisis.
2. Hypoglycemia due to insulinoma.

Pharmacokinetics:

1. **Absorption:** Oral.
2. **Metabolism:** Liver.
3. **Excretion:** Renal; effects prolonged in renal insufficiency.
4. **Onset of action:** Decreases blood pressure within seconds of IV administration; peak effect occurs at 5 min. Hyperglycemic effects occur within 1 hr of PO administration.
5. **Duration of antihypertensive effect:** 3–12 hr.
6. **Duration of antihypoglycemic effect:** 8 hr.
7. **Plasma half-life:** 28 ±8 hr.

Drug Preparations:

IV Injection: 300 mg/20 mL.
Capsules: 50 mg.
PO suspension: 50 mg/mL in 30 mL bottles.

Dosage:

1. **Hypertensive crisis:** 1–3 mg/kg IV (max. 150 mg) q 5–15 min until blood pressure controlled; repeated injections at intervals of 4–24 hr usually maintain the effect.

2. **Antihypoglycemic:** 3–8 mg/kg/day PO in two to three divided doses.

Adverse Effects:

1. **Cardiovascular:** Hypotension, angina pectoris, myocardial ischemia, arrhythmias, tachycardia, fluid retention, heart failure.
2. **GI:** Nausea/vomiting, anorexia, abdominal pain, ileus, diarrhea, pancreatitis.
3. **Metabolic:** Hyperglycemia, hyperuricemia, ketoacidosis.
4. **CNS:** Dizziness, headache, weakness, malaise, euphoria, cerebral ischemia, seizures, unconsciousness, stroke.
5. **Other:** Sodium and water retention, sweating, flushing, hypertrichosis, thrombocytopenia, neutropenia, anemia, renal insufficiency, blurred vision, skin rash.

Drug Interactions:

1. May potentiate antihypertensive effects of other antihypertensives.
2. Decreases protein binding of warfarin and bilirubin, resulting in higher blood levels.
3. Actions potentiated by diuretics.
4. Alters requirements for insulin and PO hypoglycemics.
5. Inhibition of insulin release antagonized by α-adrenergic antagonists.
6. Increases hepatic metabolism of hydantoins, reducing serum levels.

Monitoring:

1. Blood pressure, heart rate.
2. Blood glucose.
3. Urine ketones.
4. Blood cell counts.
5. BUN, creatinine.
6. Sodium, potassium.

BIBLIOGRAPHY

Diazoxide. In *Drug Facts and Comparisons,* Philadelphia, 1989, JB Lippincott, pp 411, 670.
Diazoxide. In *AMA Drug Evaluations,* ed 6, Philadelphia, 1986, WB Saunders, pp 533, 792.

DIGOXIN

Trade Name: *Lanoxin.*

Drug Action:

1. Inhibition of Na^+-K^+ ATPase in myocardial cells leads to increased intracellular Na^+. Increased Na^+ results in Na-Ca^{++} exchange, which increases intracellular Ca^{++} available for excitation-contraction coupling. The net result is increased inotropy.
2. Prolongs refractoriness in AV node and His-Purkinje system; shortens refractoriness of atria and ventricles.
3. In Purkinje cells, increases slope of phase 4 depolarization, leading to increased automaticity.
4. In Purkinje cells, increased Ca^{++} influx can lead to early or late afterdepolarization and tachyarrhythmias.
5. Indirect effects mediated through vagus nerve.

Indications:

1. Treatment of supraventricular arrhythmias:
   a. Supraventricular tachycardias.
   b. Atrial fibrillation.
   c. Atrial flutter.
2. Congestive heart failure.

Pharmacokinetics:

1. **Absorption:** PO (60%–80% absorbed), IV, IM.
2. **Onset of action:** 30–120 min after PO administration; 30 min after IM; 5–30 min after IV injection. Peak AV nodal effects may require over 1 hr.
3. **Metabolism:** Minimal hepatic.
4. **Excretion:** Renal.
5. **Protein binding:** 25%.
6. **Plasma half-life:** 36–48 hr; increased in renal insufficiency.
7. **Therapeutic level:** 0.6–1.8 ng/mL.

Drug Preparations:

Tablets: 0.125, 0.25, 0.50 mg.
Capsules: 0.05, 0.10, 0.20 mg.
Injection: 0.1 mg/1 mL, 0.5 mg/2 mL.

Dosage:

1. **Digitalizing dose:** 0.4–0.6 mg IV. Detectable effects in 5–30 min; peak effects in 1–4 hr. Additional fractions of 0.125–0.25 mg q 4–8 hr. It is usually necessary to give 0.75–1.25 mg total for desired effect.
2. **Maintenance dose:** 0.125–0.25 mg/day PO tabs or IV.

Adverse Effects:

1. Toxicity can produce almost any arrhythmia or disturbance of conduction, especially sinus bradycardia, SA block, AV block, accelerated junctional rhythms, premature ventricular contractions, ventricular tachycardia, ventricular fibrillation.
2. Anorexia, nausea, vomiting, diarrhea
3. Visual disturbances
4. Neurologic effects: Fatigue, weakness, headache, stupor, agitation.

Drug Interactions:

1. Quinidine, verapamil, amiodarone increase digoxin levels.
2. Antacids, sulfasalazine, neomycin, cholestyramine decrease intestinal digoxin absorption.
3. Sympathomimetics increase risk of cardiac arrhythmias.
4. Concurrent use of β-blockers and calcium channel blockers can lead to complete heart block.
5. Diuretics increase risk of digitalis toxicity by decreasing serum potassium and magnesium levels.

Monitoring:

1. Serum levels: 0.6–1.8 ng/mL.
2. Heart rate.
3. Clinical symptoms.

Drug Reversal: Digibind (digoxin immune Fab) for life-threatening digitalis intoxication.

BIBLIOGRAPHY

Hoffman BF, Bigger JT Jr: Digitalis and allied cardiac glycosides. In Gilman AG, Goodman LS, Gilman A (eds): *The Pharmacological Basis of Therapeutics,* ed 6, New York, 1980, Macmillan, pp 729–760.

Smith TW, Braunwald E, Kelly RA: The management of heart failure. In Braunwald E (ed): *Heart Disease,* Philadelphia, 1988, WB Saunders, pp 485–507.

DIGOXIN IMMUNE FAB

Trade Name: *Digibind.*

Drug Action: Fab fragments bind free digoxin and digitoxin in blood; affinity for digoxin is greater than that of the Na-K ATPase pump.

Indications: Severe digoxin/digitoxin intoxication (manifested by a serum K^+ $\geq$5.0 mEq/L, malignant tachyarrhythmias, and/or hemodynamically significant bradyarrhythmias unresponsive to atropine). Also useful for oleander poisoning.

Pharmacokinetics:
1. **Absorption:** Immediate (IV administration).
2. **Distribution:** Extracellular fluid.
3. **Excretion:** Renal.
4. **Plasma half-life:** 15–20 hr (normal renal function).
5. **Onset of action:** Immediate.
6. **Cardiac toxicity** begins to subside within 20–30 min., with complete response in approximately 90 min.
7. Each 40 mg Fab binds 0.6 mg digoxin.

Drug Preparations:

Vials: 40 mg (lyophilized powder—reconstitute with 4 mL sterile water).

Dosage: Administer IV over 30 min or as an IV bolus if cardiac arrest is imminent; dosage varies according to amount ingested (see specific instructions in package insert).

1. For acute toxicity when steady-state serum level and amount are unknown, give 800 mg (20 vials) in both adults and children.
2. Approximate dose for reversal of known acute ingestion in adult (70 kg).

a. 6.25 mg ingested: Give 360 mg.
b. 12.5 mg ingested: 680 mg.
c. 25 mg ingested: 1360 mg.
3. Approximate dose for reversal in 70 kg adult when steady-state serum digoxin level is known (roughly follows the formula

$$\frac{[digoxin\ ng/ml][wt \in kg]}{100} = \text{number of vials}$$

2 ng/mL: Give 80 mg (2 vials).
4 ng/mL: 120 mg (3 vials).
8 ng/mL: 240 mg (6 vials).
4. Digoxin body load (mg) = (steady-state serum concentration) (5.6) (weight in kg) ÷ 1000.
a. Dose of Fab (vials) = (body load in mg)/0.6 mg bound per vial (rounded up to next whole vial).

Adverse Effects:

1. **Cardiovascular:** Tachyarrhythmias, bradyarrhythmias, congestive heart failure.
2. **Metabolic:** Hypokalemia.
3. **Other:** Rash, hypersensitivity.

Drug Interactions: None reported.

Monitoring:

1. Serum digitoxin levels (will increase after administration from Fab-digoxin complexes, thus rendering further measurements meaningless).
2. Serum K^+ (particularly in the first 6–8 hr after digoxin immune Fab administration).
3. Blood pressure, heart rate, ECG.

BIBLIOGRAPHY

Physicians' Desk Reference, ed 49, Montvale, 1995, Medical Economics, p 755.

Committee on Injury and Poison Prevention: *Handbook of Common Poisonings in Children,* ed 3, American Academy of Pediatrics, 1994, p 18.

Howland MA: Digoxin-specific antibody fragments (Fab). In Goldfrank LR, Flomenbaum NE, Lewin NA, et al (eds): *Toxicologic Emergencies,* ed 5, Norwalk, 1994, Appleton & Lange, p 693.

DILTIAZEM

Trade Names: *Cardizem, Cardizem CD, Dilacor XR.*

Drug Action:

1. Blocks calcium entry into cells through slow calcium channels.
2. Vasodilator.
3. Depresses SA and AV nodal function.
4. Negative inotropic effect. Decreases myocardial oxygen demand.

Indications:

1. Ischemic heart disease (e.g., angina pectoris).
2. Hypertension.
3. Atrial fibrillation/flutter, paroxysmal supraventricular tachycardia (do not use in patients with accessory bypass tracts).

Pharmacokinetics:

1. **Absorption:** Well absorbed (80%–90%) PO. Onset of action: PO 30–60 min. Time to peak concentration: Short-acting tablets 2–3 hr, sustained release 6–14 hr.
2. **Metabolism:** Liver.
3. **Excretion:** Renal, bile.
4. **Plasma half-life:** 3–9 hr.

Drug Preparations:

Short-acting tablets: 30, 60, 90, 120 mg.
Sustained-release tablets (SR): 60, 90, 120, 180, 240, 500 mg.
Once daily (Cardizem CD): 120, 180, 240, 300 mg capsules.
Injection: 5 mg/ml (5 ml, 10 ml).

Dosage:

1. **Adult:**

Short-acting tablets 30 mg PO three to four times/day. Increase dosage at 1–2 day intervals until desired effect achieved; max. dose 360 mg/day.

Sustained-release (SR) tablets: Begin 60–120 mg bid (average dose 240–360 mg/day).

Once daily capsules (Cardizem CD): Give total daily dose once daily, begin 180–240 mg/day.

IV dosage: Initial bolus 0.25 mg/kg over 2 min; may repeat bolus in 15 min; continuous infusion 5–10 mg/hr, increase to 15 mg/hr.
2. Reduce dose in renal or hepatic failure.
3. Titrate dose to desired effect.

Adverse Effects:

1. **Cardiovascular:** Arrhythmias, hypotension, edema, flushing, bradycardia, conduction disturbances, heart block, angina, syncope.
2. **GI:** Nausea/vomiting, diarrhea, hepatic toxicity, constipation, anorexia.
3. **GU:** Polyuria.
4. **Dermatologic:** Rash, pruritus.
5. **CNS:** Fatigue, headache, dizziness, drowsiness, nervousness, depression, insomnia, confusion, abnormal dreams, amnesia.
6. Tremor.

Drug Interactions:

1. Congestive heart failure or conduction disturbances may be precipitated when used with β-blockers.
2. Increases digoxin, carbamazepine, cyclosporin, quinidine, theophylline levels.
3. Antagonized by calcium/vitamin D.
4. H_2 blockers decrease hepatic metabolism of diltiazem.
5. Potentiates lithium effects.

Monitoring: Blood pressure, heart rate.

BIBLIOGRAPHY

Diltiazem. In *Drug Facts and Comparisons,* Philadelphia, 1989, JB Lippincott, p 557.
Diltiazem. In *AMA Drug Evaluations,* ed 6, Philadelphia, 1986, WB Saunders, pp 474, 538.

DIPHENHYDRAMINE HYDROCHLORIDE

Trade Names: *Benadryl, Dytuss, Maximum Strength Unisom SleepGels.*

Drug Action:

1. Histamine$_1$ receptor (H$_1$) antagonist that blocks vasodilator, secretory, and bronchospastic response to histamine.
2. H$_1$ antagonist that attenuates the H$_1$ receptor–mediated increase in capillary permeability (at postcapillary venule) and therefore decreases edema formation.
3. CNS sedation and suppression of cough.
4. Anticholinergic (drying) action on mucosal surfaces and secretions.
5 Antinausea action.

Indications:

1. Exudative allergic phenomena (e.g., seasonal rhinitis, allergic conjunctivitis, some forms of urticaria, some forms of contact and atopic dermatitis).
2. Motion sickness (both treatment and prophylaxis).
3. Preoperative sedation; and drying agent.
4. For pretreatment in patients susceptible to allergic reactions (drugs such as Protamine, penicillins, etc; blood products; IV contrast).
5. Anaphylactic shock (secondary adjunct to epinephrine, fluid, and oxygen).
6. Parkinsonism.
7. Dystonic reactions to dopamine-blocking agents.
8. Bedtime hypnotic/insomnia.

Pharmacokinetics:

1. **Absorption:** Well absorbed from gut; peak effect in approximately 1 hr.
2. **Metabolism:** Hepatic.
3. **Excretion:** Renal.
4. **Plasma elimination** half-life: 8 hr.
5. **Duration of action:** 4–6 hr.

Dosage:

1. **Administration:** Can be given PO, IM/IV, topically.
2. **PO: Adult:** 25–50 mg q 6–8 hr.
3. **Parenteral:** 10–50 mg (up to 100 mg) IM (deep)/IV.

Adverse Effects: Contraindications: Neonates, nursing women, glaucoma, benign prostatic hypertrophy/urinary retention, bowel obstruction.

1. **CNS Sedation:** Dizziness, ataxia, confusion, blurred vision, tremor, tinnitus, may produce paradoxical excitation (especially in children).
2. **GI:** Anorexia, nausea/vomiting, epigastric distress, diarrhea, constipation.
3. **Hematologic:** Leukopenia, thrombocytopenia, hemolytic anemia, agranulocytosis.
4. **GU:** Urinary retention, difficulty voiding.
5. **Overdosage:** Sedation or excitation (centrally mediated), hallucinations, ataxia, incoordination, athetosis, dry mouth, mydriasis, flushing, convulsions. Small children are particularly susceptible.

Drug Interactions: Additive sedation when used with other sedatives (e.g., opiates, benzodiazepines, barbiturates).

BIBLIOGRAPHY

Benadryl. In *Physicians' Desk Reference,* ed 49, Montvale, 1995, Medical Economics, p 1818.
Gilman AG, Goodman LS, Rall TW, et al: *The Pharmacological Basis of Therapeutics,* ed 8, New York, 1990, Pergamon Press, p 582.
Stoelting RK: *Pharmacology and Physiology in Anesthetic Practice,* ed 2, Philadelphia, 1991, JB Lippincott, p 397.

DIPYRIDAMOLE

Trade Name: *Persantine.*

Drug Actions: Inhibits platelet aggregation, may cause vasodilation, may stimulate release of prostacyclin; inhibits adenosine deaminase and phosphodiesterase.

Indications:

1. Prevent thrombosis (especially after surgical grafting, including coronary arteries).

2. Prevent thromboembolism (in combination with aspirin or warfarin).

Pharmacokinetics:

1. **Absorption:** PO.
2. **Onset of action:** Peak effect 2–2.5 hr.
3. **Metabolism:** Liver.
4. **Excretion:** In feces via bile.
5. **Half-life:** 10–12 hr.

Drug Preparations:

Tablets: 25, 50, 75 mg.
Injection: 10 mg/2 mL.

Dosage:

1. Adult: 75–400 mg/day PO in three to four divided doses.
2. IV: 0.14 mg/kg/min ×4 min (max. 60 mg).

Adverse Effects:

1. Hypersensitivity reactions, rash.
2. Cardiovascular: Hypotension, angina pectoria, hypertension, tachycardia, flushing, syncope, edema.
3. Dizziness, headache.
4. GI upset, dyspnea, weakness, hyperventilation, rhinitis.
5. Bleeding.

Drug Interactions: Synergistic with other drugs that affect platelet function or coagulation (e.g., heparin, aspirin).

Monitoring: Clinical response, watch for bleeding, blood pressure, heart rate.

BIBLIOGRAPHY

Stein PD, Dalan JE, Goldman S, et al: Antithrombotic therapy in patients with saphenous vein and internal mammary artery bypass grafts, *Chest* 1995, 108(Suppl):424–430.
Verstraete M: Primary and secondary prevention of arterial thromboembolism, *Br Med Bull* 1994, 50:946–965.

DIRITHROMYCIN

Trade Name: *Dynabac.*

Drug Actions:

1. Inhibits bacterial protein synthesis by binding to the 50S ribosomal subunit.
2. Spectrum of activity is similar to that of erythromycin and includes gram-positive aerobes, *Mycoplasma pneuomniae,* and *Legionella pneumophila* (as with erythromycin, many strains of *Haemophilus influenzae* are resistant to dirithromycin).

Indications:

1. Treatment of bronchitis due to *Streptococcus pneumoniae* or *Moraxella catarrhalis* (but not *H. influenzae,* which is a common pathogen in bronchitis).
2. Community-acquired pneumonia.
3. Skin and soft tissue infections.
4. Group A streptococcal pharyngitis.

Pharmacokinetics:

1. **Absorption:** PO; slightly enhanced by food.
2. **Metabolism:** Converted to erythromycylamine, an active compound that reaches peak serum concentrations in 4–5 hr.
3. **Excretion:** In bile and feces.
4. **Half-life:** 30–44 hr.

Drug Preparations:

Tablets (enteric-coated): 250, 500 mg.

Dosage: 500 mg PO q day (advantage over erythromycin is once-daily dosing).

Adverse Effects: Abdominal pain and nausea occurred in <10% in controlled trials, but these side effects may be more common in clinical practice.

Drug Interactions:

1. Unlike clarithromycin and azithromycin (two other relatively new macrolide antibiotics), dirithromycin is not thought to bind cytochrome P-450 isozymes.

2. Other macrolides have had numerous other drug interactions, including potentially dangerous interaction with nonsedating antihistamines (torsades de pointes).

BIBLIOGRAPHY

Dirithromycin. In *Drug Facts and Comparisons,* ed 50, St. Louis, 1996, Facts and Comparisons, p 3420.
Med Lett Drugs Ther 1995, 37:109–110.

DOBUTAMINE

Trade Name: *Dobutrex.*

Drug Action:

1. Racemic mixture of D and L forms. L-isomer is predominately a potent α_1 agonist; D-isomer is a potent β_1 and β_2 receptor stimulant.
2. Increased automaticity in sinus node. Enhanced AV and intraventricular conduction.
3. Increased inotropy.
4. Mild peripheral vasodilation (β_2 effects greater than α_1 effects). Decreased wall tension by decreased left ventricular end-diastolic pressure; decreased diastolic and systolic ventricular volumes.
5. Direct acting; no dopaminergic effects on renal vessels.

Indications:

1. Congestive heart failure.
2. Mitral regurgitation: Increased contractility, decreased afterload, small increase in heart rate will increase forward flow.
3. Right ventricular failure with high pulmonary vascular resistance.
4. May have sustained action after bolus therapy.

Pharmacokinetics:

1. **Absorption:** Give IV.
2. **Metabolism:** Methylation and conjugation in liver.
3. **Excretion:** Renal.

4. **Plasma half-life:** 2 min.
5. **Onset of action:** Immediate.

Drug Preparations:

Ampules: 250 mg/20 mL.

Dosage: 2.5–10 μg/kg/min most commonly used.

Adverse Effects:

1. Tachycardia.
2. Ventricular arrhythmias.
3. Hypotension at higher doses owing to vasodilation.

Monitoring:

1. Heart rate; tachycardia.
2. Hypotension may be limiting factor.

BIBLIOGRAPHY

Colucci WS, Wright RF, Braunwald E: New positive inotropic agents in the treatment of congestive heart failure, *N Engl J Med* 1986, 314:290–297.

Makabali C, Weil MH, Henning RJ: Dobutamine and other sympathomimetic drugs for the treatment of low cardiac output failure, *Semin Anesth* 1982, 1:63–69.

DOPAMINE

Trade Name: *Intropin.*

Drug Action:

1. Direct α, β₁, and dopaminergic receptor stimulation.
   a. **DA₁ receptors:** Postsynaptic to sympathetic nerves. Stimulation results in vasodilation in renal, mesenteric, coronary, cerebral arterial blood vessels.
   b. **DA₂ receptors:** Prejunctional sympathetic nerve location stimulation results in inhibition of norepinephrine release from sympathetic nerve storage sites.
2. Indirect actions result in release of norepinephrine.

Indications:

1. Hypotension (e.g., sepsis).
2. Increase renal blood flow and urine output.
3. Increase heart rate.

Pharmacokinetics:

1. **Absorption:** Give IV.
2. **Metabolism:** Metabolized by monoamine oxidase (MAO) and catechol-*o*-methyltransferase.
3. **Excretion:** Renal.
4. **Plasma half-life:** Minutes.
5. **Onset of action:** Immediate.

Drug Preparations:

Ampules: 200, 400, 800 mg in 5 mL.

Dosage:

1. Primarily dopaminergic stimulation: 0.5–2.0 μg/kg/min.
2. Recruitment of β_1 receptors and maintained dopaminergic stimulation: 2–5 μg/kg/min.
3. α, β, dopaminergic effects: >10 μg/kg/min.

Adverse Effects:

1. Arrhythmias, tachycardia, hypertension.
2. Maldistribution of myocardial blood flow, resulting in myocardial ischemia.
3. Tachyphylaxis for inotropic effects may develop within 24 hr.
4. Venoconstriction increases wedge pressure.
5. Nausea/vomiting.

Drug Interactions:

1. MAO inhibitors potentiate effects of dopamine.
2. Haloperidol, droperidol may inhibit dopaminergic effects.
3. Antagonized by β- and α-blockers.

Monitoring:

1. Tachycardia is a limiting factor.
2. Monitor stroke volume, not overall cardiac output, to observe for tachyphylaxis.
3. Urine output; measure K^+.

BIBLIOGRAPHY

DiSesa VJ: The rational selection of inotropic drugs in cardiac surgery, *J Cardiac Surg* 1987, 2:385–406.

Goldberg LI: Dopamine and new dopamine analogs: receptors and clinical applications, *J Clin Anesth* 1988, 1:66–74.

DOXAPRAM

Trade Name: *Dopram.*

Drug Action:

1. Nonselective respiratory stimulant.
2. Stimulates peripheral carotid chemoreceptors (low dose).
3. Stimulates central medullary respiratory centers (high dose).
4. Increases tidal volume with a slight increase in respiratory rate.

Indications:

1. Postanesthesia respiratory stimulant in the absence of other causes (hypoxemia, muscle relaxants, airway obstruction).
2. Drug-induced CNS depression of respiratory and airway reflexes (along with aspiration precautions simultaneously).
3. Acute hypercapnia associated with chronic obstructive pulmonary disease (temporizing measure).
4. ? Neonatal apneic episodes.

Pharmacokinetics:

1. **Absorption:** Give slowly IV. Action begins within 20–40 sec; peak effect in 1–2 min.
2. **Distribution:** Throughout body.
3. **Metabolism:** Liver.
4. **Excretion:** Metabolites in urine (<5% excreted unchanged).
5. **Plasma half-life:** 2–4 hr; duration of action, 5–12 min.
6. Mix drug in D_5W or normal saline solution.

Drug Preparations:

Injection: 20 mg/mL.

Dosage: Adult:

1. **Ventilatory depression following anesthesia:**
   a. 0.5–1 mg/kg body weight IV as single dose; may be repeated q 5 min to max. dose 2 mg/kg.
   b. Alternatively, 5 mg/min as infusion until satisfactory respiratory response is obtained, then 1–3 mg/min. Titrated to the desired level of respiratory stimulation. Max. total dose is 4 mg/kg or 300 mg.
2. **Drug-induced CNS depression:**
   a. **Intermittent injection:** 1–2 mg/kg IV; repeat in 5 min as indicated, then q 1–2 hr until patient awakens. Max. daily dose 3 g.
   b. Alternatively, 1–2 mg/kg IV, then continuous infusion at 1–3 mg/kg/hr (max. daily dose 3 g).
3. **Chronic obstructive pulmonary disease associated with acute hypercapnia:**
   a. 1–3 mg/min, by infusion for 2 hr max. Monitor blood gases every 30 min to ensure adequate oxygenation and ventilation.

Adverse Effects: Contraindications: Hypersensitivity, hyperthyroidism, pheochromocytoma, mechanical ventilation, neonates, seizures, respiratory depression from neuromuscular or mechanical causes, asthma, hypertension, ischemic heart disease, stroke, increased intracranial pressure.

1. **CNS:** Seizures, headache, dizziness, disorientation, paresthesia, flushing, sweating, pupillary dilation, spasticity, fever, increased deep tendon reflexes.
2. **Cardiovascular:** Increased cardiac output, chest pain, arrhythmias, hypertension, tachycardia, phlebitis, myocardial ischemia.
3. **GI:** Nausea/vomiting, diarrhea, desire to defecate.
4. **GU:** Urinary retention, incontinence.
5. Pruritus, cough, sneezing, hiccups, laryngospasm, bronchospasm, rebound hypoventilation, dyspnea.
6. Increased oxygen consumption and CO_2 production.
7. Rapid infusion may cause hemolysis, thrombophlebitis.

Drug Interactions:

1. Extreme caution with sympathomimetics and monoamine oxidase inhibitors (potentiate pressor effects).

2. Halothane, cyclopropane, enflurane sensitize myocardium to catecholamines, which are released by doxapram administration.
3. May mask residual effects from neuromuscular blocking drugs.

Monitoring:

1. Respiratory rate, tidal volume, minute volume, arterial blood gases, pulse oximetry.
2. Blood pressure, heart rate, deep tendon reflexes.

BIBLIOGRAPHY

Dopram. In *Physicians' Desk Reference,* ed 49, Montvale, 1995, Medical Economics, p 2005.

Stoelting RK: Central nervous system stimulants and muscle relaxants. In: *Pharmacology and Physiology in Anesthetic Practice,* ed 2, Philadelphia, 1991, JB Lippincott, p 541.

Gilman AG, Goodman LS, Rall TW, et al (eds): *The Pharmacological Basis of Therapeutics,* ed 8, New York, 1990, Pergamon Press, p 629.

DOXYCYCLINE

Trade Names: *Doryx,* DOXY-CAPS, *Doxycycline, Vibramycin.*

Drug Actions:

1. Inhibits protein synthesis by binding to 30S ribosomal subunit.
2. Broad spectrum of activity including many aerobes and anaerobes (but **not** nosocomial pathogens or *Pseudomonas aeruginosa*) as well as *Mycoplasma pneumoniae, Chlamydia,* and *Rickettsia.*
   a. Variable activity against *Bacteroides* spp.

Indications: Infections caused by susceptible organisms:

1. **Rickettsial infections** (e.g., Rocky Mountain spotted fever, typhus): Alternative to chloramphenicol.
2. **Chlamydial infections:** Alternative to erythromycin.
3. **Mycoplasmal infections:** Alternative to erythromycin.

4. **Sexually transmitted diseases** (e.g., gonorrhea, syphilis, chlamydiosis, chancroid, granuloma inguinale, pelvic inflammatory disease).
5. **Brucellosis:** Along with streptomycin.
6. **Others,** including Lyme borreliosis, actinomycosis, acne, respiratory tract infections.

Pharmacokinetics:

1. **Absorption:** Almost complete after PO administration.
2. **Serum half-life:** 18–22 hr; no difference with normal or severely impaired renal function.
3. **Penetrates** well into most tissues.

Drug Preparations:

Capsules/tablets: 100 mg.
Suspension/syrup: 50 mg/5 mL.
Vials: 100 mg for parenteral use.

Dosage:

1. **Normal/impaired renal function:** 100 mg q 12–24 hr PO/IV.
2. **Hemodialysis:** Serum half-life not altered.

Adverse Effects:

1. **Dental damage:** Pigmentation and enamel defects if given in pregnant women, infants, children ≤8 yr.
2. **Bone damage:** Permanent binding during bone formation; do not give in pregnant women, children <12 yr.
3. **Esophageal ulcerations:** Increased with any esophageal obstructive defect.
4. **Photosensitivity.**
5. **Other:** hypersensitivity reactions (e.g., rash), GI problems (e.g., nausea, especially on empty stomach), hepatotoxicity (high-dose IV), nephrotoxicity, neutropenia.

Drug Interactions:

1. **PO anticoagulants:** Increased anticoagulant effct.
2. **Barbiturates:** Decreased doxycycline effect.
3. **Carbamazepine:** Decreased doxycycline effect.
4. **Phenytoin:** Decreased doxycycline effect.

5. **Digoxin:** Increased digoxin effect secondary to decreased gut metabolism and increased absorption.
6. **PO contraceptives:** Decreased contraceptive effect.
7. **Lithium:** Increased lithium toxicity.

DROPERIDOL

Trade Name: *Inapsine.*

Drug Actions: Butyrophenone, antiemetic, tranquilizer; alters action of dopamine in the CNS, blocks stimulation of chemotrigger zone.

Indications: Nausea/vomiting.

Pharmacokinetics:

1. **Absorption:** Give parenterally.
2. **Onset of action:** Within 30 min.
3. **Metabolism:** Liver.
4. **Excretion:** Urine (75%), feces (22%).
5. **Half-life:** 2.3 hr (duration 2–4 hr).

Drug Preparations: Injection 2.5 mg/mL (1, 2, 5, 10 mL).

Dosage: Adults 2.5–5 mg IM or IV q 3–4 hr (give by slow IV push over 2–5 min).

Adverse Effects:

1. Less sedation and hypotension than chlorpromazine or triflupromazine.
2. Hypotension (especially IV), arrhythmias, tachycardia, hypertension.
3. Tardive dyskinesia, extrapyramidal reactions, akathisia, confusion, memory loss, psychotic behavior, agitation, sedation, dizziness, seizures.
4. Anticholinergic effects.
5. Respiratory depression, bronchospasm, laryngospasm.
6. Hyperthermia.

Drug Interactions:

1. Increased toxicity when used with other CNS depressants, narcotics.

Monitoring: Blood pressure, heart rate, respiratory rate; observe for dystonias, extrapyramidal effects, and temperature changes (hyperthermia).

BIBLIOGRAPHY

Gan TJ, Collis R, Hetreed M: Double-blind comparison of ondansetron, droperidol, and saline in the prevention of postoperative nausea and vomiting, *Br J Anaesth* 1994, 72:544–547.

Pandit SK, Kothany SP, Pandit UA, Randel G, Levy L: Dose-response study of droperidol and metoclopramide as antiemetics for outpatient anesthesia, *Anesth Analg* 1989, 68:798–802.

EDROPHONIUM

Trade Names: *Enlon, Tensilon, Reversol.*

Drug Actions: Edrophonium is a rapidly reversible anticholinesterase agent. It attaches briefly to the anionic site of the neuromuscular junction, blocking binding and subsequent hydrolysis of acetylcholine. This produces a generalized cholinergic response with miosis, increased tone in intestinal and skeletal musculature, constriction of bronchi and ureters, bradycardia, and stimulation of sweat and salivary glands.

Major Indications:

1. **Myasthenia gravis:** Used as a diagnostic test for myasthenia gravis; has been reported to establish the diagnosis in 90%–95% of cases. May also be used in differentiating myasthenia from cholinergic crisis in myasthenic patients receiving treatment.
2. May be used to reverse curariform, nondepolarizing neuromuscular blocking agents; however, its short duration of action, compared with neostigmine or pyridostigmine, makes it of little clinical use.
3. Treatment of supraventricular tachyarrhythmias.

Pharmacokinetics:

1. **Absorption:** Give IV/IM.
2. **Excretion:** Primarily by renal route; rate of clearance 9.6 ± 2.7 mL/min/kg.
3. **Volume of distribution:** 1.1 ± 0.2 L/kg.
4. **Plasma half-life:** 1.8 ± 0.6 hr.
5. **Onset of action: IM,** 2–10 min; **IV,** 30–60 sec.
6. **Duration of action: IM,** 5–30 min; **IV,** approx 10 min.

Drug Preparations:

Sterile solution: 10 mg/mL for parenteral use.

Dosage:

1. **Myasthenia gravis:**
   a. **Evaluation of treatment requirements:**
      (1) **Adult:** 1–2 mg slow IV 1 hr after administration of usual anticholinesterase agent.
   b. **Diagnostic test:** IV Tensilon test:
      (1) **Adult:** Initially, 1 mg IV over 15–30 sec while monitoring for bradycardias and observing for cholinergic reaction. If no response after 45 sec, give additional 8 mg slow IV, again monitoring heart rate carefully.
         (a) Atropine should be available for treatment of symptomatic bradyarrhythmias or hazardous respiratory secretions.
      (2) **Pediatric:**
         (a) **Infants:** 0.5–1 mg IM/SQ or 0.5 mg IV.
         (b) **Children ≤34 kg body wt:** 2 mg IM may be used, but 1 mg IV, repeated after 45 sec if no response, to max. of 5 mg, is recommended.
         (c) **Children >34 kg body wt:** 5 mg IM or 2 mg IV, repeated as above, to 10 mg.
2. **Reversal of curare-type neuromuscular blockage:**
   a. 10 mg given over 30–45 sec, repeated as needed to maximum of 40 mg.
   b. Neostigmine or pyridostigmine preferred, because of longer half-life.
3. **Treatment of supraventricular tachycardias:**
   a. **Adult:** 5–10 mg IV; may be repeated once in 10 min if necessary.
   b. **Pediatric:** 2 mg slow IV.

Adverse Reactions:

1. Worsening of asthma, respiratory paralysis.
2. Intestinal or urinary obstruction may occur.
3. May precipitate symptomatic bradycardias and AV conduction block, hypotension.
4. Because of short duration of action, side effects and unpleasant cholinergic effects are short-lived and rarely need treatment.
5. Symptomatic bradycardia should be treated with atropine, which should be immediately available any time edrophonium is being used.

Drug Interactions:

1. May worsen weakness in patients in cholinergic crisis.
2. Additive vagal effects may occur in patients receiving digitalis preparations.
3. May prolong neuromuscular blockage in patients receiving depolarizing neuromuscular blockers.

BIBLIOGRAPHY

Denniston PL Jr (ed): *Physicians GenRx,* Riverside, 1995, Denniston Publishing.

Physicians' Desk Reference, ed 49, Montvale, 1995, Medical Economics Data Production.

Gilman AG, Rall TW, Nies AS, Taylor P (ed): *Goodman and Gilman's The Pharmacological Basis of Therapeutics,* ed 8, New York, 1990, Macmillan.

Miller RD (ed): *Anesthesia,* ed 4, New York, 1994, Churchill Livingstone.

Stoelting RK: *Pharmacology and Physiology in Anesthetic Practice,* ed 2, Philadelphia, JB Lippincott.

EMETINE HYDROCHLORIDE

Generic Drug: *Emetine HCl.*

Drug Action:

1. Amebicidal (against protozoa, especially *Entamoeba histolytica*).
2. Blocks protein synthesis.

Indications:

1. Amebic dysentery.
2. Amebic hepatitis or abscess.

Pharmacokinetics:

1. **Absorption:** PO absorption variable; give IM/SQ.
2. **Metabolism:** Unknown.
3. **Excretion:** Slowly by kidneys (over months).
4. **Distribution:** Concentrated in lungs, liver, kidneys, spleen, where it persists for months.

Dosage: Do not give IV.

1. **Amebic dysentery.**
   a. **Adult:** 1 mg/kg/day (up to 60 mg) in one to two doses IM/SQ for 3–5 days.
   b. **Pediatric:** 1 mg/kg/day in one to two doses IM/SQ for up to 5 days (max. dose for children <8 yr, 10 mg/day; >8 yr, 20 mg/day).
2. **Amebic hepatitis or abscess:**
   a. **Adult:** 60 mg/day in one to two doses IM/SQ for 10 days (decrease by 50% in elderly or debilitated).

Drug Preparations:

Injection: 65 mg/mL.

Adverse Reactions:

1. **Cardiovascular:** Tachycardia, hypotension, chest pain, dyspnea, arrhythmias, cardiac failure, myocarditis, pericarditis, palpitations, ECG changes (QRS widening, prolongation of PR or QT intervals, T wave inversion, ST changes, premature ventricular contractions, supraventricular tachycardias).
2. **GI:** Nausea/vomiting, diarrhea, abdominal cramps, epigastric pain, constipation.
3. **Dermatologic:** Rash, urticaria, cellulitis, tissue necrosis.
4. **Musculoskeletal:** Weakness.
5. **CNS:** Headache, dizziness, sensory deficits, central and peripheral nerve dysfunction.
6. **Other:** Edema, hypokalemia.

Drug Interactions: None reported.

Monitoring:

1. Blood pressure, heart rate, ECG.
2. Signs of toxicity: Tremors, weakness, neuritis, cardiac toxicity.

BIBLIOGRAPHY

Emetine. In *Drug Facts and Comparisons,* New York, 1989, JB Lippincott, p 1608.
Emetine hydrochloride. In *AMA Drug Evaluations,* ed 6, Philadelphia, 1986, WB Saunders, p 1577.

EPINEPHRINE

Trade Names: *Epinephrine Injection, Epinephrine in Tubex, EpiPen and EpiPen Jr, auto-injector.*

Drug Action: Binds directly to α-, β_1- and β_2-adrenergic receptors. Inotropic drugs interact with receptors on myocardial cells.

The β_1 receptor is the best characterized system. A drug with β_1-agonist activity binds to the β_1 receptor on the membrane of myocardial cells. This activation of the β_1 receptor stimulates adenylcyclase, which converts ATP to cAMP. cAMP activates a cascade system of kinases. The net result is an increased influx of calcium into the cell through the slow Ca^{++} channel during systole. cAMP is broken down by phosphodiesterases. Drugs that inhibit phosphodiesterase will thus prolong the intracellular half-life of cAMP as well as its activities (e.g., increasing intracellular calcium).

Effects of α_1 stimulation are less well known. Drugs that bind to myocardial α_1 receptors may also increase intracellular calcium through the slow Ca^{++} channel. These actions may be medicated by phosphatidyl inositol. As opposed to β_1 stimulation, α_1 stimulation develops slowly over time. The net result is an increase in intracellular calcium. This increase in intracellular calcium is part of an amplification system that results in more calcium binding to troponin C, allowing for greater interaction between actin-myosin, thus increasing developed force.

1. **Cardiac:**
   a. Increases heart rate, systolic blood pressure, cardiac output.

    b. Increases automaticity by increased rate of rise of phase 4 depolarization in SA and AV nodes.

    c. Low doses cause peripheral vasodilation. High doses cause venoconstriction and peripheral vasoconstriction.

2. **Pulmonary:** Smooth muscle bronchodilation (β_2 stimulation).

3. **Metabolic:**

    a. Increased liver glycogenolysis (β_2 stimulation).

    b. Increased adipose lipolysis (β_2 stimulation).

    c. Inhibits insulin secretion (α_1 stimulation).

    d. Hypokalemia by β_2 stimulation of muscle Na^+–K^+ pump.

4. **GI:**

    a. Relaxation of smooth muscle.

    b. β_2 stimulation relaxes bladder detrussor muscle.

    c. α stimulation contracts trigone sphincter muscle in bladder.

Indications:

1. Allergic reactions (anaphylaxis).
2. Cardiopulmonary resuscitation.
3. Severe asthma.
4. Hypotension.
5. Myocardial failure.

Pharmacokinetics:

1. **Absorption:** Give IV/SQ.
2. **Metabolism:** Monoamine oxidase + catechol-*O*-methyl transferase in liver, kidney, GI tract. Reuptake into nerve terminals helps terminate biologic actions.
3. **Excretion:** Renal.
4. **Plasma half-life:** Minutes.
5. **Onset of action:** Almost immediate after IV administration.

Drug Preparations:

    Ampules: 1 mg/1 mL for IV use.

Dosage:

1. Primarily β_1, β_2 effects: 1–10 µg/min.
2. β_1, β_2, α effects: ≥10 µg/min.

Adverse Effects:

1. Tachycardia and increased myocardial oxygen demand.
2. Arrhythmias, hypertension.

3. Hyperglycemia.
4. Decreased renal blood flow.
5. Myocardial necrosis (e.g., platelet aggregation).
6. Anxiety, agitation, tremor, fear, headache, disorientation, nausea/vomiting, diaphoresis, tissue necrosis.

Drug Interactions:

1. Additive with other drugs that sensitize heart to arrhythmias.
2. Potentiated by tricyclic antidepressants, MAO inhibitors, certain antihistamines.
3. Antagonized by α- and β-blockers.

Monitoring:

1. Heart rate and rhythm.
2. Blood pressure.
3. Urine output.
4. PA catheter when using for contractility effects (e.g., cardiac output, stroke volume).

BIBLIOGRAPHY

Colucci WS, Wright RF, Braunwald E: New positive inotropic agents in the treatment of congestive heart failure, *N Engl J Med* 1986, 314:290–297.

DiSesa VJ: The rational selection of inotropic drugs in cardiac surgery, *J Cardiac Surg* 1987, 2:385–406.

Kaplan JA: Treatment of perioperative left ventricular failure. In Kaplan JA (ed): *Cardiac Anesthesia,* Orlando, 1987, Grune & Stratton, pp 963–994.

Weiner N: Norepinephrine, epinephrine, and the sympathomimetic amines. In Gilman AG, Goodman LS, Gilman A (eds): *The Pharmacologic Basis of Therapeutics,* New York, 1980, Macmillan, pp 158–175.

ERYTHROMYCIN

Trade Names: *ERYC, Ilotycin, PCE, E-Mycin, Ilosone, E.E.S., EryPed, Erythrocin, Wyamycin S.*

Drug Action:

1. Inhibition of protein synthesis by binding to 50S ribosomal subunit (bacteriostatic).
2. Spectrum of activity includes gram-positive aerobes, *Legionella, Mycoplasma, Chlamydia, Bordetella, Campylobacter,* and others.

Indications:

1. Legionellosis
2. *Mycoplasma pneumoniae* infections.
3. Diphtheria (disease and carrier).
4. Pertussis (treatment and prophylaxis).
5. Chlamydial infections (alternative to tetracycline).
6. *Campylobacter* infections.
7. *Haemophilus ducreyi* infections (alternative to tetracycline, sulfonamides, ceftriaxone).
8. Other: Group A streptococcal and pneumococcal infections, *Haemophilus influenzae, Entamoeba histolytica, Staphylococcus aureus, Listeria* spp., *Neisseria gonorrhoeae,* syphilis, acne.

Pharmacokinetics:

1. **Absorption:** Acid salts and esters well absorbed after PO administration; other PO forms require enteric coating to prevent destruction by gastric acid.
2. **Excretion:** Hepatobiliary.
3. **Diffuses readily into most tissues** except CNS.
4. **Serum half-life:** 1.4 hr.

Drug Preparations:

1. Erythromycin base: *Gel, solution, ointment, tablet, capsule:* 250, 500 mg.
2. Erythromycin: *Enteric coated tablets:* 250, 333, 500 mg.
3. Erythromycin estolate:
   Suspension: 125, 500 mg/5 mL.
   Tablets: 125, 250, 500 mg.
4. Erythromycin ethylsuccinate:
   Suspension: 200 mg/5 mL.
   Tablets: 200, 400 mg.
5. Erythromycin gluceptate: *Vials:* 250, 500, 1000 mg for IV use.

6. Erythromycin lactobionate: IV preparations: *Vials:* 500, 1000 mg.
7. Erythromycin stearate: *Tablets:* 250, 500 mg.

Dosage:

1. **Normal/impaired renal function:** 0.25–1 g q 6 hr PO/IV.
2. **Dialysis:** No dosage change.

Adverse Effects:

1. Among the least toxic antimicrobial agents; primary side effect is GI problems (e.g., cramping, nausea).
2. **Intrahepatic cholestasis:** Fever, abdominal pain, jaundice (up to 4%) in adult patients receiving erythromycin estolate (rarely ethylsuccinate).
3. **Transient deafness:** rare with <4 g/day IV.
4. **Phlebitis** (IV); **pain** (IM).
5. **Other:** Rash, hypersensitivity reactions.

Drug Interactions:

1. **PO anticoagulant:** Hypoprothrombinemia potentiated; impairs metabolism of warfarin.
2. **Carbamazepine:** Increased carbamazepine toxicity.
3. **Digoxin:** Increased digoxin effect.
4. **Theophylline:** Increased theophylline effect.
5. **Cyclosporin:** Increased effect.

ERYTHROPOIETIN

Trade Names: *Epogen, Procrit.*

Drug Actions: Induces erythropoiesis by stimulating erythroid progenitor cells; induces release of reticulocytes from bone marrow; requires adequate iron stores, folate, vitamin B_{12}.

Indications:

1. Anemia associated with end-stage renal disease, neoplasia, zidovudine-treated HIV infection.
2. Autologous blood donation.
3. Anemia associated with inappropriately low endogenous erythropoietin levels.

Pharmacokinetics:

1. **Absorption:** Give SQ or IV.
2. **Onset of action:** 7–10 days (reticulocyte response); hemoglobin rise appears over 2–6 wk.
3. **Metabolism:** Liver, kidneys, bone marrow.
4. **Excretion: 10% unchanged in urine.**
5. **Half-life:** 2–12 hr in normal renal function; 4–13 hr in chronic renal failure.
6. **Therapeutic level:** >500 mIU/mL (levels in patients with normal hematocrit are 4–26 m IU/mL)

Drug Preparations:

1. 1 mL single use vials (2000–10,000 units/mL).
2. 2 mL multidose vials 10,000 units/mL.

Dosage:

1. Chronic Renal Failure: 50–100 units/kg 3 times/wk IV or SQ, reduce dose when hematocrit 30%–36% or rise in hematocrit >4% over 2 wk; if response inadequate, increase dose (25–50 units/kg increments 3 times/wk) at 4–6 wk intervals; individualize maintenance dose for the desired hematocrit (range 12.5–500 units/kg 3 times/wk).
2. Zidovudine-treated HIV patients: Initial dose in patients with serum erythropoietin levels <500 mIU/mL–100 units/kg IV or SQ three times weekly; hold dose if hematocrit >40% or there is >4% rise in 2 wk; increase dose by 50–100 units/kg increments if response not adequate at 4–8 wk intervals; titrate to effect (i.e., target hematocrit of 36%–40%).
3. Cancer patients on chemotherapy: Begin with 150 units/kg IV or SQ three times/wk. Taper dose to desired hematocrit (see above).

Adverse Effects:

1. Cardiovascular: Hypertension, chest pain, edema, infarction.
2. CNS: Fatigue, headache, asthenia, dizziness, seizures, CVA/TIA.
3. Rash, nausea, vomiting, diarrhea, fever, arthralgias, hypersensitivity reactions (especially to albumin).
4. Polycythemia.
5. Thrombotic events (patients may require increased dose of anticoagulants).

6. Blood pressure should be controlled before initiation of therapy.

Drug Interactions: May need to increase dose of antihypertensives and anticoagulants (especially during dialysis).

Monitoring:

1. Pretherapy parameters: Serum ferritin >100 ng/dL, transferrin saturation >20%; iron supplementation (325 mg ferrous sulfate two to three times/day) should be given during therapy to ensure adequate iron supplies.
2. During therapy: Hematocrit (twice weekly), blood pressure, monthly ferritin (>100 ng/dL), transferrin saturation monthly (>20%).
3. Serum erythropoietin levels >300–500 mIU/mL—patients unlikely to respond to therapy since levels produce maximal stimulation of erythropoiesis.
4. CBC with differential and platelet count at regular intervals.
5. Monitor electrolytes, BUN, creatinine in renal failure patients.

BIBLIOGRAPHY

Egne JC, Strickland TW, Lane J, et al: Characterization and biological effects of recombinant human erythropoietin, *Immunology* 1986, 72:213–224.

Eschbach JW, Egne JC, Downing MR, et al: Correction of the anemia of end-stage renal disease, *N Engl J Med* 1987, 316:73–78.

Egne JC, Eschbach JW, McGuire T, Adamson JW: Pharmacokinetics of recombinant human erythropoietin (r-HuEPo). Administered to hemodialysis (HD) patients, *Kidney Intern* 1988, 33:262.

ESMOLOL

Trade Name: *Brevibloc.*

Drug Action:

1. β_1 selective adrenergic receptor blockade.
2. Inhibition of β_2 receptors at higher dose.
3. Electrophysiologic effects.

Major Indications:

1. Treatment of supraventricular tachycardia: More effective than propranol in controlling ventricular response rate in atrial fibrillation and flutter.
2. Very effective at converting recent-onset atrial fibrillation to sinus rhythm.
3. Postoperative hypertension.
4. Reinstitution of β-blockers postoperatively.
5. Acute stress situations (e.g., intubation, suctioning).

Pharmacokinetics:

1. **Absorption:** Give IV.
2. **Metabolism:** Red blood cell esterase.
3. **Excretion:** Renal.
4. **Onset of action:** Immediate.
5. **Plasma half-life:** 9 min.

Drug Preparations:

Vials: 2.5 g/10 mL, 100 mg/10 mL.

Dosage:

1. **Bolus** 0.5–1.0 mg/kg, followed by infusion at 50 μg/kg/min. If inadequate effect within 5 min, repeat bolus and increase maintenance to 100 μg/kg/min. Can repeat procedure, to 200–300 μg/kg/min.
2. Maintenance infusions of 50–200 μg/kg/min are commonly used.

Adverse Reactions:

1. Hypotension, bradycardia, chest pain.
2. Congestive heart failure.
3. Bronchospasm.
4. Nausea/vomiting.

Drug Interactions:

1. Use with verapamil may result in AV block.
2. Digoxin blood level increased by 10%–20%.
3. Esmolol levels increased in presence of morphine.
4. Esmolol prolongs neuromuscular blocking action of metocurine, pancuronium (nondepolarizing agents).
5. Hypertension when used with MAO inhibitors.

Monitoring: Limiting factors are blood pressure and heart rate.

BIBLIOGRAPHY

Davis RF: Etiology and treatment of perioperative cardiac dys-rhythmias. In Kaplan JA (ed): *Cardiac Anesthesia,* Orlando, 1987, Grune & Stratton, pp 411–450.

Kates RA: Antianginal drug therapy. In Kaplan JA (ed): *Cardiac Anesthesia,* vol 1, Orlando, 1987, Grune & Stratton, pp 451–517.

Stoelting RK: Alpha- and beta-adrenergic receptor antagonists. In *Pharmacology and Physiology in Anesthetic Practice,* Philadelphia, 1987, JB Lippincott, pp 280–293.

ESTAZOLAM

Trade Name: *ProSom.*

Drug Actions: Oral triazolobenzodiazepine derivative with hypnotic properties.

Indications: Short-term therapy of insomnia (up to 12 wk).

Pharmacokinetics:

1. **Absorption:** Well absorbed orally.
2. **Onset of action:** Peak activity 2 hr after oral dose.
3. **Metabolism:** Extensive hepatic metabolites.
4. **Excretion:** Metabolites excreted primarily in urine.
5. **Half-life:** 10–20 hr.
6. **Therapeutic level:** Not established.

Drug Preparations:

Tablets: 1, 2 mg.

Dosage:

1. 1 mg PO at bedtime.
2. May increase to 2 mg if needed.

Adverse Effects: Daytime somnolence, hypokinesia, dizziness, poor coordination.

Drug Interactions: Additive effect with other CNS depressants.

Monitoring: Sedation, somnolence, risk of habituation.

BIBLIOGRAPHY

Miller LG, Galpern WR, Byrnes JJ, Greenblatt DJ: Benzodiazepine receptor binding of benzodiazepine hynotus-receptor and ligand specificity, *Pharmacol Biochem Behav* 1992, 43:413–416.

Vogel GW, Morris D: The effects of estazolam on sleep, performance, and memory—a long-term sleep laboratory study of elderly insomniacs, *J Clin Pharmacol* 1992, 32:647–651.

ETHACRYNIC ACID

Trade Name: *Edecrin.*

Drug Action:

1. Inhibits absorption of sodium and chloride in ascending limb of loop of Henle, by inhibiting the sodium-potassium-chloride transport system.

Indications:

1. **Acute oliguria:** Possible adjunct in therapy for oliguria when attempting to prevent acute oliguric renal failure. Other measures must also be taken to ensure adequate circulating blood volume and renal perfusion.
2. **Edema:** Indicated for treatment of edema associated with congestive heart failure, liver failure, renal disease, including nephrotic syndrome. Short-term management of ascites due to malignancy, lymphedema, idiopathic edema.
3. **Pulmonary edema:** Indicated as adjunctive therapy in treatment of acute pulmonary edema.
4. **Hypertension:** May be useful in short-term management of hypertension or as adjunct in management of mild to moderate hypertension. Not considered the drug of choice in treatment of chronic essential hypertension.
5. **Hypercalcemia:** Can be used in therapy for severe hypercalcemia by promoting diuresis and calcium wasting.

Pharmacokinetics:

1. **Metabolism:** Hepatic.
2. **Excretion:** 67% renal, 33% biliary, 20% excreted unchanged.

3. **Volume of distribution:** 0.10 L/kg.
4. **Protein binding:** >90%.
5. **Plasma half-life:** 60 min.
6. **Absorption:** mF100% after PO dose.

Dosage:

1. **Adult:**
   a. **Diuretic IV:** 50 mg (0.5–1 mg/kg), repeated in 2–4 hr, then q 4–6 hr if urinary output increased. May give up to 200 mg.
   b. **Diuretic PO:** 50–200 mg/day in single or divided doses; increase 25–50 mg/day until desired effect obtained. Usually given in divided doses.
      (1) Maintenance usually achieved at 50–200 mg/day. Not recommended to exceed 400 mg/day.
2. **Pediatric:** Insufficient experience precludes recommendations for this age group.

Drug Preparations:

Powder: 50 mg for dilution and IV administration.
Tablets: 25, 50 mg.

Adverse Effects:

1. **Common:** Hyponatremia, hypokalemia, dizziness, glucose tolerance, hypomagnesemia, hypovolemia, hyperuricemia, prerenal azotemia, metabolic alkalosis, hypotension.
2. **Uncommon:** Pancreatitis, ototoxicity, exacerbation of lupus erythematosus, syncope, hyperosmolality, thromboembolic complications, rash, agranulocytosis.

Drug Interactions:

1. Increased hypokalemia: Adrenocorticoids, other potassium-depleting diuretics, amphotericin B.
2. Increased effects: Nondepolarizing neuromuscular blocking agents, lithium.
3. Decreased effects: Allopurinol, PO hypoglycemics, insulin.
4. Nephrotoxicity increased: Aminoglycosides.
5. Ototoxicity increased: Aminoglycosides, cisplatin.
6. Digoxin toxicity: secondary to hypokalemia.

Monitoring:

1. Follow urinary output and taper drug to desired effect.
2. Monitor for adverse effects:

a. Blood pressure.
b. Serum electrolyte determinations.
c. BUN, creatinine, serum uric acid.
d. Hearing examinations.
e. Hepatic function.
f. Renal function.

BIBLIOGRAPHY

Diuretics and cardiovasculars. In *Drug Facts and Comparisons,* Philadelphia, 1995, JB Lippincott, pp 607–613.

Diuretics, loop (systemic). In *Drug Information for the Health Care Provider,* vol 1, ed 15, Rockville, 1995, US Pharmacopeial Convention, pp 1144–1151.

Diuretics. In *AMA Drug Evaluations,* Annual 1995, 1995, American Medical Association, pp 849–620.

Weiner IM, Mudge GH: Diuretics and other agents employed in the mobilization of edema fluid. In Gilman A, Goodman L, Rall T, et al (eds): *Goodman and Gilman's The Pharmacologic Basis of Therapeutics,* ed 7, New York, 1985, Macmillan, pp 896–900.

ETHAMBUTOL

Trade Name: *Myambutol.*

Drug Action:

1. Inhibits synthesis of RNA, protein.
2. Spectrum of activity limited to *mycobacteria.*

Indications: Tuberculosis.

Pharmacokinetics:

1. **Absorption:** Rapid from GI tract.
2. **Distribution:** Most tissues, including brain and CSF.
3. **Metabolism:** Partial hepatic.
4. **Excretion:** Renal, feces.
5. **Serum half-life:** 4–6 hr, removed by dialysis.

Drug Preparations:

Tablets: 100, 400 mg.

Dosage:

1. **Normal renal function:** 15–25 mg/kg/day PO.
2. **Impaired renal function:**

Dose (mg/kg)	Creatinine Clearance	Interval
15	>80	Daily
15	80–50	Daily
7.5–15	50–10	Daily
5	<10 (anuria)	Daily

3. **Hemodialysis/peritoneal dialysis:** Supplemental dose 15 mg/kg on day of dialysis.

Adverse Effects:

1. **Optic neuritis:** Decreased visual acuity, central scotomata, loss of green and red color perception (usually reversible).
2. Occasionally hypersensitivity reactions (e.g., rash), hyperuricemia, GI upset, headache, mental confusion, peripheral neuritis, hepatic toxicity.

Monitoring: Serial ophthalmoscopy, finger perimetry, testing for color discrimination, uric acid, renal/hepatic function.

ETHOSUXIMIDE

Trade Name: *Zarontin.*

Drug Action: Elevates seizure thresholds and thereby suppresses spontaneous seizure activity.

Indications: Considered the drug of choice in controlling absence seizures; some reports show efficacy in myoclonic and partial seizures as well.

Pharmacokinetics:

1. **Absorption:** Rapid PO.
2. **Metabolism:** Rapidly absorbed from GI tract. Peak concentrations reached 4 hr after dosing; 4–7 days of therapy at stable doses required to reach steady state. Metabolized in liver.

3. **Excretion:** Slowly in urine. Approximately 20% of dose excreted unchanged; up to 50% has hydroxylated metabolite or glucuronide. Small amounts excreted in bile or feces.
4. **Volume of distribution:** No substantial degree of plasma binding. Distribution of volume is 0.72 ±0.16 L/kg.
5. **Basal clearance:** 0.19 ±0.04 mL/min/kg; may be higher in younger children.
6. **Plasma half-life:** 60 hr in adults; 30 hr in children.
7. **Compatibilities:** Significant drug interactions with other drugs are rare.

Drug Preparations:

> *Capsules:* 250 mg.
> *Syrup:* 250 mg/5 mL.

Dosage:

1. **Adult:** 30 mg/kg/day PO in two to four divided doses.
2. **Pediatric:** 15–40 mg/kg/day PO in two to four divided doses.

Adverse Reactions: Associated with skin rashes, systemic lupus erythematosus–type reactions with myocarditis and pericarditis, nausea/vomiting, abdominal pain, leukopenia, thrombocytopenia, eosinophilia, aplastic anemia, drowsiness, sleep disturbances, anxiety, dizziness, Parkinson symptoms, acute confusional states, hallucinations, photophobia, rare nephrotic syndrome, hiccups.

Drug Interactions: Additive CNS depression with other CNS depressants.

Monitoring: Drug levels readily available in most hospitals and commercial laboratories. Usual therapeutic range is 40–100 mg/L. Because of long half-life, precise sampling times are not required, although for consistency, drug levels should be drawn at similar times.

BIBLIOGRAPHY

Cohen S, Armstrong M: *Drug Interactions: A Handbook for Clinical Use,* Baltimore, 1974, Williams & Wilkins.

Drug Information for the Health Care Professional, ed 8, Rockville, 1988, US Pharmacopeial Convention.

Evans WE, Oellerich M: *Therapeutic Drug Monitoring Clinical Guide,* ed 2, Irving, 1984, Abbott Laboratories Publications.

Gilman A, Goodman L, Rall T, et al (eds): *The Pharmacological Basis of Therapeutics,* ed 7, New York, 1985, Macmillan.

Johnson G: *Blue Book of Pharmacologic Therapeutics,* Philadelphia, 1985, WB Saunders.

McEvoy GK: *Drug Information 88,* Bethesda, 1988, American Society of Hospital Pharmacists.

ETIDRONATE DISODIUM

Trade Names: *Didronel, Didronel IV.*

Drug Action:

1. Hypocalcemic agent.
2. Inhibits bone resorption and formation.

Indications:

1. Hypercalcemia of malignancy (IV).
2. Paget's disease of bone (PO).
3. Heterotopic ossification.

Pharmacokinetics:

1. **Absorption:** 1%–6% of PO dose.
2. **Distribution:** Bone.
3. **Metabolism:** Not metabolized.
4. **Excretion:** Renal (unchanged). Reduce dosage for renal impairment.
5. **Plasma half-life:** 6 hr.
6. **Bone half-life:** 3–6 mo.

Drug Preparations:

Tablets: 200, 400 mg.
Ampules: 300 mg/6 mL for IV use.

Dosage:

1. **Paget's disease of bone:** 5–10 mg/kg/day PO. Do not use for more than 6 mo.
2. **Hypercalcemia of malignancy:** Maintain adequate hydration. Avoid in renal failure. Give 7.5 mg/kg/day for 3 successive days; dilute dose in 250 mL saline solution and administer over 2 hr.

3. **Heterotopic ossification** (spinal cord injury): 20 mg/kg/day
   PO for 2 wk, then 10 mg/kg/day for 10 wk.

Adverse Effects:

1. **GI:** Diarrhea, nausea/vomiting.
2. **Elevated serum phosphate levels.** Increased renal tubular reabsorption of phosphate.
3. **Fractures,** especially with prolonged use.
4. **Hypersensitivity reactions:** Urticaria, angioedema, rash, pruritus are rare.
5. **Renal function:** May result in deterioration.

Drug Interactions: Absorption decreased by food, high calcium
agents such as milk or milk products, mineral supplements, antacids.

Monitoring:

1. Serum calcium (ionized calcium best).
2. Serum phosphate.
3. Alkaline phosphatase and urine hydroxyproline excretion in
   Paget's disease of bone.
4. BUN, creatinine with IV form.

BIBLIOGRAPHY

Zaloga GP, Chernow B: Divalent ions: Calcium, magnesium, and
   phosphorus. In Chernow B (ed): *The Pharmacologic Approach
   to the Critically Ill Patient,* ed 3, Baltimore, 1993, Williams &
   Wilkins, pp 777–804.
Stevenson JC: Current management of malignant hypercalcemia,
   Drugs 1988, 36:229–238.
Dunn CJ, Fitton A, Sorkin EM: Etidronic acid. A review of its
   pharmacological properties and therapeutic efficacy in resorp-
   tive bone disease, *Drugs Aging* 1994, 5:446–474.

ETOMIDATE

Trade Name: *Amidate.*

Drug Actions: Ultra-short-acting IV hypnotic.

Indications:

1. Induction of general anesthesia.
2. Brief sedation for painful procedures (e.g., cardioversion).

Pharmacokinetics:

1. **Absorption:** Intravenous formulation in 35% propylene glycol.
2. **Onset of action:** Within 1 min; duration: 5–15 min for awakening
3. **Metabolism:** Liver hydrolysis and dealkylation.
4. **Excretion:** Renal (metabolites).
5. **Half-life:** Terminal half-life 1.5 hr.
6. **Therapeutic level:** Titrated IV dose "to effect."

Drug Preparations:

Injection solution, intravenous: 2 mg/mL (20 mL).

Dosage: Induction of anesthesia: 0.1–0.4 mg/kg IV (over 30–60 sec) (administer smaller doses to maintain effect); reduce in patients with hepatic insufficiency and elderly.

Adverse Effects: Respiratory depression, reduced cortisol levels and aldosterone (avoid prolonged administration), transient venous pain and skeletal muscle myoclonic movements; cardiovascular: occasional hypotension, tachycardia/bradycardia, rarely arrhythmias; GI: nausea/vomiting frequently.

Drug Interactions: Formulated in 35% propylene glycol. Potentiation with other CNS depressants.

Monitoring: Respiratory and CV status, CNS status; monitor for signs of adrenal insufficiency.

BIBLIOGRAPHY

Wagner RL, White PF, Kan PB, et al: Inhibition of adrenal steroidogenesis by the anesthetic etomidate, *N Engl J Med* 1984, 310:1415–1421.

Levine RL: Pharmacology of intravenous sedatives and opioids in critically ill patients, *Crit Care Clin* 1994, 10:709–731.

FAMCICLOVIR

Trade Name: *Famvir.*

Drug Actions:

1. Famciclovir (a prodrug) undergoes rapid biotransformation to the active antiviral agent penciclovir. Penciclovir inhibits viral replication after a series of biochemical steps: It is first converted by viral thymidine kinase to a monophosphate, and then cellular kinases further convert the drug to its triphosphate form, which inhibits viral DNA polymerase competitively with deoxyguanosine triphosphate. (The cytochrome P-450 system does not play an important role in famciclovir metabolism.)
2. Spectrum of activity: Herpes simplex virus (HSV) types 1 and 2, and varicella-zoster virus (VZV).

Indications:

1. Acute herpes zoster (shingles).
2. Treatment of recurrent episodes of genital herpes.

Pharmacokinetics:

1. **Absorption:** PO; high oral availability (77%); may be taken without regard to meals.
2. **Excretion:** Renal.
3. **Half-life:** 2.3 hr in healthy individuals, increased in renal failure.

Drug Preparations:

Tablets: 125, 250, 500 mg.

Dosage:

1. Herpes zoster: 500 mg PO q 8 hr for 7 days (more useful if started within the first 48 hr of onset of rash).
2. Recurrent genital herpes: 125 mg PO bid for 5 days (should be initiated within 6 hr of onset of symptoms).
3. Reduction in dosage is recommended for patients with renal insufficiency.

Adverse Effects:

1. Headache (23.6%), nausea (10%), fatigue (6.3%), dizziness (5.5%), nausea (4.5%), and others.
2. Confusion has occurred rarely, mostly reported in the elderly.

Drug Interactions: None yet of note.

BIBLIOGRAPHY

Physicians' Desk Reference, ed 50, Montvale, 1996, Medical Economics Co.

FELBAMATE

Trade Names: *Felbatol, Felbamyl, Taloxa.*

Drug Actions: Anticonvulsant, antiepileptic, mechanism of action unknown.

Indications: Monotherapy or adjunctive therapy in treatment of partial seizures with or without generalized seizure activity.

Pharmacokinetics:
1. **Absorption:** Well absorbed after oral administration, both tablet and suspension.
2. **Metabolism:** Mostly excreted unchanged.
3. **Excretion:** 90% urine, inactive metabolites.
4. **Half-life:** 20–23 hr, not altered by multiple doses.
5. **Therapeutic level:** Monitoring levels is not required.

Drug Preparations:
   Suspension: 600 mg/5 mL
   Tablets: 400, 600 mg.

Dosage: Initially 1200 mg/day in three or four doses, gradually increasing to 3600 mg/day.

Adverse Effects: May increase heart rate slightly. Anorexia, vomiting, insomnia, nausea, headache.

Drug Interactions: Felbamate alters the serum concentrations of most other antiepileptic drugs. Reduce other drugs by 20%–33% when starting felbamate.

Monitoring: Routine laboratory monitoring is not necessary. Liver enzymes may rise slightly. Drug levels have not been established.

BIBLIOGRAPHY

Walker MC, Patsalos PN: Clinical pharmacokinetics of new antiepileptic drugs. *Pharmacol Ther* 1995, 67:351–384.

Mutani R, Cantello R, Gianelli M, Civardi C: Antiepileptic drugs and mechanisms of epileptogenesis. A review, *Ital J Neurol Sci* 1995, 16:217–222.

FENTANYL

Trade Name: *Sublimaze*; generics also available. *Duragesic patches.*

Drug Action: Similar to morphine but 75–125 times more potent. Narcotic analgesic.

Indications:

1. Adjunct to local, regional, or inhalational anesthesia.
2. Useful in pain management in potentially hemodynamically unstable patients.
3. A primary component in nitrous oxide–narcotic–relaxant anesthesia, and can be the predominant anesthetic when used in "high-dose" techniques, as in cardiac anesthesia.
4. Now being used in the epidural space for postoperative pain therapy as either bolus or continuous infusion. Fentanyl is very lipid soluble, resulting in brief duration of action except when large doses are used; its suitability for pain control is limited when given parenterally.
5. Sedation.

Pharmacokinetics:

1. **Absorption:** Well absorbed IM, with onset of action in 10–15 min and duration of approximately 1 hr.
2. **Onset:** Rapid (within minutes) after IV administration. Duration 1–2 hr. Patches may take 12–24 hr to reach steady-state blood levels.
3. **Distribution:** More lipophilic than morphine, which accounts for its more rapid onset of action. It rapidly redistributes to fat

as well as muscle, and this accounts for its relatively short duration of action compared with morphine.
4. **Metabolism:** Hydroxylation, hydrolysis, oxidation in the liver.
5. **Excretion:** Predominantly in urine, with approximately 10%
   eliminated in the feces.
6. **Half-life:** Elimination half-life approximately 220 min, which
   is greater than for morphine. However, effects are of shorter
   duration, owing to extensive redistribution to lipid and skeletal
   muscle stores except when used in doses >10–20 μg/kg.

   Patches: After removal of fentanyl patches the elimination
   half-life is prolonged to approximately 17 hr owing to continued slow absorbance of fentanyl from the skin and into the
   bloodstream.

Drug Preparations:

   Vials: 50 μg/mL in 2, 5, 10, 20 mL vials.
   Patches: 25, 50, 75 and 100 μg/hr patches.
   100 μg fentanyl = 10 mg morphine = 75 mg meperidine.

Dosage:

1. **Sedation/analgesia:** 1 μg/kg IM/IV every 1–2 hr as needed.
2. **General anesthesia:** 10–30 μg/kg IV.
3. **Cardiac surgery:** 75–150 μg/kg.
4. **Epidural analgesia:** Bolus 50–100 μg, followed by infusion
   of 0.3–2 μg/kg/hr.

Adverse Effects:

1. Respiratory depression, nausea/vomiting, dysphoria, potential
   for elevation in intracranial pressure, CNS depression,
   seizures. Patches delivering ≥50 μg/hr should be used only in
   opioid-tolerant patients.
2. Bradycardia frequently occurs, but hemodynamic compromise
   is seldom a problem, except occasionally in large doses used
   for cardiac anesthesia; hypotension, shock.
3. Skeletal muscle rigidity of presumed CNS origin occasionally
   occurs, resulting in decreased chest wall compliance and difficulty in ventilation. Concurrent administration of skeletal muscle relaxants diminishes the significance of this adverse effect.
4. Unlike morphine, no histamine release even when large
   amounts of fentanyl are used.

5. Other: Urinary retention, dry mouth, biliary tract spasm, ileus, nausea/vomiting, constipation, rash, pruritus.

Drug Interactions: As with morphine and other narcotics, may potentiate or be potentiated by other drugs that produce sedation, somnolence, respiratory depression. Potentiated by agents that affect hepatic metabolism (e.g., phenytoin).

Monitoring: Respiratory rate, heart rate, blood pressure, mental status.

BIBLIOGRAPHY

Gilman AG, Goodman LS, Rall TW, et al (ed): *Goodman and Gilman's The Pharmacological Basis of Therapeutics,* ed 7, New York, 1985, Macmillan.

McEvoy GK (ed): *AHFS Drug Information 89,* Bethesda, MD, 1989, American Society of Hospital Pharmacists.

Physicians' Desk Reference, ed 42, Oradell, 1988, Medical Economics Co.

Stoelting RK: *Pharmacology and Physiology in Anesthetic Practice,* Philadelphia, 1987, JB Lippincott.

FLUCONAZOLE

Trade Name: *Diflucan.*

Drug Actions:

1. Inhibits 14-α-demethylation of lanosterol in fungi. This leads to accumulation of 14-α-methylsterols and reduced concentrations of ergosterol, a sterol needed in fungal cytoplasmic membranes.
2. Spectrum of activity includes: *Candida* spp. (*not C. krusei*), *Cryptococcus neoformans, Coccidioides immitis, Histoplasma capsulatum,* dermatophytes, and others. *C. glabrata* (formerly *Torulopsis glabrata*) is relatively resistant.

Indications:

1. Oropharyngeal, esophageal, and vaginal candidiasis.
2. Candidal urinary tract infections and peritonitis.

3. Systemic candidal infections, including candidemia, disseminated candidiasis, and pneumonia.
4. Cryptococcal meningitis—treatment; life-long suppression after treatment in AIDS patients.
5. Prophylaxis of candidiasis in bone marrow transplantation patients.
6. Prophylaxis in surgical ICU patients is controversial.
7. Fluconazole should not be used as treatment of aspergillosis, mucormycosis, or pseudallescheriasis.

Pharmacokinetics:

1. **Absorption:** PO/IV. Acid not required for oral absorption (as it is for ketoconazole and itraconazole). >50% penetration into CNS.
2. **Excretion:** Primarily renal (80% appears in urine as unchanged drug, and 11% is excreted as fluconazole metabolites). The dosage of fluconazole should be reduced in patients with renal impairment.
3. **Half-life:** 30 hr.

Drug Preparations:

Tablets: 50, 100, 150, and 200 mg.
Oral suspension: 10 mg/mL or 40 mg/mL.
Injections in glass bottles of Viaflex plastic containers (2 mg/mL solutions): 100 mL (200 mg), 200 mL (400 mg).

Dosage:

1. Oropharyngeal candidiasis: 100 mg PO q day for 7–10 days.
2. Esophageal candidiasis: 100–400 mg/day for 3 wks.
3. Vaginal candidiasis (nonimmunocompromised women): 150 mg PO once.
4. Candidal urinary tract infections and peritonitis: 50–400 mg/day.
5. Systemic candidal infections: up to 1600 mg/day.
6. Cryptococcal meningitis: 200–800 mg/day until 10–12 wk after CSF cultures become negative. (Studies comparing fluconazole with amphotericin B in non–HIV-infected patients with cryptococcal meningitis have not been published.) 600–800 mg/day for 6–8 wk in AIDS patients·(and see 7 on next page).

7. Suppression of relapse of cryptococcal meningitis: 200 mg PO q day.
8. Prophylaxis of candidiasis in patients undergoing bone marrow transplantation: 400 mg/day beginning several days before anticipated neutropenia (absolute neutrophil count <500 neutrophils/mm³) and continued until 7 days after neutrophil count rises above 1000 neutrophils/mm³.

Adverse Effects:

1. Nausea (3.7%), headache (1.9%), rash (1.8%), and others.
2. Rare but potentially very serious: Hepatic reactions, exfoliative skin disorders including Stevens-Johnson syndrome, and toxic epidermal necrolysis.

Drug Interactions:

1. Fluconazole increases levels of oral hypoglycemics, phenytoin, and cyclosporine.
2. Prothrombin times in patients taking coumarin-type anticoagulants may be increased when fluconazole is given concomitantly.
3. Metabolism of fluconazole is enhanced by rifampin.
4. Serious cardiac dysrhythmias (including torsades de pointes) have occurred in patients taking other azole antifungals (ketoconazole and itraconazole) and terfenadine (Seldane). This drug interaction has not been shown to occur with fluconazole, but caution and close monitoring is advised if fluconazole and terfenadine (or other nonsedating antihistamines) are to be coadministered.

BIBLIOGRAPHY

Physicians' Desk Reference, ed 50, Montvale, 1996, Medical Economics Co.

Sanford JP, Gilbert DN, Sande MA (eds): *The Sanford Guide to Antimicrobial Therapy,* ed 26, Dallas, 1996, Antimicrobial Therapy, Inc.

FLUCYTOSINE

Trade Name: *Ancobon.*

Drug Action:

1. Deamination to 5-fluorouracil with interference of synthesis of pyrimidines and resultant defective RNA and cell death. Human cells lack the enzyme to deaminate the drug.
2. Spectrum of activity includes cryptococci and *Candida* spp.

Indications:

1. Cryptococcosis (with amphotericin B).
2. Candidal infections.

Pharmacokinetics:

1. **Absorption:** Readily absorbed PO.
2. **Excretion:** Renal.
3. **Distributes well,** including into CSF.
4. **Serum half-life:** 4–6 hr.
5. **Metabolism:** Minimal.

Drug Preparations:

Capsules: 250, 500 mg.

Dosage:

1. **Normal renal function:** 150 mg/kg/day PO in four divided doses.
2. **Impaired renal function:**

Dose (mg/kg)	Creatinine Clearance	Interval (hr)
12.5–37.5	>80	6
	80–50	6
	50–10	12–24
15–25 mg/kg	<10 (anuria)	24 (or by plasma level = 50–75)

3. **With each dialysis:** Supplemental dose of 37.5 mg/kg.

Adverse Effects: Overall 30%; all increased with renal insufficiency.

1. **Hepatic abnormalities:** 5%; generally asymptomatic and reversible.
2. **Leukopenia, thrombocytopenia:** 22%.
3. **GI intolerance:** 6%; usually nausea/vomiting, anorexia, diarrhea (rare case of perforation).
4. **Skin rash:** 7%.
5. **Other:** Drowsiness, confusion, renal toxicity.

Monitoring: Serum levels, therapeutic range 25–120 mg/mL; renal/hepatic function; blood cell counts.

FLUDROCORTISONE

Trade Name: *Florinef.*

Drug Action:

1. Mineralocorticoid; regulates sodium, potassium, and hydrogen homeostasis.
2. Acts in distal renal tubule to enhance reabsorption of sodium and excretion of potassium and hydrogen.

Indications:

1. Primary adrenal insufficiency.
2. Salt-losing congenital adrenal hyperplasia.
3. Hypoaldosteronism.
4. Severe orthostatic hypotension.

Pharmacokinetics:

1. **Absorption:** Well absorbed from GI tract; peak 1.5 hr.
2. **Distribution:** Body tissues; crosses placenta.
3. **Plasma half-life:** 30 min.
4. **Biologic half-life:** 18–36 hr.
5. **Metabolism:** Liver.
6. **Excretion:** Kidneys, breast milk.

Drug Preparations:

Tablets: 0.1 mg.

Dosage:

1. **Adjust to clinical response.**
2. **Adrenal insufficiency:**
   Adults: 0.05–0.2 mg/day PO. Children: 0.05–0.1 mg/day.
3. **Congenital adrenal hyperplasia:**
   Adults: 0.05–0.2 mg/day PO. Children: 0.05–0.1 mg/day.

Adverse Effects:

1. Sodium and water retention, hypertension, edema, cardiac failure, weight gain.
2. Potassium loss.
3. **CNS:** Headache, dizziness, decreased mentation, seizures, paresthesias.
4. Arthralgias, weakness (low potassium), arrhythmias, numbness, fatigue, anorexia, nausea/vomiting, metabolic alkalosis, acne, rash.

Drug Interactions:

1. Sodium retention, potassium loss with high sodium intake.
2. Decreased effect due to increased hepatic metabolism of drug with barbiturates, phenytoin, rifampin.
3. Enhances hypokalemia with diuretics, amphotericin B.
4. Fludrocortisone increases metabolism of isoniazid and salicylates.
5. Antagonizes effects of anticholinesterases.

Monitoring:

1. Serum sodium, potassium, bicarbonate.
2. Fluid status, weight.
3. Clinical features of salt and water retention (e.g., congestive heart failure, edema).
4. Plasma renin activity.
5. Blood pressure, heart rate.

BIBLIOGRAPHY

Desoxycorticosterone and fludrocortisone. In *AMA Drug Evaluations,* ed 6, Philadelphia, 1986, WB Saunders, pp 672–673.

Mineralocorticoids. In *Drug Facts and Comparisons,* Philadelphia, 1989, JB Lippincott, pp 363–365.

Whitworth JA, et al: 9-α-fluorocortisol-induced hypertension: a review, *J Hypertens* 1986, 4:133–139.

FLUMAZENIL

Trade Name: *Romazicon* (formerly known as *Mazicon*).

Drug Actions: Competitive benzodiazepine receptor-antagonist. Inhibits activity at the GABA/benzodiazepine receptor complex, to selectively reverse the effects of benzodiazepines.

Indications: Management of benzodiazepine overdose, or excess sedation due to benzodiazepines.

Pharmacokinetics:

1. **Absorption:** IV formulation
2. **Onset of action:** 1–2 min; peak effect 6–10 min.
3. **Metabolism:** Hepatic; <1% unchanged in urine.
4. **Excretion:** 90%–95% renal; 5%–10% fecal.
5. **Half-life:** Initial t½ 7–15 min, terminal t½ 41–79 min
6. **Therapeutic level:** Partial antagonism 3–6 ng/mL; complete antagonism 12–28 ng/mL (after normal sedating dose of benzodiazepine).

Drug Preparations:

Vials: 5, 10 mL multi-injection containing 0.1 mg/mL.

Dosage: Doses of 0.1–0.2 mg produce partial antagonism. Repeated doses to total 3–5 mg (at 0.2–0.4 mg/min), may be needed in large overdoses. Decrease dose in patients with hepatic insufficiency. Compatible with 5% dextrose in water, normal saline.

Adverse Effects: Precipitates withdrawal seizures in patients physically dependent on benzodiazepines. Resedation possible when drug effect dissipates. Confusion, emotional lability, perceptual distortion, panic attacks, dizziness, headaches, blurred vision, persistent hypoventilation, rare cardiac dysrhythmias; vasodilation (flushing), nausea/vomiting also possible.

Drug Interactions: Metabolism increased by ingestion of food (increased hepatic blood flow)

Monitoring: Rate and depth respirations; level of sedation (Ramsay Sedation Score).

BIBLIOGRAPHY

Brogden RN, Goa KL: Flumazenil. A reappraisal of its pharmacologic properties and therapeutic efficacy as a benzodiazepine antagonist, *Drugs* 1991, 42:1061–1089.

FLUPHENAZINE

Trade Names: *Prolixin, Permitil.*

Drug Action: Antipsychotic effect thought to be caused by blockade of dopamine receptors in the forebrain and basal ganglia.

Indications: Treatment of psychotic symptoms and/or agitation resulting from a variety of psychiatric/medical illnesses.

Drug Preparations:

Tablets: 1, 2.5, 5, 10 mg.
Elixir: 2.5 mg/5 mL.
IM injection: 2.5 mg/mL.
Depot injection: 25 mg/mL.

Dosage: Acute active psychosis:

1. **Adult:** 1.25–2.5 mg IM q 6–8 hr until symptoms are controlled; (usually <10 mg/day) or 2.5–10 mg/day PO in divided doses.
2. **Elderly/debilitated patients:** 1–2.5 mg/day PO.

Pharmacokinetics:

1. **Absorption:** PO/IM.
2. **Metabolism:** (?)Hepatic.
3. **Half-life:** About 12 hr.
4. **Excretion:** (?)Renal and hepatic.
5. **Dialyzable**(?): (?)Limited.
6. **Renal failure:** Reduce dosage.
7. **Hepatic failure:** Use with extreme caution, at reduced dosage.

Adverse Effects:

1. Sedation, extrapyramidal reactions (e.g., dystonias, akathisia, parkinsonism), anticholinergic effects (e.g., dry mouth, blurred vision, urinary retention, constipation), orthostatic hypotension, asystole, tachycardia, dysrhythmias.
2. Rare allergic, hematologic, hepatic, neuroendocrine, respiratory, cardiac effects.
3. Neuroleptic malignant syndrome.
4. Tardive dyskinesia.

Drug Interactions:

1. Enhances effects of other CNS depressants.
2. Additive effect with other anticholinergic drugs.
3. Antagonizes antihypertensive effect of guanethidine, pressor effects of sympathomimetics.

Monitoring: Blood levels for routine therapeutic monitoring are currently unavailable.

BIBLIOGRAPHY

Antipsychotic drugs. In *AMA Drug Evaluations,* ed 6, Philadelphia, 1986, WB Saunders, pp 111–130.
Antipsychotic drugs. In Schatzberg A, Cole J (ed): *Manual of Clinical Psychopharmacology,* Washington, 1986, American Psychiatric Press, pp 67–106.

FOLATE/FOLIC ACID

Trade Name: *Folvite.*

Drug Actions: Cofactor for enzymes involved in many metabolic pathways (e.g., purine and pyrimidine synthesis); required for erythropoiesis.

Indications:

1. Treatment of megaloblastic and macrocytic anemias due to folate deficiency; rule out vitamin B_{12} deficiency. Folate admin-

istration may obscure pernicious anemia with continuing irreversible nerve damage.
2. Dietary supplement to prevent neural tube defects.

Pharmacokinetics:

1. **Absorption:** Well absorbed from GI tract.
2. **Onset of action:** 0.5–1 hr.
3. **Metabolism:** Liver, tissues.
4. **Excretion: bile** (enterohepatic circulation), urine.
5. **Therapeutic level:** 6–20 mg/mL in plasma.

Drug Preparations:

Tablets: 0.1, 0.4, 0.8, 1 mg.
Injection: 5, 10 mg/mL.

Dosage: Oral, IM, IV or SQ. Infants: 0.1 mg/day. Children: initial 1 mg/day; maintenance < 4 yr 0.1–0.3 mg/day, > 4 yr 0.4 mg/day. Adults: Initial 1 mg/day, maintenance 0.5 mg/day.

Adverse Effects:

1. Flushing, malaise, pruritus, rash, bronchospasm, hypersensitivity reactions.
2. May correct macrocytosis of vitamin B_{12} deficiency while nerve damage continues.

Drug Interactions:

1. Decreased effect: Phenytoin, primidone, para-aminosalicylic acid, sulfasalazine, oral contraceptives, chloramphenicol.
2. Increases metabolism of phenytoin.

Monitoring: Folate level: 6–20 ng/mL.

BIBLIOGRAPHY

Hillman RS: Hematopoietic agents: growth factors, minerals, and vitamins. In Gilman AG, et al (eds): *The Pharmacological Basis of Therapeutics,* ed 8, New York, 1993, McGraw-Hill, pp 1302–1306.

Bortenschlager L, Zaloga GP: Vitamins. In Chernow B (ed): *The Pharmacological Approach to the Critically Ill Patient,* ed 3, Baltimore, 1994, Williams & Wilkins, pp 805–819.

FOSCARNET

Trade Name: *Foscavir.*

Drug Actions:

1. Organic analog of inorganic phosphate that exerts antiviral activity by a selective inhibition at the pyrophosphate binding site on virus-specific DNA polymerases and reverse transcriptases at concentrations that do not affect cellular DNA polymerases. Foscarnet does not require activation by thymidine kinase or other kinases and thus shows *in vitro* activity against herpes simplex virus (HSV) mutants deficient in thymidine kinase (and may be effective against ganciclovir-resistant cytomegalovirus [CMV]strains).
2. Spectrum of activity: CMV, HSV 1 and 2, human herpesvirus 6 (HHV-6), Epstein-Barr virus (EBV), varicella-zoster virus (VZV), and possibly HIV to some degree.

Indications:

1. CMV retinitis in patients with AIDS.
2. Possible alternative to acyclovir for treatment of acyclovir-resistant HSV or VZV in HIV positive patients.

Pharmacokinetics:

1. **Absorption:** IV.
2. **Metabolism:** Renal.
3. **Excretion:** 80%–90% of foscarnet is excreted unchanged in urine.
4. **Half-life:** 3 hr.

Drug Preparations:

Injections in glass bottles (in 24 mg/mL concentrations): 250, 500 mL.

Dosage:

1. CMV retinitis.
   Induction: 90 mg/kg (range 90–100 mg/kg) IV (infuse over 2 hr) q 12 hr for 14–21 days).
   Maintenance: 90–120 mg/kg (infuse over 2 hr) q day.
2. HSV and VZV: 40 mg/kg IV q 8 hr.

Adverse Effects:

1. Renal impairment—occurs to some degree in most patients receiving foscarnet. 33% of 189 patients in clinical studies developed significant renal insufficiency manifested by a rise in serum creatinine to 2.0 mg/dL or greater. Elevations in creatinine are usually, but not uniformly, reversible.
2. Forcarnet has the potential to chelate divalent metal ions (e.g., Ca^{2+}, Mg^{2+}) and may cause hypocalcemia (15%) and hypomagnesemia (15%). Other possible electrolyte abnormalities: Hypokalemia (16%), hypophosphatemia (8%), hyperphosphatemia (6%).
3. Fever (65%), nausea (47%), anemia (33%), diarrhea (30%), vomiting (26%), headache (26%), seizures (10%), and others.
4. Genital ulcerations.

Drug Interactions:

1. Pentamidine: Concomitant treatment with foscarnet and pentamidine (IV formulation only) may result in severe hypocalcemia.
2. Owing to tendency of foscarnet to cause renal impairment, avoid using with other potentially nephrotoxic drugs such as aminoglycosides, amphotericin B, and IV pentamidine if possible.

Monitoring: Creatinine (with measured or estimated creatinine clearance) and electrolytes (to include potassium, calcium, magnesium, and phosphorus) two to three times/wk during induction therapy and at least once every 1–2 wk during maintenance therapy.

BIBLIOGRAPHY

Physicians' Desk Reference, ed 50, Montvale, 1996, Medical Economics Co.
Sanford JP, Gilbert DN, Sande MA (eds): *The Sanford Guide to Antimicrobial Therapy,* ed 26, Dallas, 1996, Antimicrobial Therapy, Inc.

FUROSEMIDE

Trade Names: *Lasix, Furomide, Uritol,* generics.

Drug Action:

1. Inhibits absorption of sodium and chloride in the ascending limb of the loop of Henle by blocking the chloride site of the sodium-potassium-chloride pump.

Indications:

1. **Acute oliguria:** Possible adjunct in treatment of oliguria when attempting to prevent oliguric acute renal failure. Other measures must also be taken to ensure adequate circulating blood volume and renal perfusion.
2. **Edematous states:** Treatment of edema associated with congestive heart failure, liver failure with ascites, renal disease (including nephrotic syndrome).
3. **Pulmonary edema:** Adjunctive therapy in treatment of acute cardiogenic pulmonary edema.
4. **Hypertension:** May be useful in acute management of hypertension or as adjunct in management of mild to moderate hypertension. Not considered the drug of choice in treatment of chronic essential hypertension.
5. **Hypercalcemia:** Can be used as part of therapy for severe hypercalcemia by promoting diuresis and calcium wasting.
6. **Acute oliguric renal failure:** May convert acute oliguric renal failure to acute nonoliguric renal failure.

Pharmacokinetics:

1. **Metabolism:** Hepatic.
2. **Excretion:** 88% renal, 12% biliary.
3. **Volume of distribution:** 0.1 L/kg.
4. **Protein binding:** 95%–99% (mainly to albumin).
5. **Plasma half-life:** Wide variation, normally 0.5–1.5 hr. Increases to 75–155 min in anuric patients and to 11–20 hr in combined renal and hepatic failure.
6. **Absorption:** 60%–70% of PO dose absorbed; may be less in patients with end-stage renal disease or congestive heart failure.

Dosage:

1. **Adult:**
   a. **Diuretic (IV/IM):** 10–200 mg, adjusted as necessary until desired response obtained. Upper range doses required in renal failure. Higher doses should be infused ≤4 mg/min to avoid ototoxicity.
   b. **Diuretic (PO):** 20–160 mg as single dose, then at 6–8-hr intervals until desired effect achieved.
   c. **Diuretic (continuous infusion):** 5–40 mg/hr by continuous infusion may result in greater diuresis than bolus dosing by avoiding phenomenon of "postdiuretic sodium retention." Infusions may allow more gradual and titratable diuresis in unstable patients. Furthermore, infusions may avoid the ototoxicity sometimes encountered following large bolus doses, since ototoxicity is associated with high peaks. Ototoxicity seldom seen when infusion rates <4 mg/min are used.
   d. **Antihypertensive** (IV): 10–80 mg.
   e. **Antihypertensive** (PO): 20–40 mg q/day or bid (dose adjusted based on response).

   Up to 6 g/day has been given by slow continuous infusion.

2. **Pediatric:**
   a. **Diuretic** (IM/IV: 1.0 mg/kg body weight, increased by 1.0 mg/kg at 2-hr intervals until desired response has been achieved.
   b. **Diuretic** (PO): 2.0 mg/kg body weight as single dose, increased by 1–2 mg/kg in 6–8 hr until desired response is obtained.

   Doses >6 mg/kg not recommended.

Drug Preparations:

Solution: 10 mg/mL.
Tablets: 20, 40, 80 mg.

Adverse Effects:

1. Common: Hyponatremia, hypokalemia, dizziness, glucose intolerance, hypomagnesemia, hypovolemia, hyperuricemia, prerenal azotemia, metabolic alkalosis, muscle spasm, cramps.

2. Uncommon: Tinnitus, bone marrow depression, erythema multiforme, hypoacusis, exfoliative dermatitis, exacerbation of
   lupus erythematosus, pancreatitis, syncope, hyperosmolality,
   thromboembolic complications. Hearing loss (related to
   peak concentrations and may be avoided with continuous
   infusion).

Drug Interactions:

1. Increased hypokalemia:
   a. Adrenocorticoids.
   b. Antihypertensives.
   c. Amphotericin B.
2. Increased effects:
   a. Nondepolarizing neuromuscular blocking agents.
   b. Lithium. Concomitant use may elevate lithium levels and is
      generally not recommended.
3. Decreased effects:
   a. Allopurinol.
   b. PO hypoglycemics, insulin.
4. Nephrotoxicity increased:
   a. Aminoglycosides.
5. Ototoxicity increased:
   a. Aminoglycosides.
   b. Cisplatin.
6. Digoxin toxicity (secondary to hypokalemia).

Monitoring:

1. Follow urinary output and taper to desired effect.
2. Monitor for adverse effects:
   a. Blood pressure.
   b. Serum electrolyte determinations.
   c. BUN, creatinine, serum uric acid.
   d. Hearing examinations.
   e. Hepatic function.

BIBLIOGRAPHY

Diuretics. In *AMA Drug Evaluations,* Annual 1995, 1995, Ameri-
can Medical Association, pp 620, 848, 839.
Diuretics and cardiovasculars. In *Drug Facts and Comparisons,*
Philadelphia, 1995, JB Lippincott, pp 607–613.

Diuretics, loop (systemic). In *Drug Information for the Health Care Provider,* ed 15, Rockville, 1995, US Pharmacopeial Convention, pp 1144–1151.

Furosemide. In Bocher F, Carruthers G, Kampmann J, et al (eds): *Handbook of Clinical Pharmacology,* ed 1, Boston, 1978, Little, Brown, pp 177–179.

GABAPENTIN

Trade Name: *Neurontin.*

Drug Actions: Decreases seizure threshold. Increases brain levels of gamma-aminobutyric acid.

Indications: Antiepileptic drug used in combination with other anticonvulsants for treatment of partial (focal) seizures with or without generalization

Pharmacokinetics:

1. **Absorption:** Rapidly absorbed with or without food. Higher doses are less completely absorbed.
2. **Onset of action:** Maximum plasma levels reached in 2–3 hr.
3. **Metabolism:** Not metabolized
4. **Excretion:** Renal
5. **Half-life:** 5–7 hr.

Drug Preparations:

   Capsules: 100, 300, 400 mg

Dosage: 300 mg at bedtime, then 300 mg bid on day 2 and 300 mg tid thereafter. Doses up to 1800 mg/day have been used.

Adverse Effects: Somnolence, dizziness, nystagmus, ataxia, GI distress.

Drug Interactions: Does not alter the metabolism of other anticonvulsants and does not induce hepatic microenzymes.

Monitoring: Clinical response.

BIBLIOGRAPHY

Walker MC, Patsalos PN: Clinical pharmacokinetics of new-antiepileptic drugs, *Pharmacol Ther* 1995, 67:351–384.

Leach JP, Brodie MJ: New antiepileptic drugs—an explosion of activity, *Seizure* 1995, 4:5–17.

GANCICLOVIR

Trade Name: *Cytovene.*

Drug Actions:

1. Inhibits replication of viruses in the Herpesviridae family through actions as an acyclic nucleoside analog of 2'-deoxyguanosine. In cytomegalovirus (CMV)-infected cells, ganciclovir-triphosphate (formed by phosphorylation of ganciclovir by one or more CMV-induced cellular thymidine kinases) impairs viral DNA synthesis. Levels of ganciclovir-triphosphate are as much as 100-fold greater in CMV-infected cells than in uninfected cells.
2. Spectrum of activity: CMV, herpes simplex viruses 1 and 2, human herpesvirus 6, Epstein-Barr virus (EBV), varicella-zoster virus (VZV), and hepatitis B virus.

Indications:

1. Treatment of CMV retinitis (induction and maintenance) in immunocompromised patients, primarily patients with AIDS.
2. Prevention of CMV disease in transplant recipients at risk for CMV disease.
3. Treatment of CMV disease in immunocompromised patients (includes AIDS patients and transplant recipients).
4. Viruses in the Herpesviridae family resistant to acyclovir are also resistant to ganciclovir.

Pharmacokinetics:

1. **Absorption:** IV/PO. Capsules are poorly absorbed (5% when fasting and 6%–9% when taken after food).
2. **Metabolism:** Renal (major) and hepatic.
3. **Excretion:** With IV ganciclovir, 91% is recovered unmetabolized in the urine. With oral ^{14}C-labeled ganciclovir, 86% was recovered in feces and 5% was recovered in urine. No metabolites measured greater than 1%–2% in feces or urine.
4. **Half-life:** IV, 3.5 hr; PO, 4.8 hr.

Drug Preparations:

Vials: 10 mL (contains ganciclovir sodium equivalent to 500 mg of ganciclovir).

Capsules: 250 mg.

Dosage: There are a *variety of strategies* for prevention, treatment, and suppression (maintenance therapy) of CMV disease. Some reasonable approaches are listed below.

1. HIV-infected patients.
   CMV retinitis:
   > Induction: 5 mg/kg (range 5–10 mg/kg) IV q 12 hr for 14–21 days.
   > Maintenance: 6 mg/kg (range 5–10 mg/kg) IV q day 5 days/wk (if using capsules, 1000 mg PO tid with food).

   Other CMV disease (encephalitis, esophagitis, gastritis, etc.):
   > Induction: 5 mg/kg (range 5–10 mg/kg) IV q 12 hr for 14–21 days. (Unlike CMV retinitis, maintenance therapy may not be needed.)

2. Solid organ transplant patients.
   Prevention—there are numerous regimens for the different transplanted organs, but generally the data best support ganciclovir use in heart and liver transplants.
   > Heart: 5 mg/kg IV q 12 hr for ≥2 wk, then 6 mg/kg IV 5 days/wk, for ≥2 wk.
   > Liver: 5 mg/kg IV q 12 hr for ≥2 wk (followed by acyclovir 3200 mg/day for 3 mo).
   > Treatment: 5 mg/kg IV q 12 hr for 2 wk, then 5 mg/kg IV q day for 1 wk.

3. Bone marrow transplant patients.
   Prevention: 5 mg/kg IV q 12 hr for 2 wk (begun if a BAL at day 35 or blood culture positive for CMV), then 5 mg/kg IV q 12 hr 5 days/wk until day 120.
   Allogeneic recipients receive IV immunoglobulin (IVIG) routinely as part of graft-versus-host disease prophylaxis, which may decrease incidence of CMV disease as well.
   > Treatment: 2.5 mg/kg IV q 8 hr or 5 mg/kg IV q 12 hr for 14–21 days (and used with IVIG (400–500 mg/kg qod for 14–21 day) with tapers of both agents thereafter.

Ganciclovir dosages must be reduced in patients with renal impairment, neutropenia, or thrombocytopenia.

Adverse Effects:

1. Neutropenia, anemia, thrombocytopenia, fever, diarrhea, nausea, rash, and others.
2. Carcinogenic, mutagenic, embryotoxic, and teratogenic in laboratory animals at dosages somewhat higher than used in humans. Use in pregnancy only if potential benefits justify potential risks to the fetus. Animal data also indicate that ganciclovir causes impairment of fertility.

Drug Interactions:

1. Didanosine (ddI) levels increased when given concurrently with ganciclovir capsules.
2. Caution should be exercised if zidovudine (AZT) and ganciclovir are given together (both have potential to cause neutropenia and anemia).
3. Seizures have been reported in patients receiving ganciclovir and imipenem-cilastatin.

Monitoring: Frequent CBC with differential and creatinine determinations.

BIBLIOGRAPHY

Physicians' Desk Reference, 3d 50, Montvale, 1996, Medical Economics Co.

Schmidt GM, Horak DA, Niland JC, et al: A randomized, controlled trial of prophylactic ganciclovir for cytomegalovirus pulmonary infection in recipients of allogeneic bone marrow transplants, *N Engl J Med* 1991, 324:1005–1011.

GENTAMICIN

Trade Names: *Garamycin*, generics.

Drug Action:

1. Inhibition of protein biosynthesis through binding to 30S ribosomal subunits.

2. Spectrum of activity includes staphylococci (not streptococci), enterococci (only with penicillin or vancomycin), and most gram-negative aerobes (including *Pseudomonas aeruginosa*); **no** anti-anaerobic activity.

Indications:

1. Infections caused by susceptible organisms, primarily gram-negative bacilli.
2. Enterococcal infections in combination with penicillins or vancomycin.

Pharmacokinetics:

1. **Absorption:** Not appreciably absorbed PO.
2. **Excretion:** Renal.
3. **Penetrates** CNS poorly.
4. **Half-life:** 2–3 hr.

Drug Preparations:

Ointment/cream: 0.1%.
IV: 40 mg/mL.

Dosage:

1. **Normal renal function:** 1–1.7 mg/kg q 8 hr IV.
2. **Alternate dosing:** 5–7 mg/kg q 24 hr IV.
3. **Impaired renal function:**

Dose (mg/kg)	Creatinine Clearance	Interval (hr)
1.5	>80	8
	80–50	8–12
	50–10	12–24
	<10 (anuria)	24–48

3. **Dialysis:** Supplemental dose of 1–1.5 mg/kg after each hemodialysis or 1 mg/2L dialysate removed.

Adverse Effects:

1. **Nephrotoxicity:** Proximal tubular necrosis with excessive levels, concurrent use of other nephrotoxic drugs, dehydration, prolonged therapy.

2. **Ototoxicity:** Increased in renal insufficiency, elderly, excessive serum levels, and concomitant use of loop diuretics (e.g., ethacrynic acid, furosemide).
3. **Neuromuscular blocking effect:** Use cautiously in patients being weaned from mechanical ventilators; with myasthenia gravis, parkinsonism, botulism; in children with low calcium; in adults with low magnesium; or in patients massively transfused with citrated blood.
4. **Other:** Headache, diarrhea, hypomagnesemia, hypersensitivity.

Drug Interactions:

1. **Amphotericin B:** Increased nephrotoxicity.
2. **Loop diuretics:** Increased ototoxicity.
3. **Antipseudomonal penicillins** (e.g., carbenicillin): Decreased aminoglycoside effect due to inactivation.
4. **Cephalosporins** (cephalothin): Increased nephrotoxicity.
5. **Magnesium sulfate:** Increased neuromuscular blockage.

Monitoring:

1. **Serum gentamicin levels:** Peak (<10–12 μg/mL) and trough (<1–2 μg/mL).
2. **Serial renal function studies:** BUN, serum creatinine, creatinine clearance.
3. **Signs and symptoms of ototoxicity:** Tinnitus, dizziness, vertigo.
4. **Audiometry:** Loss of acuity at 4000–8000 cycles typically occurs before subjective hearing loss.

GLUCAGON

Trade Name: *Glucagon.*

Drug Action:

1. Antihypoglycemic; increases blood glucose by stimulating hepatic glucose output via glycogenolysis and gluconeogenesis. Also decreased glycogen synthesis and increased lipolysis. Acute hyperglycemic effect requires glycogen stores.

2. Smooth muscle relaxant (e.g., GI tract).
3. Positive inotrope and chronotrope.
4. Decreases gastric and pancreatic secretions.

Indications:

1. Hypoglycemia
2. Diagnostic aid for radiologic examination of GI tract (hypotonic agent).
3. Treatment of bradycardia from β-blocker overdose or slow calcium channel toxicity.
4. Meat impaction of esophagus (smooth muscle relaxant).

Pharmacokinetics:

1. **Absorption:** Must give parenterally.
   a. Hyperglycemic activity peaks 30 min after IV injection.
   b. GI muscle relaxation occurs 1 min after IV injection, 10 min after IM injection.
2. **Metabolism:** Liver, kidneys, plasma, tissues.
3. **Excretion:** Metabolic products excreted in urine.
4. **Plasma half-life:** 3–10 min.
5. **Duration of action:** IM injection, 32 min; IV injection, 20–25 min.

Dosage:

1. **Hypoglycemia:** Adults: 0.5–1 mg SQ/IM/IV; may repeat in 15 min. Also give glucose (especially if coma persists). Children: 20–30 µg/kg.
2. **Radiologic evaluation:** 0.5–2 mg IV/IM.
3. **Bradycardia:** 1–20 mg/hr IV as intermittent bolus or continuous infusion.

Drug Preparations:

Powder: 1 mg/vial, 10 mg/vial; use diluent provided.

Adverse Effects:

1. Hyperglycemia, hypokalemia, tachycardia, nausea/vomiting, dizziness, skin hypersensitivity reactions.
2. May release insulin and cause severe hypoglycemia in patients with insulinoma.

3. May release catecholamines and cause severe hypertension/tachycardia in patients with pheochromocytoma.
4. Decreased hyperglycemic effect in patients with depleted hepatic glycogen (e.g., starvation, adrenal insufficiency, chronic hypoglycemia).
5. Large doses of diluent can be toxic (contains phenol preservative).

Drug Interactions:

1. Glucagon increases effect of PO anticoagulants.
2. Phenytoin inhibits glucagon-induced insulin release.

Monitoring:

1. Serum glucose; potassium.
2. Blood pressure, heart rate.

BIBLIOGRAPHY

Zaloga GP: Hormones—vasopressin, growth hormone, glucagon, somatostatin, prolactin, G-CSF, GM-CSF. In Chernow B (ed): *The Pharmacologic Approach to the Critically Ill Patient,* ed 3, Baltimore, 1994, Williams & Wilkins, pp 700–714.

Picazo J (ed): Glucagon in acute medicine, Boston, 1993, Kluwer Academic, pp 1–172.

Pollack CV: Utility of glucagon in the emergency department, *J Emerg Med* 1993, 11:195–205.

GLUCOCORTICOIDS

Trade Names:

Betamethasone: *Betnesol, Benoson, Celestone, Prelestone, Selestoject, Uticort.*

Cortisone: *Cortone Acetate.*

Dexamethasone: *Decadron, Dexone, Hexadrol.*

Hydrocortisone: *Cortef, Hydrocortone, Solu-Cortef.*

Methylprednisolone: *Medrol, Depo-Medrol, Solu-Medrol.*

Prednisolone: *Delta-Cortef, Sterane, Cortalone.*

Prednisone: *Deltasone, Meticorten, Orasone, SK-Prednisone.*

Triamcinolone: *Aristocort, Kenacort, Kenalog, Kenalone.*

Drug Action:

1. Binds to cytoplasmic receptors, migrates to nucleus, regulates transcription of DNA; essential for life.
2. Regulates carbohydrate, lipid, protein metabolism.
3. Anti-inflammatory.
4. Controls catecholamine sensitivity.
5. Stabilizes membranes (e.g., lysosomal).
6. Immunosuppressive.
7. Mineralocorticoid activity.
8. Diminishes vasogenic edema (some causes of cerebral edema).
9. Antihypercalcemic; antagonizes vitamins D and A.
10. Antineoplastic.
11. Bronchodilation.

Indications:

1. Adrenal insufficiency, congenital adrenal hyperplasia.
2. Anti-inflammatory (many diseases).
3. Vasogenic cerebral edema (e.g., from tumor), spinal cord injury.
4. Immunosuppression (many diseases, e.g., rheumatic).
5. Asthma, sarcoidosis, chronic obstructive pulmonary disease.
6. Allergic reactions.
7. Hypercalcemia.
8. Dermatologic diseases.
9. Idiopathic thrombocytopenic purpura, autoimmune hemolytic anemia.
10. Neoplastic diseases.
11. Spinal cord injury (methylprednisolone).

Pharmacokinetics: *see* Table 9.

1. **Metabolism:** Hepatic.
2. **Excretion:** Renal.
3. **Distribution:** All tissues, breast milk, placenta.

Drug Preparations:

1. **Betamethasone sodium phosphate:**
   Tablets: 0.5 mg.
   Vials (5 mL): 4 mg/mL for injection.

TABLE 9.

Glucocorticoids: Pharmacologic Parameters

Drug	Glucocorticoid Potency	Mineralocorticoid Potency	Peak Effects (hr)	Plasma t½ (min)	Biologic t½ (hr)	Dose (mg)	Route
Betamethasone	25	0	1–2	300	36–54	0.75	PO, IV, IM, T, I
Dexamethasone	25	0	1–2	110–210	36–54	0.75	PO, IV, IM, T, O, I
Triamcinolone	5	0	Varied	200	18–36	4	PO, IM*, T, I
Methylprednisolone	5	0.5	1–2	80–180	18–36	4	PO, IV, IM, T
Prednisolone	4	0.8	1–2	115–212	18–36	5	PO, IV, IM, O
Prednisone	4	0.8	1–2	60	18–36	5	PO
Cortisol	1	1.0			8–12	20	
Hydrocortisone	0.8	1.0	1–2	80–120	8–12	20	PO, IV, IM, enema, T, I
Cortisone	0.8	1.0	1–2	30	8–12	25	PO, IM*

PO, Oral; IV, intravenous; IM, intramuscular; T, topical; O, ophthalmic suspension; I, inhalant.
*IM only; **not for IV use.**

2. **Dexamethasone:**
   0.25, 0,5 0.75, 1.0, 1.5, 2, 4, 6 mg.
   Elixir: 0.05 mg/5 mL.
   Suspension: 8, 16 mg/mL for injection. 4, 10, 20, 24 mg/mL as
         sodium phosphate for IV/IM.

3. **Hydrocortisone:**
   Tablets: 5, 10, 20 mg.
   Suspension: 10, 25, 50 mg/mL. 50 mg/mL as sodium phos-
         phate salt for IV/IM.
   Powder: 100, 250, 500, 1000 mg as sodium succinate salt for
         injection.
   Enema: 100 mg/60 mL.
   Suppositories: 10, 25 mg.

4. **Cortisone:**
   Tablets: 5, 10, 25 mg.
   Suspension: 25, 50 mg/mL.

5. **Prednisolone:**
   Tablets: 5 mg.
   Syrup: 15 mg/5 mL.
   Suspension: 25, 50, 100 mg/mL as acetate salt; **not** for IV. 20
         mg/mL as sodium phosphate salt for IV/IM.

6. **Prednisone:**
   Tablets: 1, 2.5, 5, 10, 20, 25, 50 mg.
   Syrup: 5 mg/5 mL.
   Solution, oral: 5 mg/mL, 5 mg/5 mL.

7. **Methylprednisolone:**
   Tablets: 2, 4, 8, 16, 24, 32 mg.
   Suspension: 20, 40, 80 mg/mL as acetate salt; **not** for IV. 40,
         125, 500, 1000, 2000 mg as sodium succinate salt
         for injection.

8. **Triamcinolone:**
   Tablets: 1, 2, 4, 8 mg.
   Syrup: 2, 4 mg/mL.
   Vials: 10, 40 mg/mL for injection.

Dosage:

1. **Replacement for adrenal insufficiency:** 12–15 mg/m^2/day
   hydrocortisone; give two thirds in AM and one third in PM; individualize dose.

2. **Acute stress with adrenal insufficiency:** 100 mg hydrocortisone q 8 hr; taper to replacement dose as condition improves.
3. **Congenital adrenal hyperplasia:** 25 mg/m^2/day hydrocortisone in divided doses q 8 hr.
4. **Cerebral edema:** Dexamethasone sodium phosphate 10 mg IV initially, followed by 4–6 mg IV q 6 hr.
5. **Inflammatory diseases:** Dosage requirements are variable and must be individualized. Common doses dexamethasone 0.5–10 mg q 6–12 hr; hydrocortisone 20–2000 mg/day in two to four divided doses; methylprednisolone 30–60 mg q 6 hr, prednisone 30–60 mg q 12–24 hr.
6. **Spinal cord injury:** Methylprednisolone 30 mg/kg bolus plus 5.4 mg/kg/hr for 23 hr.
7. **Asthma:** Hydrocortisone 1–2 mg/kg q 5 hr, methylprednisolone 0.5–1 mg/kg q 6 hr, prednisone 1–2 mg/kg q 12–24 hr.

Adverse Effects:

1. Cushingoid features, e.g., moon facies, central obesity, striae, petechiae, ecchymosis, purpura, fat atrophy, hirsutism, acne, hypertension, osteoporosis, muscle atrophy, sexual dysfunction, diabetes mellitus, cataracts, glaucoma, hyperlipidemia, peptic ulcer, dermal thinning.
2. Immunosuppression; increased risk of infection.
3. Sodium and fluid retention, worsening of hypertension, attenuation of febrile response, leukocytosis, congestive heart failure, edema, hypokalemia, metabolic alkalosis.
4. Loss of body calcium, osteoporosis, fractures, arthropathy.
5. CNS: Euphoria, insomnia, headache, psychosis, pseudotumor cerebri, mental status changes, nervousness, seizures, behavioral disturbances.
6. Pancreatitis, nausea/vomiting, peptic ulcer, GI upset, esophagitis.
7. Decreased growth, protein wasting, muscle atrophy, weakness, poor wound healing.
8. Adrenal suppression.
9. Thromboembolism, aseptic necrosis of femoral heads.
10. Glucose intolerance, hyperglycemia.
11. Myopathy.
12. Causes anergy.

Drug Interactions:

1. May decrease effects of PO anticoagulants.
2. May increase metabolism of isoniazid and salicylates.
3. Increased need for insulin, PO hypoglycemics.
4. Increased metabolism of glucocorticoids: Barbiturates, phenytoin, rifampin.
5. Decreased absorption of glucocorticoids: Cholestyramine, colestipol, antacids.
6. Glucocorticoids enhance hypokalemia from amphotericin B and diuretics.
7. Estrogens, cyclosporin, and erythromycin decrease glucocorticoid metabolism.
8. Increased risk of GI bleeding from nonsteroidal anti-inflammatory drugs.
9. Attenuated virus vaccines contraindicated in patients receiving immunosuppressive doses of glucocorticoids.
10. Diminished effect of growth hormone.

Monitoring:

1. Blood pressure.
2. Sodium, potassium, glucose.
3. Weight, edema.
4. Clinical signs of hypercortisolism.
5. Normal levels: cortisol 5–25 μg/dL (AM), 2–9 μg/dL (PM).

BIBLIOGRAPHY

Chen R, Eagerton DC, Salem M: Corticosteroids. In Chernow B (ed): *The Pharmacologic Approach to the Critically Ill Patient,* ed 3, Baltimore, 1994, Williams & Wilkins, pp 715–740.

Haynes RC: Adrenocorticotropic hormone; adrenocortical steroids and their synthetic analogs; inhibitors of the synthesis and actions of adrenocortical hormones. In Gilman AG, et al (eds): *The Pharmacological Basis of Therapeutics,* ed 8, McGraw-Hill, New York, 1993, pp 1431–1462.

Yanovski JA, Culter GB: Glucocorticoid action and the clinical features of Cushing's syndrome, *Endocrinol Metab Clin North Am* 1994, 23:487–509.

Jackson RV, Bowman RV: Corticosteroids, *Med J Aust* 1995, 162:663–665.

GRANISETRON

Trade Name: *Kytril.*

Drug Actions: Antiemetic, selective 5-HT$_3$ receptor antagonist; blocks serotonin on vagal nerve and in central chemoreceptor zone

Indications: Nausea/vomiting (especially during chemotherapy)

Pharmacokinetics:

1. **Absorption:** May give orally, faster with IV.
2. **Onset of action:** 1–3 min; duration <24 hr.
3. **Metabolism:** Liver.
4. **Excretion:** Primarily nonrenal (8%–15% unchanged in urine).
5. **Half-life:** Healthy, 3–4 hr; cancer patients, 10–12 hr.

Drug Preparations:

Injection: 1 mg/mL.
Tablet: 1 mg.

Dosage:

1. IV: 10 μg/kg over 5–60 min for one to three doses; give prior to chemotherapy.
2. Oral: 1 mg bid.

Adverse Effects:

1. CNS: Headache, asthenia, dizziness, insomnia, anxiety, somnolence, agitation, weakness.
2. GI: Constipation, abdominal pain, diarrhea, elevated liver enzymes.
3. Cardiovascular: Transient blood pressure changes, arrhythmias.
4. Hot flashes, hypersensitivity reactions.

Drug Interactions: None reported.

Monitoring: Clinical response.

REFERENCES

1. Blower P: A pharmacologic profile of oral granisetron (Kytril tablets), *Semin Oncol* 1995, 22(suppl):3–5.

2. Nodoushani M: Granisetron, *Conn Med* 1995, 59:209–211.
3. Yarker YE, McTavish D: Granisetron—an update of therapeutic use in nausea and vomiting induced by antineoplastic therapy, *Drugs* 1994, 48:761–793.

GROWTH HORMONE

Trade Names: *Protropin, Humatrope, Nutropin, Recombinant DNA. Somatropin:* Pituitary derived.

Drug Action:

1. Stimulates growth (skeletal and tissue) and repair via somatomedins.
2. Anabolic hormone (increases protein synthesis, increases glucose output, increases lipid mobilization, causes retention of potassium and phosphorus).

Indications:

1. Growth hormone deficiency.
2. Experimental: Anabolic hormone to improve nitrogen balance, wound repair, muscle strength.

Pharmacokinetics:

1. **Absorption:** Destroyed in GI tract; give IM/SQ.
2. **Metabolism:** Liver (90%), tissues.
3. **Excretion:** 0.1% unchanged in urine.
4. **Serum half-life:** 20–30 min; cellular effects are long-lasting (>3 days).

Dosage:

1. **Growth in children:** Up to 0.1 mg/kg IM/SQ three times/wk or 0.05 mg/kg/day IM/SQ.
2. **Anabolic action:** 2.5–7.5 mg/day IM/SQ.

Drug Preparations:

Lyophilized powder: 5 and 10 mg (13–26 IU)/vial.

Adverse Effects:

1. Hyperglycemia, insulin resistance, hypoglycemia.
2. Pain and swelling at injection site.
3. Headache, muscle pain, weakness.
4. Hypersensitivity reactions.
5. May stimulate tumor growth (caution with intracranial tumors)
6. Long term: Acromegaly, gigantism.
7. Joint pain, nerve entrapment.

Drug Interactions:

1. Effects diminished by glucocorticoids, hypothyroidism, insulin deficiency.
2. Effects accelerated by anabolic steroids, androgens, estrogens, thyroid hormones.

Monitor:

1. Serum and urine glucose.
2. Urine nitrogen, somatomedin-C (IGF-1) levels.
3. Growth. Clinical response.

BIBLIOGRAPHY

Zaloga GP: Hormones—vasopressin, growth hormone, glucagon, somatostatin, prolactin, G-CSF, GM-CSF. In Chernow B (ed): *The Pharmacologic Approach to the Critically Ill Patient,* ed 3, Baltimore, 1994, Williams & Wilkins.

Kuret JA, Murad F: Adrenohypophyseal hormones and related substances. In Gilman AG, et al (eds): *The Pharmacological Basis of Therapeutics,* ed 8, New York, 1993, McGraw-Hill, pp 1334–1360.

HALOPERIDOL

Trade Name: *Haldol.*

Drug Action: Antipsychotic effect thought to be caused by blockade of dopamine receptors in the forebrain and basal ganglia.

Indications: Treatment of psychotic symptoms and/or agitation resulting from a variety of psychiatric/medical illnesses.

Drug Preparations:

Tablets: 0.5, 1, 2.5, 10, 20 mg.
Injection: 5 mg/mL, 50 mg/mL, 100 mg/mL.
PO concentrate: 2 mg/mL.

Dosage:

1. **Adult:**
   a. **Acute psychosis with marked agitation:** Initial dose 2–5 mg IM up to every hour until symptoms are controlled, usually <10–15 mg/day. Also has been given IV.
   b. **Active psychosis:** 0.5–5 mg q 8–12 hr IM/PO, usually <10 mg/day.
2. **Elderly/debilitated patients:** 0.5–2 mg/day PO, with gradual increase in 0.5 mg increments.

Pharmacokinetics:

1. **Absorption:** PO/IV/IM.
2. **Metabolism:** Hepatic.
3. **Half-life:** 12–38 hr.
4. **Excretion:** <1% unchanged in urine.
5. **Dialyzable(?):** Limited.
6. **Renal failure:** Reduce dosage.
7. **Hepatic failure:** Use with extreme caution, at reduced dosage.

Adverse Effects:

1. Sedation, extrapyramidal reactions (e.g., dystonias, akathisia, parkinsonism), anticholinergic effects (e.g., dry mouth, blurred vision, urinary retention, constipation), orthostatic hypotension. Haloperidol has been implicated as a factor contributing to the development of torsades de pointes cardiac arrhythmias. Use with caution in patients who have prolonged QT segments on ECG.
2. Rarer allergic, hematologic, neuroendocrine, respiratory, cardiac effects.
3. Neuroleptic malignant syndrome.
4. Tardive dyskinesia.

Drug Interactions:

1. Enhances effects of other CNS depressants.
2. Additive effect with other anticholinergic drugs.
3. Antagonizes antihypertensive effect of guanethidine.

Monitoring: Blood levels for routine therapeutic monitoring are currently unavailable.

BIBLIOGRAPHY

Zeifman CWE, Friedman B: Torsades de points: potential consequence of intravenous haloperidol in the intensive care unit, *Intensive Care World* 11:109–112, 1994.

Antipsychotic drugs. In *AMA Drug Evaluations,* ed 6, Philadelphia, 1986, WB Saunders, pp 111–130.

Antipsychotic drugs. In Schatzberg A, Cole J: *Manual of Clinical Psychopharmacology,* Washington, DC, 1986, American Psychiatric Press, pp 67–106.

HEPARIN AND LOW-MOLECULAR-WEIGHT HEPARIN (LMW HEPARIN)

Trade Names:

> Heparin sodium:
>> From porcine intestinal mucosa
>>> *Liquaemin.*
>>> *Tubex Heparin Injection.*
>> From beef lung sources
> Heparin calcium:
>> *Calciparine.*
> Heparin plus dihydroergotamine (DHE) mesylate with lidocaine:
>> *Embolex.*
> LMW Heparin
>> Enoxaparin: *Lovenox.*
>> Dalteparin: *Fragmin.*

Drug Action: Heparin is a potent anticoagulant. Its primary anticoagulant action occurs via acceleration of formation of complexes between antithrombin III and activated factor II (thrombin) and activated factor X. Partial inhibition of factors XIIa, XIa, and IXa, and platelet function also contribute to total anticoagulant effect. Most of the anticoagulant effect is from the lower-molecular-weight component of heparin. The newer LMW heparin compounds generally have better anticoagulation with fewer side effects.

Used exclusively for anticoagulant effects, generally in one of five clinical settings.

1. Prophylaxis against deep venous thromboembolism (DVT).
2. Therapy for DVT or pulmonary embolism.
3. Anticoagulation during vascular/cardiac surgery and hemodialysis.
4. To maintain patency of intravascular catheters (e.g., total parenteral nutrition).
5. Therapy for some types of disseminated intravascular coagulation (DIC).

Pharmacokinetics:

1. **Metabolism:** Liver, by heparinase.
2. **Excretion:** Renal.
3. **Onset of action:** Almost instantaneous after IV administration.
4. **Endogenous secretion:** Heparin is present in high concentrations in liver and mast cells (of uncertain physiologic significance).
5. **Plasma half-life:** Dependent on patient temperature and dose administered. When 100 U/kg is injected IV, circulating half-life approximately 60 min (standard heparin). LMW heparin has an elimination half-life of approximately 4.5 hr and thus can be given bid.

Drug Preparations: *See* Table 10. Major source is beef lung or porcine intestinal mucosa. Standardization of potency is based on in vitro comparison with known USP reference standards. Guidelines state sodium heparin contains 120 USP U/mg, but manufacturers are allowed ±10% margin of error. Standard heparin doses are correctly ordered only in **units,** not milligrams, whereas LMW heparin is dosed in milligrams.

Dosage:

1. LMW heparin: The dose for all indications is 30 mg SQ bid (enoxaparin).
2. Standard heparin (bovine or porcine):
    a. **DVT prophylaxis:** 5000 U heparin SQ 2 hr before surgery, then 5000 U q 8–12 hr until the patient is fully mobilized.
    b. **DVT/pulmonary emboli therapy:** IV bolus load with 100 U/kg heparin (5000–10,000 USP units), followed by contin-

TABLE 10.
Heparin Preparations

Preparation	Concentration (U/mL)	Route of Administration*	Heparin Source	Hypothetical Advantage
Calciparine	25,000 USP	SQ/IV	Porcine intestinal mucosa site hematoma	Decreased incidence of injection
Embolex	5000 USP +DHE mesylate 0.5 mg	Deep SQ only (intrafat)	Porcine intestinal mucosa	DHE venoconstrictor properties **may** decrease venous stasis
Heparin USP	1000 5000 10,000	SQ/IV	Beef lung sources	**May** have increased incidence of thrombocytopenia compared with porcine preparations
Liquaemin	1000 5000 10,000 20,000 40,000	SQ/IV	Porcine intestinal mucosa	Preservative-free formulations also available

*IM injections are painful and should be avoided with all preparations. Heparin is poorly lipid soluble and therefore is not effective via PO administration.
DHE, Dihydroergotamine.

uous hourly infusion of 800–1200 U/hr, titrated to maintain activated partial thromboplastin time (aPTT) approximately 1½–2 times baseline control.

c. **Cardiac surgery:** In adults, 300–350 U/kg bolus before bypass. Monitor with activated coagulation time (ACT) to maintain ACT >400 sec before/during cardiopulmonary bypass (Bull et al, 1975).

d. **Vascular catheters:** Continuous flush of solutions with heparin 2 U/mL helps maintain catheter patency.

e. **DIC:** Controversial and variable; hematology consultation recommended for specific guidelines in this setting.

Adverse Effects:

1. **Hemorrhage:** Most serious complication, with risk 1%–33%. Heparin is generally contraindicated in patients with recent neurotrauma or neurosurgery, intraocular surgery, thrombocytopenia, known coagulation disorders, or known hypersensitivity to pork/beef heparin preparations. The risk of bleeding is considerably less with LMW heparins (<2%).
   a. **Warning:** Concomitant administration with other drugs that affect coagulation (e.g., antiplatelet drugs, warfarin) may result in serious or life-threatening bleeding.

2. **Thrombocytopenia:** Generally mild to moderate, frequently seen, and occurs 6–10 days after initiation of therapy. Rarely, serious and severe heparin-induced platelet aggregation (thrombotic thrombocytopenia) may occur, precipitating arterial thrombosis with limb-threatening consequences.

3. **Hypotension:** With large bolus injections used for cardiac surgery (300 U/kg), a decrease in systemic vascular resistance is frequently noted, resulting in transient hypotension.

4. **Other:** Allergic reactions; altered erythrocyte morphology; osteoporosis with long-term use; elevation of serum aminotransferase levels.

Monitoring:

1. **DVT prophylaxis** with low-dose heparin usually does not require laboratory testing (except periodic platelet counts).

2. **DVT/pulmonary emboli:** Therapy is monitored by following aPTT, aiming to keep laboratory values at 1½–2 times normal.

3. **Cardiac surgery:** ACT is maintained at $\geq$400 sec (Bull et al, 1975).

4. **Heparin levels:** Because ACT is a *functional* test, a number of clotting parameters (e.g., platelet count, temperature, protein C, pH) have an impact on ACT in addition to the presence of heparin. Thus, a specific heparin assay may be desirable to delineate whether prolonged ACT is actually secondary to heparin or to some other factor. Two specific quantitative heparin assays (titration of USP heparin activity with protamine and heparin dye binding) can be performed and are not cost prohibitive. Resolution of one such assay system (Hepcon Assay System, Hemotec, Inc, Englewood, CO) is 50 U heparin/kg.

5. All patients receiving heparin should have periodic platelet counts, hematocrits, and test for occult blood in stool in addition to specific coagulation tests noted above.

Drug Reversal: *Protamine:*

1. Low mol wt, strongly basic fish proteins that combine ionically with heparin to form a neutralizing salt.

2. Dose to neutralize heparin is calculated as 1 mg protamine/ 100 U heparin **remaining** in the patient, estimated by heparin plasma half-life of approximately 60 min in a normothermic patient.

3. Administration is by slow infusion over $\geq$10 min to avoid hypotension.

4. Anaphylaxis to protamine (foreign fish protein) is possible.

BIBLIOGRAPHY

Agents used for anticoagulant therapy. In *AMA Drug Evaluations,* ed 6, Philadelphia, 1986, WB Saunders, pp 603–616.

Anticoagulants. In Stoelting RK: *Pharmacology and Physiology in Anesthetic Practice,* Philadelphia, 1987, JB Lippincott, pp 444–453.

Bull BS, Huse WM, Brauer FS, et al: Heparin therapy during extracorporeal circulation: the use of a dose-response curve to individualize heparin and protamine dosage, *J Thorac Cardiovasc Surg* 1975, 69:685–689.

Nanfro J: Anticoagulants in critical care medicine. In Chernow B (ed): *The Pharmacologic Approach to the Critically Ill Patient,* ed 2, Baltimore, 1988, Williams & Wilkins, pp 511–535.

O'Reilly R: Anticoagulant, antithrombotic, and thrombolytic drugs. In Gilman AG, Goodman LS, Rall TW, et al (eds): *The Pharmacologic Basis of Therapeutics,* ed 7, New York, 1985, Macmillan, pp 1338–1359.

HEPATIC ENCEPHALOPATHY MEDICATIONS

Trade Names:

Neomycin: *Mycifradin.*
Lactulose: *Cephulac, Chronulac.*
Bromocriptine: *Parlodel.*
Levodopa: *Larodopa, Dopar.*

Drug Action:

1. **Neomycin** is an aminoglycoside antibiotic that suppresses growth of bowel bacteria, including those that produce ammonia. Because it is not absorbed in significant quantities, there are few systemic side effects.
2. **Lactulose** is a synthetic disaccharide that acidifies the colonic contents after being degraded by colon bacteria. The decreased colonic pH "traps" ammonia by forming ammonium ion, which cannot cross the lipid interface of the bowel mucosa. Lactulose also inhibits ammonia production by substituting for proteins as the preferred substrate for colonic bacteria. The osmotic laxative actions of this drug also promote colonic clearance of nitrogenous waste products.
3. **Bromocriptine** is a specific dopamine receptor agonist; **levodopa** is a dopamine precursor. Both are thought to favorably influence cerebral neurotransmitter levels, and have been shown to improve cerebral glucose metabolism and hemodynamics and normalize EEG patterns.

Indications: *See* Table 11.

1. **Neomycin:** Management of acute hepatic encephalopathy.
2. **Lactulose:** Management of acute and chronic hepatic encephalopathy. Acts synergistically with neomycin; thus, the two agents can be used simultaneously.

TABLE 11.

Indications for Management of Hepatic Encephalopathy

Drug	Acute	Chronic	Other Uses
Neomycin	Yes	No	Preoperative bowel preparation
Lactulose	Yes	Yes	Laxative
Bromocriptine	No	Yes	Parkinson's disease, hyperprolactinemia
Levodopa	No	Yes	Parkinson's disease

3. **Bromocriptine and levodopa:** Principally used as antiparkinsonian agents. Bromocriptine is also effective in controlling galactorrhea secondary to hyperprolactinemia. Both agents are effective in management of chronic hepatic encephalopathy in selected patients.

Pharmacokinetics: *See* Table 12.

Drug Preparations: No parenteral forms are available.

Drug	Tabs/Caps	Syrup
Neomycin	500 mg	125 mg/15 mL
Lactulose	—	10 g/15 mL
Bromocriptine	2.5, 5 mg	—
Levodopa	100, 250, 500 mg	—

Dosage:

1. **Neomycin:** 1.5–6 g/day PO in divided doses q 6–8 hr (can be given per NG).

TABLE 12.

Pharmacokinetics

Drug	Absorption	Metabolism	t½	Duration	Excretion
Neomycin	3%	—	—	—	Fecal
Lactulose	Poor	—	—	—	Fecal
Bromocriptine	30%	Hepatic	4 hr	8–24 hr	95% biliary
Levodopa	Good	95% Hepatic	1–3 hr	To 5 hr	Renal

2. **Lactulose:**
   a. Acute: 30–45 mL PO/NG q hr until laxative effect noted, then 30–45 mL PO tid/qid.
   b. Chronic: Adjust dose to induce two to three soft stools/day.
   c. Alternatively, can be given as retention enema, 300 mL lactulose in 700 mL water or saline solution via rectal balloon catheter, retained for 30–60 min q 4–6 hr.
3. **Bromocriptine:** 2.5 mg/day PO, increased by 2.5 mg q 3 days until improvement, adverse effects, or max. daily dose of 15 mg/day.
4. **Levodopa:** 250 mg PO bid–qid, increased by additional 100–750 mg at q 3–7 days as tolerated until improvement, adverse effects, or max. daily dose of 8 g/day in divided doses.

Adverse Effects:

1. **Neomycin:** Ototoxicity (auditory, vestibular), nephrotoxicity, diarrhea, occasional skin rash.
2. **Lactulose:** Excessive diarrhea, electrolyte abnormalities, abdominal distention, flatulence, nausea.
3. **Bromocriptine:** Orthostasis with dizziness on postural changes, drowsiness, nausea, headache.
4. **Levodopa:** Nausea/vomiting is often dose limiting; dizziness, depression, and arrhythmias have been reported.

Drug Interactions:

1. **Neomycin:** Ototoxicity/nephrotoxicity is additive with other systemic aminoglycosides. Absorption of digitalis and penicillin is decreased.
2. **Lactulose:** Additive effect with other laxatives and stool softeners. Decreases drug absorption because of laxative action.
3. **Bromocriptine:** Additive with antihypertensives.
4. **Levodopa:** Antacids increase absorption. General anesthetics in combination with levodopa are arrhythmogenic. High-protein diet decreases absorption.

Comments and Recommendations: Hepatic or portasystemic encephalopathy is a well-known complication of acute/chronic liver disease. Cerebral toxins incriminated in this disease are multiple and include ammonia, fatty acids, amino acids (increased aromatic vs. branch chain), and altered neurochemical transmitters. Most compounds are thought to arise from GI bacterial action on gut proteins.

Hepatic encephalopathy is characterized by confusion, flapping tremor, hypertonicity, somnolence, and coma. EEG shows nonspecific slow wave activity. Acute precipitating events include alcoholic hepatitis, GI hemorrhage, infection, surgery, dietary indiscretion, and metabolic alkalosis secondary to overaggressive diuresis and paracentesis.

Short-term acute management includes identifying and correcting precipitating factors, evacuation of the bowels to remove nitrogen-containing material, decreasing protein intake to basal requirements, and decreasing or altering colonic flora with neomycin and/or lactulose. Electrolytes should be balanced and calories maintained as much as possible with carbohydrates. Lactulose is recommended as initial therapy for acute encephalopathy, because it decreases ammonia absorption and production and functions as a laxative to empty the bowel. Neomycin is added if necessary. Protein is slowly reintroduced with recovery.

Long-term management includes limiting dietary protein to 50 g/day, with high-fiber foods encouraged. Prolonged lactulose therapy should be adjusted to ensure two to three soft bowel movements/day. In chronic liver disease not responding to standard treatment, a trial of bromocriptine or levodopa can be instituted.

Alternative antibiotics that can be used to decrease GI ammonia formation are tetracyclines and metronidazole 200 mg PO qid. Like neomycin, neither should be used long term.

BIBLIOGRAPHY

AMA Drug Evaluations, ed 6, Philadelphia, 1986, WB Saunders.
Drug Information for the Health Care Provider, ed 6, Rockville, 1986, US Pharmacopeial Convention.
Sherlock DS: Acute fulminant hepatic failure. In *Diseases of the Liver and Biliary System,* ed 7, London, 1985, Blackwell Scientific Publications.

HISTAMINE H₂ RECEPTOR ANTAGONISTS

Trade Names:

Cimetidine: *Tagamet.*
Ranitidine: *Zantac.*
Famotidine: *Pepcid.*
Nizatidine: *Axid.*

Drug Action:

1. Competitive H₂ receptor antagonist.
2. Decreases basal and nocturnal acid secretion.
3. Decreases acid output stimulated by food and medications.

Indications:

1. Acute and chronic therapy for peptic ulcer disease (PUD).
2. Acute and chronic therapy for gastroesophageal reflux disease (GERD).
3. Hypersecretory conditions (Zollinger-Ellison syndrome, systemic mastocytosis).
4. Stress ulcer prophylaxis.

Pharmacokinetics: *See* Table 13.

Drug Preparations:

Drug	Tablets (mg)	Oral liquid	Injection (IM/IV) (mg/2 mL)
Cimetidine	200, 300, 400, 800	300	300
Ranitidine	150, 300	NA	50
Famotidine	20, 40	40	20
Nizatidine	150, 300	NA	NA

Dosage: *See* Table 14.

1. Dosage should be adjusted on basis of gastric PH.
2. Dosage of cimetidine should be decreased in patients with hepatic/renal disease. Dosage of ranitidine, famotidine, and nizatidine should be decreased in patients with renal disease. Give

TABLE 13.
Pharmacokinetics

Drug	Absorption (%)	Metabolism	t½ (hr)	Excretion (%)	Duration (hr)
Cimetidine	60–70	Hepatic (30%–40%)	2–3	Renal (30–75)	4–5
Ranitidine	50	Hepatic (10%)	2–3	Renal (30–70)	4–12
Famotidine	40–45	Min hepatic	2.3–3.5	Renal (30–70)	10–12
Nizatidine	90	Min hepatic	1–2	Renal (90)	4–10

TABLE 14.
Dosage

	Cimetidine	Ranitidine	Famotidine	Nizatidine
PUD				
Acute (6–8 wk)	300 mg PO qid or 400 mg bid or 800 mg qhs; 300 mg IV q6hr 35–40 mg/hr continuous IV infusion	150 mg PO bid or 300 mg qhs; 50 mg IV q6–8hr 6.25 mg/hr continuous IV	20 mg bid PO or 40 mg qhs; 20 mg IV q12hr	150 mg bid PO or 300 mg qhs
Chronic	400 mg qhs PO	150 mg qhs PO	20 mg qhs PO	150 mg qhs
GERD	400 mg bid PO	150 mg bid PO	20 mg bid PO	150 mg bid
Stress ulcer	300 mg IV q6hr	50 mg IV q8hr	20 mg IV q12hr	150 mg bid
Renal disease	300 mg PO/IV q12hr	150 mg PO q24hr	20 mg PO/IV q24–36hr	150 mg PO qod

50%–75% of dose for creatinine clearance 20–40 mL/min; 25%–50% of dose for creatinine clearance 0–20 mL/min.
3. Zollinger-Ellison syndrome poses a unique clinical situation in which extremely high doses (three to four times recommendations) of H$_2$ blockers may be required q 3–6 hr to control hypersecretion and acid output.

Adverse Effects:

1. Cimetidine: Dizziness, agitation, confusion, headache, drowsiness, diarrhea, nausea, vomiting, hypotension, bradycardia, tachycardia, fever, rash, gynecomastia, swelling of breasts, decreased sexual ability, bone marrow suppression, renal toxicity, hepatic toxicity, myalgias.
2. Ranitidine: Dizziness, sedation, malaise, headache, drowsiness, confusion, fever, rash, gynecomastia, arthralgias, diarrhea, nausea, vomiting, bradycardia, tachycardia, bone marrow suppression.
3. Famotidine: Dizziness, headache, drowsiness, weakness, fatigue, seizures, diarrhea, flatulence, anorexia, acne, pruritus, urticaria, bradycardia, tachycardia, hypertension, bone marrow depression, hepatic and renal toxicity, paresthesia, bronchospasm, hypersensitivity reactions.
4. Nizatidine: Dizziness, headache, weakness, drowsiness, fatigue, seizures, insomnia, diarrhea, flatulence, anorexia, bradycardia, tachycardia, hypertension, acne, pruritus, urticaria, bone marrow depression, hepatic and renal toxicity, hypersensitivity reactions, paresthesias.

Adverse Effects:

Drug	Antiandrogenic	Confusion	Bone Marrow Suppression
Cimetidine	Yes	In elderly	Rare
Ranitidine	Yes	In elderly	Rare
Famotidine	No	No	Rare thrombocytopenia
Nizatidine	No	No	Rare

Drug Interactions:

Drug	Increased Toxicity	Decreased Absorption
Cimetidine	Theophyline, phenytoin, β-blockers, warfarin sodium, lidocaine, procainamide, quinidine, benzodiazepines, metronidazole, triamterene, cyclosporin, tricyclics	Ketoconazole
Ranitidine	Cyclosporine, glipizide, glybruride, midazolam, metoprolol, gentamicin, pentoxifylline, phenytoin, quinidine	Ketoconazole
Famotidine	None	Ketoconazole
Nizatidine	None	Ketoconazole

1. Concomitant administration of PO H$_2$ blockers and antacids decreases H$_2$ blocker absorption; administration should be separated by 2 hr, if possible.

Monitoring: Gastric pH, blood pressure (IV push), CBC, renal function, clinical features of peptic ulcer disease and GI bleeding.

Test Interactions: May elevate creatinine, AST, ALT measurements (false-positives).

BIBLIOGRAPHY

Agents used in disorders of the upper gastrointestinal tract. *AMA Drug Evaluations,* ed 6, Philadelphia, 1986, WB Saunders, pp 943–946.

Clearfield H, et al: International perspectives on acid-peptic disorders, *Pract Gastroenterol* 1988, (suppl):1–40.

Ostro M, Russel J, Soldin S, et al: Control of gastric pH with cimetidine: boluses versus primed infusions, *Gastroenterology* 1985, 89:532–537.

Siepler J, Prindiville T, Nishikawa R, et al: Prophylaxis of stress ulceration in the ICU: a comparison of cimetidine and ranitidine constant infusion, *AGA Abst* May 1987, 1639.

Tryba M, Zevounou F, Torok M, et al: Prevention of acute stress bleeding with sucralfate, antacids, or cimetidine, *Am J Intern Med* 1985, 79(suppl 2C):55–61.

HYDRALAZINE

Trade Name: *Apresoline.*

Drug Action:

1. Direct action on vascular smooth muscle, producing greater vasodilation of arterioles than in venous system. Exact mechanism not known but thought to involve inhibition of intracellular calcium.
2. Vasodilation usually lowers diastolic blood pressure more than systolic blood pressure.
3. Decrease in peripheral vascular resistance with concomitant reflex increase in heart rate, stroke volume, and cardiac output.
4. Increase in splanchnic, coronary, cerebral, and renal blood flow unless blood pressure fall is marked.
5. Increases plasma renin activity.
6. Retention of Na$^+$, H$_2$O, and decrease in urine production.

Indications:

1. Chronic hypertension.
2. Can be used for acute lowering of blood pressure in mild to moderate hypertension.

Pharmacokinetics:

1. **Absorption:** PO/IV.
2. **Metabolism:** Acetylation in liver.
3. **Excretion:** Metabolites excreted renally.
4. **Plasma half-life:** Approximately 3 hr.
5. **Onset of action:** 10–20 min IV; 20–30 min PO.

Drug Preparations:

    Tablets: 10, 25, 50, 100 mg.
    Ampules: 20 mg/mL for IV.

Dosage:

1. **PO:** 25–50 mg qid.
2. **IV:** 5 mg bolus. Repeat prn after 15–20 min; may require 20–40 mg. **Maintenance dose** 5–10 mg IV q 6 hr.

Adverse Effects:

1. Exacerbation of angina pectoris caused by increase in heart rate with shorter diastolic time and lower diastolic blood pressure (reduction in coronary perfusion pressure and shorter time for coronary blood flow).
2. Headache, nausea/vomiting, diarrhea.
3. Constipation.
4. Hypotension.
5. Peripheral neuropathy: Corrected by pyridoxine.
6. Lupus-like syndrome.

Drug Interactions: Use with caution in patients receiving MAO inhibitors or other antihypertensives.

Monitoring:

1. Blood pressure, heart rate.
2. ST segments.

BIBLIOGRAPHY

Blaschlee TF, Melmon KL: Antihypertensive agents and the drug therapy of hypertension. In Gilman AG, Goodman LS, Gilman A (eds): *The Pharmacological Basis of Therapeutics,* ed 6, New York, 1980, Macmillan, pp 799–801.

HYDROMORPHONE

Trade Name: *Dilaudid:* Generic brands.

Drug Action:

1. Approximately eight times more potent than morphine but may produce less nausea/vomiting and euphoria.
2. Centrally acting antitussive.

Indications:

1. Moderate to severe pain.
2. Can be used to control persistent, nonproductive cough.

Pharmacokinetics:

1. **Absorption:** Well absorbed after PO/IM/SQ administration.
2. **Metabolism:** Glucuronide conjugation in liver.
3. **Excretion:** Renal.
4. **Plasma half-life:** Approximately 2.5 hr.

Drug Preparations:

Ampules: 1, 2, 3, 4, 10 mg/mL.
Tablets: 1, 2, 3, 4, mg.
Cough syrup: 1 mg/5 mL.
Suppositories: 3 mg.

Dosage:

1. **Pain control:**
   a. **IM/SC:** 1–2 mg q 4–6 hr.
   b. **IV:** 1–2 mg slowly over 2–3 min q 4–6 hr.
   c. **PO:** 2–4 mg q 4–6 hr.
   d. **PR:** 3 mg q 6–8 hr.
2. **Antitussive:**
   a. **PO:** 5 mL (1 mg) Dilaudid cough syrup q 3–4 hr. Similar doses of other drug forms can also be used.

Adverse Effects: Similar to those from morphine, including dysphoria, lethargy, nausea/vomiting, urinary retention, potential for elevated intracranial pressure in patients at risk, sedation, confusion, respiratory depression, constipation, anorexia, hypotension, tachycardia.

Drug Interactions: CNS depression may be augmented with concomitant administration of phenothiazines, tricyclic antidepressants, hypnotics, sedatives, alcohol, other CNS depressants.

Monitoring:

1. Respiratory rate.
2. Blood pressure, heart rate.
3. Mental status.

BIBLIOGRAPHY

AMA Drug Evaluations, ed 6, Philadelphia, 1986, WB Saunders.
McEvoy GK (ed): *AHFS Drug Information 88,* Bethesda, 1989,
  American Society of Hospital Pharmacists.
Physicians' Desk Reference, ed 42, Oradell, 1988, Medical Eco-
  nomics Co.

HYDROXYZINE HYDROCHLORIDE

Trade Names: *Atarax, Hydroxyzine, Vistaril.*

Drug Actions: CNS depressant activity, bronchodilator, antihistamine (H_1 receptors), analgesic, antiemetic.

Indications: Anxiety and tension (especially psychoneurosis),
pruritus due to allergic conditions, urticaria, atopic and contact
dermatoses, sedative, nausea and vomiting.

Pharmacokinetics:

1. **Absorption:** Rapidly absorbed from GI tract.
2. **Onset of action:** 15–30 min after PO, duration 4–6 hr.
3. **Metabolism:** Exact fate unknown.
4. **Half-life:** 3–7 hr.

Drug Preparations:

  Tablets: 10, 25, 50, 100 mg.
  Syrup: 10 mg/5 mL.
  IM solution: 25, 50 mg/mL.

Dosage: Oral: Sedation and anxiety—50–100 mg qid; children
over 6 yr, 50–100 mg daily in divided doses; allergy—25 mg
tid–qid, children less than 6, 50 mg daily in divided doses; IM: sedation and antianxiety, 50–100 mg q 4–6 hr, nausea/vomiting,
25–100 mg IM (children 0.5 mg/pound).

Adverse Effects: CNS depression, drowsiness, headache, fatigue, nervousness, dizziness, urinary retention, rare tremor and
convulsions, anticholinergic—dry mouth. Intraarterial, SQ, or IV
administration can cause thrombosis and gangrene. Rare—hypotension, edema, angioedema, paradoxical excitement.

Drug Interactions: SQ injection—tissue damage, may potentiate actions of narcotics and barbiturates and other CNS depressants, counteracts pressor effects of epinephrine, synergistic with other anticholinergics.

Monitoring: Degree of sedation, relief of symptoms, mental status, blood pressure.

BIBLIOGRAPHY

Simons FE: H$_1$-receptor antagonists. Comparative tolerability and safety, *Drug Safety* 1994, 10:350–380.

Monroe EW: Relative efficacy and safety of loratadine, hydroxyzine, and placebo in chronic idiopathic urticaria and atopic dermatitis, *Clin Ther* 1992, 14:17–21.

IBUPROFEN

Trade Names:

Prescription: *Motrin, Rufen.*
Over-the-counter: *Advil, Haltran, Medipren, Midol 200, Nuprin.*

Drug Action:

1. Like aspirin, inhibits cyclooxygenase and therefore has similar antipyretic, anti-inflammatory, and analgesic actions.
2. Produces platelet dysfunction, with subsequently prolonged bleeding time.

Indications:

1. As effective as aspirin in treatment of rheumatoid arthritis and osteoarthritis.
2. Effective in mild-to-moderate pain, myalgias, arthralgias.
3. Fever.

Pharmacokinetics:

1. **Absorption:** Rapid and almost complete after PO administration.
2. **Distribution:** High degree (>95%) of protein binding.
3. **Metabolism:** Rapidly metabolized by hepatic hydroxylation and carboxylation as well as conjugation.

4. **Excretion:** >90% of drug renally excreted as inactive metabolites; only approximately 1% excreted unchanged in urine.
5. **Half-life:** Plasma half-life approximately 2 hr.

Drug Preparations:

Tablets: 200, 300, 400, 600, 800 mg.
Suspension: 100 mg/5 mL.

Dosage:

1. **Pain, headache, dysmenorrhea, fever:** 200–400 mg q 4–6 hr.
2. **Rheumatoid arthritis, osteoarthritis:** 1200–3200 mg/day in divided doses.

Adverse Effects: Probably better tolerated than aspirin or agents such as phenylbutazone or indomethacin.

1. **GI:**
   a. Nausea/vomiting, heartburn, epigastric pain, about 10% of the time.
   b. Ulceration and bleeding less common than with aspirin, but use with caution in patients with history of peptic ulcer disease.
2. Patients with known sensitivity reactions (e.g., rash, anaphylaxis) to aspirin or other nonsteroidal anti-inflammatory drugs (NSAIDs) should use ibuprofen with caution, if at all.
3. Less frequently, fluid retention and edema, elevated liver function tests, visual disturbances, dizziness, headache.
4. Acute renal failure precipitated by NSAIDs has been reported in patients with preexisting conditions such as heart failure and impaired renal/hepatic function.
5. Acute interstitial nephritis has been reported.

Drug Interactions:

1. Since it is highly bound to plasma proteins, ibuprofen can displace other similarly bound drugs. Specifically, use of warfarin and PO hypoglycemics should be closely monitored.
2. Renal effects of furosemide and thiazide diuretics may be diminished, presumably as a result of inhibition of prostaglandin synthesis.

BIBLIOGRAPHY

AMA Drug Evaluations, ed 6, Philadelphia, 1986, WB Saunders.

Geffner ES, Best ML, Mittman M, et al (ed): *Compendium of Drug Therapy,* New York, 1987, Biomedical Information Corporation.

McEvoy GK (ed): *AHFS Drug Information 89,* Bethesda, 1989, American Society of Hospital Pharmacists.

Physicians' Desk Reference, ed 42, Oradell, 1988, Medical Economics Co.

IMIPENEM AND CILASTATIN

Trade Name: *Primaxin.*

Drug Action:

1. Inhibits cell wall synthesis (carbapenem).
2. Very broad spectrum of activity, including most gram-positive and gram-negative aerobes and anaerobes plus *Campylobacter, Yersinia, Nocardia, Mycobacterium,* and others.
   a. Intermediate activity against enterococci and methicillin-resistant *Staphylococcus aureus* (MRSA) (not clinically useful).
   b. **No** activity against *Pseudomonas maltophilia* and *P. cepacia.*

Indications: Infections caused by susceptible organisms, including *Staphylococcus, Streptococcus, Escherichia coli, Klebsiella, Proteus, Enterobacter, P. aeruginosa, Bacteroides;* reserved for nosocomial and other infections caused by resistant pathogens or mixed aerobic/anaerobic organisms.

1. Useful at multiple sites.

Pharmacokinetics:

1. **Absorption:** IV, IM.
2. **Metabolism:** Renal.
3. **Excretion:** Renal; removed by hemodialysis.
4. **Serum half-life:** 1 hr.

5. **Cilastatin** acts as renal dipeptidase inhibitor and protects against potential nephrotoxicity if imipenem used alone.

Drug Preparations:

Vials: 250, 500 mg for IV use.
IM use: 500, 750 mg (mix with 1% lidocaine)

Dosage:

1. **Normal renal function:** 0.5–1 g q 6–8 hr IV; 500–750 mg q 12 hr IM.
2. Impaired renal function:

IV Dose (g)	Creatinine Clearance	Interval (hr)
0.5–1	>80	6–8
	80–50	6–8
	50–10	6–12
	<10 (anuria)	12–24

3. **Hemodialysis:** No more than 2 g/day, with one dose after each dialysis.

Adverse Effects:

1. Similar to other β-lactams, includes hypersensitivity reactions (e.g., rash), GI problems (increased nausea/vomiting with rapid infusion), phlebitis, hypotension.
2. (?)Increase in seizure activity with certain risk factors, including history of seizure disorder, renal insufficiency, advanced age.
   a. Hyperventilation and shakiness may occur with rapid infusion and be confused with minor seizure disorder.

Monitoring: Serial renal function studies.

INSULIN

Trade Names:

1. **Rapid-acting:**
   a. **Regular, crystalline zinc:** *Regular Iletin* I (beef-pork), Regular (Concentrated) *Iletin II, U-500* (pork), *Humulin R*

(human), *Regular Insulin* (pork), *Regular Purified Pork Insulin,* Velosulin (human), *Novolin R* (human).
b. **Insulin zinc suspension:** *Semilente Iletin I, Semilente Insulin, Semilente Purified Pork Prompt Insulin.*

2. **Intermediate-acting:**
   a. **Isophane (NPH) 70%, regular insulin 30%:** *Mixtard.*
   b. **Isophane (NPH) insulin suspension:** *NPH Iletin I* (beef-pork), *Humulin N* (human), *NPH Insulin* (beef), *NPH Purified Pork Isophane Insulin, Novolin N* (human), *Insulatard NPH Human.*
   c. **Insulin zinc suspension:** *Lente Iletin I* (beef-pork), *Humulin L* (human), *Lente Insulin* (beef), *Lente L* (pork), *Lente Ilentin II* (pork), *Lente Purified Pork Insulin, Novolin L* (human).

3. **Long-acting:**
   a. **Protamine zinc insulin suspension:** *Protamine, Zinc & Iletin I* (beef-pork).
   b. **Extended insulin zinc suspension:** *Ultralente Iletin I* (beef-pork), *Ultralente Insulin, Ultralente Purified Beef Extended Insulin, Humulin U Ultralente* (human).

Drug Action:

1. **Lowers blood glucose:** Increases glucose transport across cell membranes, prevents glycogenolysis, increases glycogen synthesis, suppresses gluconeogenesis.
2. **Decreases production of ketones:** Suppresses lipolysis and hepatic ketogenesis, stimulates fat synthesis.
3. **Inhibits protein degradation.**

Indications:

1. Treatment of hyperglycemic and/or ketoacidotic syndromes in patients with diabetes mellitus or glucose intolerance.
2. Hyperkalemia.

Pharmacokinetics: *See* Table 15.

1. **Metabolism:** Hepatic and renal.
2. **Excretion:** Renal. Decrease dosage in patients with renal insufficiency. Not removed by dialysis.
3. **Volume of distribution:** Extracellular fluid.
4. **Basal secretion:** 20 μg/hr.

TABLE 15.
Pharmacokinetics

		Hours After Injection*					
		Onset		Max Effect		Duration	
Preparation	Concentration (U/mL)	SQ	IV	SQ	IV	SQ	IV
Rapid-acting insulin:							
Regular	40, 100, 500	0.5–1	0.1–0.5	2–5	0.5	6–8	1
Semilente	40, 100	1–3		5–10		10–16	
Intermediate-acting insulin:							
Isophane (NPH) 70%, regular 30% (*Mixtard*)	100	0.5		4–8		24	
NPH	40, 100	2–4		6–12		18–24	
Lente	40, 100	2–4		6–15		18–24	
Long-acting insulin:							
Protamine zinc	40, 100	4–8		14–24		28–36	
Ultralente	40, 100	4–8		10–30		28–36	

*Time varies among patients and is influenced by concentration, volume, site, and depth of injection.

5. **Basal circulating level:** 500 pg/mL (12 μU/mL).
6. **Plasma half-life:** 9 min.
7. **Compatibilities:**
   a. Regular insulin may be mixed with NPH.
   b. Action of regular insulin may be delayed when mixed with Lente.
   c. Semilente, Lente, and Ultralente may be mixed.

Drug Preparations:

1. Insulins are available as human insulin (*Humulin, Novolin*), pork insulin, beef insulin, and beef-pork insulin, in 40, 100 (standard), 500 U/mL concentrations. Insulins are supplied as short-, intermediate-, and long-acting forms.
2. Only regular insulin should be administered IV/IM; all forms may be given SQ.
3. Insulin is supplied in 10 mL containers and should be refrigerated for storage (but not frozen). If refrigeration is not available, store in a cool place away from sunlight and heat. Freezing should be avoided.
4. Insulin may adhere to IV tubing and filters. Flush lines with 100–200 mL insulin solution or add albumin to minimize loss.

Dosage: Varies greatly from patient to patient and may vary with form of insulin used.

1. **Insulin-dependent diabetes mellitus:** In absence of ketosis or other complications, begin with 10–20 U intermediate-acting insulin SQ plus 4–10 U short-acting insulin SQ in the morning before breakfast. Adjust dosage on basis of blood glucose results. Increasing the morning dose of intermediate-acting insulin generally corrects hyperglycemia occurring before the evening meal or at bedtime; prebreakfast hyperglycemia is usually treated by reducing the bedtime snack and/or giving additional intermediate-acting insulin before the evening meal or at bedtime (make sure that prebreakfast hyperglycemia is not a sequela of nocturnal hypoglycemia). Regular insulin is often added to intermediate-acting insulin to control postprandial hyperglycemia and hyperglycemia occurring before the intermediate-acting insulin becomes effective.
2. **Diabetic ketoacidosis/hyperglycemic nonketotic syndromes:** Begin with 5–10 U/hr (0.1 U/kg/hr) regular insulin IV/IM. Adjust dosage on basis of blood glucose and ketosis.

3. **Insulin requirements are increased** in pregnancy, hyperthyroidism, obesity, stress, trauma, infection.
4. **Insulin requirements are decreased** in renal failure, hepatic failure, hypothyroidism, malnutrition.
5. **Hyperkalemia:** 1 unit insulin for every 4–5 g dextrose given; if hyperglycemia is present, may give 2–5 units regular insulin IV; monitor serum K and glucose.

Adverse Effects: Hypoglycemia, hypokalemia, hypophosphatemia, hypomagnesemia, hypersensitivity/allergic reactions (e.g., skin erythema/induration, urticaria, angioedema, anaphylaxis), lipodystrophies (e.g., atrophy, hypertrophy), visual deterioration, peripheral edema.

Hypoglycemia may be manifested by perspiration, palpitations, tachycardia, fatigue, mental confusion, coma, headache, hypothermia, hunger, numbness, nausea, weakness, tremor, blurred vision, speech disturbances, anxiety.

Drug Interactions:

1. **May increase blood glucose and/or antagonize insulin:** Glucocorticoids, ACTH, estrogens, progesterone, growth hormone, glucagon, epinephrine, dobutamine, amphetamines, ritodrine, thyroid hormone, dextrothyroxine, thiazides, phenytoin, triamterene, danazol, baclofen, diazoxide, acetazolamide, niacin.
2. **May enhance hypoglycemic effect of insulin:** MAO inhibitors, anabolic steroids, captopril, disopyramide, fenfluramine, propranolol, alcohol, sulfonylureas, guanethidine, nicotine, chloramphenicol, tetracycline, salicylates, nonsteroidal anti-inflammatory drugs, α-blockers, clofibrate, pentamidine.

Monitoring:

1. Blood/serum glucose (arterial/venous/capillary); may use lab or reagent strip (Dipstix) techniques.
2. Serum/urine ketones.
3. Urine glucose (poor predictor of blood glucose level).
4. Glycosylated hemoglobin (reflects average blood glucose over preceding 2–3 mo).
5. Plasma insulin levels.
6. Serum electrolytes (i.e., K, Mg, PO_4).

BIBLIOGRAPHY

Zaloga GP, Chernow B: Insulin and oral hypoglycemics. In Chernow B (ed): *The Pharmacologic Approach to the Critically Ill Patient,* ed 3, Baltimore, 1994, Williams & Wilkins, pp 758–776.

Kahn CR, Shechter Y: Insulin, oral hypoglycemic agents, and the pharmacology of the endocrine pancreas. In Gilman AG, et al (eds): *The Pharmacologic Basis of Therapeutics,* ed 8, New York, 1993, McGraw-Hill, pp 1463–1495.

Nolte MS: Insulin therapy in insulin-dependent (type I) diabetes mellitus, *Endocrinol Metab Clin North Am* 1992, 21:281–305.

INTERFERON

Trade Names: *Roferon-A* (interferon alfa-2a), *Intron A* (interferon alfa-2b), *Alferon N* (interferon alfa-n3), *Betaseron* (interferon beta-1b), *Actimmune* (interferon gamma-1b).

Drug Actions: Binds to specific membrane receptors on cell surfaces, initiating complex sequences of intracellular events (inhibition of viral replication, suppression of cell proliferation, and immunomodulation).

Indications:

1. Refractory condyloma acuminatum.
2. Chronic hepatitis B.
3. Chronic hepatitis C.
4. Chronic non-A, non-B/C hepatitis.
5. HIV-related, zidovudine-unresponsive, severe thrombocytopenia.
6. Hairy cell leukemia.
7. AIDS-related Kaposi's sarcoma.
8. Multiple sclerosis (interferon beta-1b).
9. Chronic granulomatous disease (interferon gamma-1b).

Pharmacokinetics:

1. Absorption: Given SQ, IM, or intralesionally.

Drug Preparations:

Roferon-A (interferon alfa-2a)
  Injectable solution: 3, 9, 18, and 36 million IU/vial.
  Powder for injection: 18 million IU/vial.

Intron A (interferon alfa-2b)
  Powder for injection: 3, 5, 10, 18, 25, and 50 million IU/vial.

Alferon N (interferon alfa-n3)
  Injectable solution: 5 million IU (1 mL of 5 million IU/mL in each vial).

Betaseron (interferon beta-1b)
  Powder: 0.3 mg (= 9.6 million IU) — after reconstitution with 1.2 mL diluent, vials contain 0.25 mg (8 million units)/mL.

Actimmune (interferon gamma-1b)
  Single-dose vials (0.5 mL): 100 μg (3 million units).

Dosage:

1. Condyloma acuminatum: 1 million units (0.1 mL) into lesion three times/wk for 3 wk (use 10 million IU/1 mL vial).
2. Chronic hepatitis B: 5 million units SQ or IM q day or 10 million units SQ or IM three times/wk for 4 mo.
3. Chronic hepatitis C: 3 million units SQ or IM three times/wk for 6–18 mo.
4. Chronic non-A, non-B/C hepatitis: 3 million units SQ or IM 3 times/wk (duration individualized).
5. HIV-related, zidovudine-unresponsive, severe thrombocytopenia: 3 million units SQ or IM three times/wk for 4 mo.
6. Hairy cell leukemia:
     Induction: 3 million units SQ or IM q day for 16–24 wk.
     Maintenance: 3 million units SQ or IM 3 times/wk.
7. AIDS-related Kaposi's sarcoma: 30 million IU/m^2 SQ or IM three times/wk.
8. Multiple sclerosis—use interferon beta-1b: 0.25 mg (8 million IU) SQ qod.
9. Chronic granulomatous disease—use interferon gamma-1b: 50 μg/m^2 (1.5 million units/m^2) if body surface >0.5 m^2, or 1.5 μg/kg/dose if body surface area ≤0.5 m^2. With both dosages, administration is three times/wk.

Adverse Effects: Influenza-like syndrome (especially in first week of therapy), myelosuppression (high dosages and/or chronic use), fatigue, myalgias, headache, dizziness, anorexia, diarrhea, rash, alopecia, thyroid dysfunction, autoantibody formation, menstrual cycle changes in women, possible cardiotoxicity, and others.

Drug Interactions: Caution advised if administering with other myelosuppressive agents (e.g., zidovudine).

Monitoring: Periodic hematologic tests (CBC with differential and platelet count), chemistries including liver function tests, and thyroid-stimulating hormone levels.

BIBLIOGRAPHY

Physicians' Desk Reference, ed 50, Montvale, 1996, Medical Economics Co.

Sanford JP, Gilbert DN, Sande MA (eds): *The Sanford Guide to Antimicrobial Therapy,* ed 26, Dallas, 1996, Antimicrobial Therapy.

IODIDE

Trade Names:

Potassium iodide: *Pima, Losat, Thyro-Block, SSKI.*
Potassium iodide solution.
Sodium iodide: *Various.*
Strong iodine solution: *Lugol solution.*

Drug Action:

1. Antithyroid agent.
2. Inhibits synthesis and release of thyroid hormone.
3. Blocks accumulation of radioiodine by thyroid gland (e.g., after nuclear accident).
4. Expectorant.

Indications:

1. Treatment of hyperthyroidism.
2. Preparation of hyperthyroid patients for thyroidectomy.
3. Nuclear radiation protection.
4. Expectorant.

Pharmacokinetics:

1. Crosses placenta.
2. Secreted in breast milk.
3. **Onset of action:** 24–48 hr.
4. **Peak effect:** 10–15 days.

Drug Preparations:

1. **Potassium iodide:**
   Tablets: 130 mg.
   Syrup: 325 mg/5 mL.
   Solution: 500 mg/15 mL.
   Saturated solution (SSKI): 1 g/mL.
   Strong iodine solution (Lugol solution): Iodine 50 mg/mL,
   potassium iodide 100 mg/mL.
2. **Sodium iodide:**
   10% solution for injection.

Dosage:

1. **Hyperthyroidism:** Give 1 hr after propylthiouracil (PTU) or
   methimazole:
   a. Strong iodine (Lugol's) solution, 1 mL tid; or potassium
      iodide solution, 300–500 mg tid PO.
   b. Sodium iodide, 750–1000 mg/day IV.
2. **Preparation of hyperthyroid patient for surgery:** 50–250
   mg (1–5 drops) SSKI tid PO, or 0.1–0.3 mL (3–5 drops) Lugol
   solution tid; give drug for 10–14 days before surgery.
3. **Nuclear radiation protection:** 0.13 mL (130 mg) SSKI PO
   immediately before exposure or for 10 days after.
4. **Expectorant:**
   a. **Adult:** Potassium iodide 300–650 mg bid–qid.
   b. **Pediatric:** 60–250 mg qid.
5. **RDA for iodine:** 150 μg/day.

Adverse Effects:

1. **SKIN:** Rash, acne, urticaria, angioedema.
2. **GI:** Nausea/vomiting, diarrhea, epigastric pain, bleeding, perforation, obstruction, unpleasant taste, burning in mouth, hy-
   persalivation, painful sialadenitis.
3. **Metabolic:** Goiter, hyperthyroidism (adenoma), hypothyroidism, collagen disease–like syndrome.

4. Soreness of mouth, coryza, sneezing, eyelid swelling, angioedema, serum sickness reaction, fever, headache, arthralgia.
5. Hyperkalemia. May cause muscle weakness, ECG abnormalities, cardiac toxicity.

Drug Interactions:

1. Lithium potentiates effects on thyroid gland.
2. Potassium-sparing diuretics may lead to hyperkalemia.

Monitoring:

1. Thyroxine, triiodothyronine, thyroid-stimulating hormone.
2. Potassium level.

Acute Poisoning: Gastric lavage with soluble starch solution; sodium thiosulfate is a specific antidote.

BIBLIOGRAPHY

Haynes RC: Thyroid and antithyroid drugs. In Gilman AG, et al (ed): *The Pharmacological Basis of Therapeutics,* ed 8, New York, 1993, McGraw-Hill, pp 1361–1383.

Wolff J: Excess iodide inhibits the thyroid by multiple mechanisms, *Adv Exp Med Biol* 1989, 261:211–244.

Tan TT, Morat P, Ng ML, Khalid BA: Effects of Lugol's solution on thyroid function in normals and patients with untreated thyrotoxicosis, *Clin Endocrinol* 1989, 30:645–649.

IPECAC

Trade Name: *Syrup of Ipecac.*

Drug Action: Emetic; peripheral GI irritant; also triggers central chemoreceptor zone.

Indications: To induce vomiting in selected cases of overdose/poisoning (primarily for home use under advice from the local Poison Control Center).

Pharmacokinetics:

1. **Absorption:** Enteral (minimal).
2. **Metabolism:** Unknown.

3. **Excretion:** Slowly in urine.
4. **Onset of action:** 20–30 min after PO administration.
5. **Duration of action:** 20–60 min after PO administration (may persist for up to 2 hr).

Drug Preparations:

Syrup: Contains 16–21 mg of Cephalin and emetine per 15-mL dose.

Dosage:

1. **Adult:** 30 mL PO, followed by 200–300 mL water (not required for efficacy); may repeat dose if vomiting does not occur in 30 min. If vomiting does not occur after an additional 30 min, perform gastric lavage as clinically indicated.
2. **Pediatric:** >5 yrs: 30 mL PO; ≥1–5 yr: 15 mL PO. <6 mo–1 yr: 10 mL. Each dose may be followed by 3–4 mL/kg of H_2O (not required for efficacy) and can be repeated in 30 min if vomiting does not occur.

Adverse Effects (very rarely in setting of acute one-time use):

1. **Cardiovascular:** Bradycardia, arrhythmias, conduction disturbances, hypotension, myocarditis.
2. **GI:** Diarrhea, gastric herniation (undiagnosed diaphragmatic hernia), upper GI bleeding (Mallory-Weiss tear).
3. **CNS:** Lethargy, irritability, intracranial hemorrhage.
4. **Pulmonary** aspiration, pneumomediastinum.
5. **Musculoskeletal:** Hypotonia, myopathies.

Drug Interactions:

1. Contraindications
   a. Age <6 mo.
   b. CNS depression/seizures.
   c. Clinical instability present or anticipated.
   d. Prior emesis.
   e. Nontoxic ingestion.
   f. Sharp or dangerous foreign bodies (e.g., glass, camera batteries).
   g. Petroleum distillates.
   h. Caustics.

    i. Delayed charcoal or oral antidote administration.
    j. Bleeding disorders.
2. Emetic action possibly delayed by milk products and anti-emetics.

Monitoring:

1. Blood pressure, pulse, respiratory rate.
2. Airway patency/protection.
3. Mental status.
4. GI tract for protracted emesis, possible bleeding.

BIBLIOGRAPHY

Flomenbaum NE, Goldfrank LR, Weisman RS, et al: General management of the poisoned or overdosed patient. In Goldfrank LR, Flomenbaum NE, Lewin NA, et al (eds): *Toxicologic Emergencies,* ed 5, Norwalk, 1994, Appleton & Lange, p 25.

Smilkstein MJ, Flomenbaum NE: Techniques used to prevent absorption of toxic compounds. In Goldfrank LR, Flomenbaum NE, Lewin NA, et al (eds): *Toxicologic Emergencies,* ed 5, Norwalk, 1994, Appleton & Lange, p 47.

Committee on Injury and Poison Prevention, American Academy of Pediatrics: *Handbook of Common Poisonings in Children,* ed 3, 1994, American Academy of Pediatrics, p 6.

IPRATROPIUM DERIVATIVES

Trade Name: *Atrovent.*

Drug Action:

1. Antagonizes action on acetylcholine (ACh) at its membrane-bound receptor site.
2. Blocks bronchoconstrictor effects of vagal efferent impulses within the airway.

Indications:

1. Treatment of bronchospasm (by inhalation).

Pharmacokinetics:

1. **Metabolism:** Hepatic (for systemically absorbed).
2. **Excretion:** Kidney, feces, bile.
3. **Absorption:** Ipratropium poorly absorbed.
4. **Half-life:** Ipratropium, 2 hr.
5. **Onset of action:** 1–3 min for bronchodilation; peak effect 1.5–2 hr; duration 4–6 hr.

Drug Preparations:

Ipratropium bromide: 18 μg/spray (metered dose inhaler). Nebulizer solution 0.02% (2.5 mL = 500 μg).

Dosage:

1. **For bronchospasm:**
   a. Ipratropium bromide: two to three puffs (0.04–0.06 mg) by metered dose inhaler q 6 hr. Onset of action is slow and max. effect may not be noted for 45–60 min.

Adverse Effects:

1. **Cardiovascular:** Palpitations, hypotension.
2. **CNS:** Nervousness, dizziness, fatigue, headache, insomnia.
3. **Urinary** retention.
4. **Other:** Nausea, dry mouth, gastric upset, muscle tremors, blurred vision, cough, nasal congestion, skin rash, hives; use with caution in patients with narrow-angle glaucoma, prostate hypertrophy.

Drug Interactions: Additive with other anticholinergic drugs.

Monitoring: FEV_1, spirometry, clinical response.

BIBLIOGRAPHY

Petty TL: The combination of ipratropium and albuterol is more effective than either agent alone, *Chest* 1995, 107(suppl):183–1865.

Greiger-Bronsky MJ: Anticholinergic therapy in the critically ill patient with bronchospasm, *AACN Clin Issues* 1995, 6:287–296.

Symposium: Anticholinergic therapy—the state of the art, *Postgrad Med J* 1987, 63(suppl):1–86.

ISONIAZID

Trade Names: *INH, Isoniazid, Laniazid.*

Drug Action:

1. Inhibition of synthesis of mycolic acid, an important component of mycobacterial cell walls.
2. Active against mycobacteria.

Indication: Tuberculosis.

Pharmacokinetics:

1. **Absorption:** Well absorbed PO/IM.
2. **Penetrates** throughout body, including CNS.
3. **Metabolism:** Primarily by acetylation and dehydrazination.
   a. **Slow acetylators/inactivators** (50% blacks and whites): Rarely leads to high levels and increased toxicity.
   b. **Rapid acetylators** (majority of Eskimos and Asians): (?)Fare less well with weekly intermittent therapy.
4. **Serum half-life:** 0.5–4 hr, depending on acetylation.

Dosage:

1. **Normal renal function:** 5 mg/kg/day PO/IM; may be given as single dose.
2. **Renal impairment:** No dose modification. Dose reduction to 200 mg/day in anuric slow acetylators.
3. **Severe hepatic insufficiency:** May need to adjust dose downward.
4. **Hemodialysis:** Supplemental dose of 5 mg/kg after each dialysis.

Drug Preparations:

Tablets: 50, 100, 300 mg.
Syrup: 50 mg/5 mL.
Injection: 100 mg/mL.

Adverse Effects:

1. **Hepatitis:** 10% with transaminitis; hepatitis (rarely death) associated with AST more than five times normal, alcoholism, older patients (>30 yr), concurrent use of rifampin.

2. **Peripheral neuropathy:** Increased in patients with poor nutrition or underlying neuropathy resulting from alcoholism, diabetes, uremia; more frequent in slow acetylators who have higher serum levels of unaltered drug.
   a. Prevented with daily pyridoxine therapy.
3. **Others:** Hypersensitivity reaction (e.g., fever, rash, positive antinuclear antibodies), minor disulfiram reaction, other neurologic problems (e.g., seizures), flushing after Swiss cheese ingestion, hypotension, nausea/vomiting, agranulocytosis, aplastic anemia.

Drug Interactions:

1. **Alcohol:** Increased hepatotoxicity.
2. **Aluminum antacids:** Decreased isoniazid effect with decreased absorption.
3. **PO anticoagulants:** Possible increased anticoagulant effect.
4. **Benzodiazepines:** Increased benzodiazepine effect.
5. **Carbamazepine:** Increased toxicity of both drugs secondary to altered metabolism.
6. **Corticosteroids:** Decreased INH serum concentration.
7. **Cycloserine:** CNS effects, dizziness, drowsiness.
8. **Disulfiram:** Psychotic episodes, ataxia secondary to altered dopamine metabolism.
9. **Phenytoin:** Increased phenytoin toxicity.
10. **Rifampin:** Possible increased hepatotoxicity.

Monitoring:

1. Baseline liver function studies; repeat with symptoms of hepatitis (fatigue, malaise, anorexia, weakness, nausea/vomiting) and serially at 2, 4, and 6 mo, especially in elderly.
2. Monthly clinical evaluation.

ISOPROTERENOL

Trade Name: *Isuprel.*

Drug Action: Primarily β_1- and β_2-receptor stimulant.

1. Increased heart rate, contractility, automaticity.
2. Decreased diastolic blood pressure, increased systolic blood pressure.

3. Decreased peripheral vascular resistance by producing vaso-dilation in skeletal muscle.
4. Increased myocardial O_2 demand secondary to increased heart rate, contractility.
5. Decreased O_2 supply by reducing diastolic blood pressure and lowering coronary perfusion pressure.
6. Bronchodilation.

Indications:

1. Bronchodilator: As IV infusion/aerosol.
2. Bradycardia.
3. AV heart block.
4. Cardiac transplantation.
5. Pulmonary hypertension.

Pharmacokinetics:

1. **Metabolism:** Catechol-*O*-methyltransferase in liver.
2. **Excretion:** Renal.
3. **Plasma half-life:** Very short, <5 min.
4. **Onset of action:** Immediate.

Drug Preparations:

Ampules: 1 mg/5 mL for IV/SQ.
Inhaler: 0.25%, 0.5%, 1%.
Tablets: 10, 15 mg.

Dosage:

1. **Adult:** Infusion 1–10 μg/min. Most commonly, 0.05–0.1 μg/kg/min.
2. **In bronchospasm:** Via inhaler, one to two inhalations q 3–4 hr.
3. **Sublingual:** 10–30 mg q 4–6 hr.

Adverse Effects:

1. Tachycardia, palpitations, angina.
2. Ventricular arrhythmias.
3. Myocardial necrosis after prolonged therapy.
4. CNS effects: Anxiety, fear, headache, dizziness, tremor.
5. **Other:** Nausea/vomiting, hyperglycemia, hypokalemia, diaphoresis.

Monitoring:

1. Heart rate, rhythm.
2. Blood pressure may decrease because of vasodilation.

BIBLIOGRAPHY

DiSesa VJ: The rational selection of inotropic drugs in cardiac surgery, *J Cardiac Surg* 1987, 2:385–406.

Kaplan JA: Treatment of perioperative left ventricular failure. In Kaplan JA (ed): *Cardiac Anesthesia,* Orlando, 1987, Grune & Stratton, pp 963–994.

Weiner N: Norepinephrine, epinephrine, and the sympathomimetic amines. In Gilman AG, Goodman LS, Gilman A (eds): *The Pharmacologic Basis of Therapeutics,* New York, 1980, Macmillan, pp 158–175.

ISOSORBIDE DINITRATE

Trade Names: *Isordil, sorbitrate*

Drug Actions: Organic nitrate, used primarily in patients with coronary artery disease; stimulates production of cGMP, resulting in vasodilation. Dilates coronary arteries. Relaxes esophageal muscle.

Indications:

1. Angina pectoris.
2. Congestive heart failure.
3. Relief of esophageal spasm.

Pharmacokinetics:

1. **Absorption:** Very rapid with sublingual; orally absorbed.
2. **Onset of action:** 2–4 min; duration 1–2 hr (sublingual), 4–6 hr (oral tablet), 6–12 hr (sustained-release tablet).
3. **Metabolism:** Liver.
4. **Excretion:** Urine, feces.
5. **Half-life:** 20–60 min.

Drug Preparations:

Sublingual tablets: 2.5, 5, 10 mg.
Tablets: 5, 10, 20, 30, 40 mg.
Sustained-release tablets: 40 mg.

Dosage:

1. Sublingual 2.5–5 mg to control acute symptoms, titrated to effect.
2. Oral tablets 5–40 mg q 6 hr.
3. Sustained-release tablets 40 mg q 8–12 hr.

Adverse Effects:

1. Hypotension, flushing, dizziness, palpitations, headache (average reported occurrence 25%).
2. Methemoglobinemia is reported with toxic doses.
3. Weakness, nausea/vomiting.
4. Rash.
5. Tolerance.

Drug Interactions: Alcohol and other vasodilating substances may substantially worsen the hypotension and dizziness induced by organic nitrates.

Monitoring: Cardiac evaluation is obviously recommended for any patient experiencing angina pectoris. Blood pressure, heart rate.

BIBLIOGRAPHY

Bomber JW, DeTullio PL: Oral nitrate preparations: an update, *Am Fam Physician* 1995, 52:2331–2337.

Abrams J: The role of nitrates in coronary heart disease, *Arch Intern Med* 1995, 155:357–364.

ISRADIPINE

Trade Name: *DynaCirc.*

Drug Actions: Slow calcium channel antagonist; vasodilator.

Indications:

1. Hypertension.
2. Congestive heart failure.
3. Migraine prophylaxis.

Pharmacokinetics:

1. **Absorption:** Rapid and nearly complete absorption following PO dosing.
2. **Onset of action:** 20 min, peak 2–3 hr.
3. **Metabolism:** Extensive first-pass metabolism in liver.
4. **Excretion:** Two thirds renal, one third excreted in feces.
5. **Half-life:** Terminal half-life is approximately 8 hr.

Drug Preparations:

Capsules: 2.5, 5 mg.

Dosage: 2.5 mg PO bid; increase by 5 mg/day q 2 wk to a maximum of 20 mg/day.

Adverse Effects:

1. Unlike other calcium channel blockers, isradipine has little effect on the cardiac conducting system. Hypotension, bradycardia, AV block, edema, palpitations, tachycardia, chest pain, arrhythmias.
2. Dizziness, fatigue, weakness, dyspnea, cough, headache, confusion.
3. Nausea/vomiting, diarrhea.
4. Rash, leukopenia, paresthesias.

Drug Interactions:

1. Potentiates antihypertensive effects of other vasodilators.
2. Increased effect when used with H_2 blockers.
3. Increased levels of carbamazepine, cyclosporine, digitalis, quinidine, theophylline.

Monitoring: Blood pressure, heart rate.

BIBLIOGRAPHY

1. Brogden RN, Sorken EM: Isradipine—an update of its pharmacodynamic and pharmacokinetic properties and therapeutic efficacy in the treatment of mild to moderate hypertension, *Drugs* 1995, 49:618–649.
2. Marty J: Role of isradipine and other antihypertensive agents in the treatment of peri- and postoperative hypertension, *Acta Anaesth Scand* 1993, 99:53–55.

ITRACONAZOLE

Trade Name: *Sporanox.*

Drug Actions:

1. Inhibits cytochrome P-450–dependent synthesis of ergosterol. (Like fluconazole, itraconazole has a lower binding affinity for mammalian P-450 enzymes than for fungal cytochrome enzymes.) Ergosterol is a sterol needed in fungal cytoplasmic membranes.
2. Spectrum of activity includes: *Blastomyces dermatitidis, Histoplasma capsulatum, H. duboisii, Aspergillus fumigatus, A. flavus,* and others (*Coccidiodes immitis, Paracoccidioides brasiliensis, Cryptococcus neoformans*). Itraconazole has varying activity against *Sporothrix schenckii, Trichophyton* spp., and *Candida* spp.

Indications:

1. Pulmonary and extrapulmonary blastomycosis.
2. Histoplasmosis, including pulmonary and disseminated *nonmeningeal* disease.
3. Pulmonary and extrapulmonary aspergillosis in patients who are intolerant of or refractory to treatment with amphotericin B. (Itraconazole is the only oral agent currently available with activity against *Aspergillus* spp.)
4. Although not an FDA-approved indication, patients with candidal infections may respond to itraconazole (including occasional cases of "azole-resistant thrush" where only fluconazole has been given).

Pharmacokinetics:

1. **Absorption:** PO. 55% availability after a meal (30% in fasting state), so should be taken with food or, better yet, an acidic beverage (cola) where absorption may approach 100%. Concentrations of itraconazole in fatty tissues, omentum, liver, kidney, and skin are two to twenty times plasma concentrations. There is essentially *no* penetration of itraconazole into the CSF.
2. **Excretion:** Fecal excretion of the parent drug is 3%–18%.
3. **Half-life:** Approximately 64 hr.

4. **Therapeutic level:** In treatment of aspergillosis, serum levels of 2–4 μg/mL are recommended.

Drug Preparations:

Capsules: 100 mg.

Dosage:

1. Blastomycosis and histoplasmosis: 200 mg PO q day (may give up to 200 mg bid if there is no improvement or if there is evidence of progression).
2. Aspergillosis: 200–400 mg/day (200 mg PO q day or 200 mg PO bid).
3. In life-threatening infections, a loading dose of 600 mg/day (200 mg PO tid) for the first 3 days should be considered.

Adverse Effects:

1. Nausea (10.6%), vomiting (5.1%), headache (3.8%), edema (3.5%), diarrhea (3.3%), hypokalemia (2.0%), and others.
2. Rash, although not common, occurs more frequently in immunocompromised patients receiving immunosuppressive medications.
3. Itraconazole does not have the significant risks of hepatotoxicity and adrenal or testicular function suppression seen with ketoconazole.

Drug Interactions:

1. Itraconazole elevates plasma concentrations of terfenadine (Seldane); serious cardiac dysrhythmias (including torsades de pointes) and death have occurred in patients taking these two drugs concomitantly. Additionally, another oral azole antifungal, ketoconazole, elevates plasma concentrations of astemizole (Hismanal) and its active metabolite desmethylastemizole, which may result in prolonged QT intervals. *Coadministration of itraconazole with terfenadine or astemizole (and possibly also loratadine) is contraindicated.*
2. Itraconazole may also increase levels of digoxin, cyclosporine, and oral hypoglycemics, and the anticoagulant effects of coumarin-like drugs may be enhanced.
3. Phenytoin, rifampin, H_2 antagonists, and isoniazid have decreased itraconazole plasma concentrations.

BIBLIOGRAPHY

Physicians' Desk Reference, ed 50, Montvale, 1996, Medical Economics Co.

Sanford JP, Gilbert DN, Sande MA (eds): *The Sanford Guide to Antimicrobial Therapy,* ed 26, Dallas, 1996, Antimicrobial Therapy.

KETAMINE

Trade Names: *Ketalar, Ketamine.*

Drug Actions: Rapid-acting general anesthetic with analgesic properties.

Indications: Anesthetic/analgesic for diagnostic and surgical procedures (laryngeal and pharyngeal reflexes usually maintained).

Pharmacokinetics:

1. **Absorption:** Give parenterally.
2. **Onset of action:** Seconds to minutes after IV dose (3–4 min after IM dose); duration of anesthesia after single dose IV 10–15 min.
3. **Metabolism:** Hepatic biotransformation.
4. **Excretion:** Urine (as metabolites).
5. **Half-life:** 10–15 min (alpha phase), beta phase 2.5 hr.

Drug Preparations:

Solution, IM injection: 10, 50, 100 mg/mL
Solution, IV injection: 10, 50 mg/mL.

Dosage: Titrate to effect; initial doses for induction of anesthesia: IV: 1–4 mg/kg (over 60 sec); for maintenance give one half initial dose as needed; IM: 6–13 mg/kg; smaller doses have been used for sedation/analgesia.

Adverse Effects: Emergence phenomena (dreamlike states, vivid imagery, hallucinations, delirium, confusion, excitement, irrational behavior); dissociative anesthesia, respiratory depression, apnea, laryngospasm, cardiovascular: blood pressure elevation, increased heart rate, arrhythmias, hypotension, bradycardia, diplopia, nystagmus, *tonic-clonic* movements, anorexia, nausea/vomiting, local pain at injection site.

Drug Interactions: Potentiates and prolongs action: Barbiturates, narcotics, other sedatives.

Monitoring: Cardiovascular function (blood pressure, heart rate), respiratory function (rate, O_2 saturation).

BIBLIOGRAPHY

Gilman AG, Rall TW, Nies AS, Taylor P (eds): *Goodman and Gilman's The Pharmacological Basis of Therapeutics,* ed 8, New York, 1990, Macmillan.

Denniston PL Jr (ed): *1995 Physicians GenRx,* Riverside, 1995, Denniston Publishing.

Physicians' Desk Reference, ed 49, Montvale, 1995, Medical Economics Data Production.

Miller RD (ed): *Anesthesia,* ed 4, New York, 1994, Churchill Livingstone.

Stoelting RK: *Pharmacology and Physiology in Anesthetic Practice,* ed 2, Philadelphia, 1991, JB Lippincott.

KETOCONAZOLE

Trade Name: *Nizoral.*

Drug Action:

1. Interferes with formation of membrane sterols and other membrane lipids.
2. Antifungal spectrum of activity includes *Candida, Blastomyces, Coccidioides, Histoplasma,* dermatophytes, etc.

Indications:

1. Chronic mucocutaneous candidiasis.
2. Dermatophyte infections recalcitrant to topical therapy or oral griseofulvin.
3. Selected candidal infections:
   a. Oral (and esophageal) involvement in HIV and other infections.
   b. Recurrent (chronic) vaginitis.

4. Systemic fungal infections, **excluding CSF involvement.**
   a. Paracoccidioiodomycosis, coccidioiodomycosis, blastomy-
      cosis, histoplasmosis, cryptococcosis, and others.

Pharmacokinetics:

1. **Absorption:** PO absorption variable but decreased without
   gastric acid.
   a. In achlorhydria, dissolve tablet in 4 mL 0.2N HCl; drink
      through glass straw.
2. **Metabolism:** Hepatic.
3. **Penetrates** poorly into CNS.
4. **Serum half-life:** 6.5–9.6 hr.

Drug Preparations:

Tablets: 200 mg.
Cream: 2%.

Dosage:

1. **Normal/impaired renal function:** 200–400 mg q 24 hr PO.

Adverse Effects:

1. **Nausea/vomiting:** Decreased if administered with meals.
2. **Hepatic dysfunction:** Usually reversible; rarely, fatal.
3. **Neurotoxicity:** Headache, dizziness, somnolence, hyposthesia.
4. **Hypersensitivity reaction:** Urticaria.
5. **Suppression** of serum testosterone levels (gynecomastia) and
   of cortisol production.
   a. Can block steroidogenesis in precocious puberty, and ec-
      topic hormone production in carcinomas.
6. Impotence, decreased libido, azospermia (with doses
   >800 mg/day).
7. Pruritus.
8. Thrombocytopenia, leukopenia, hemolytic anemia.

Drug Interactions:

1. **PO antacids:** Decreased absorption and antifungal effect.
2. **H$_2$ agonists** (e.g., cimetidine): Decreased absorption and antifungal effect.
3. **Rifampin:** Possible decreased fungistatic activity secondary to
   increased metabolism.
4. **Phenytoin:** Altered metabolism of both (monitor levels).

5. **PO anticoagulants:** Increased anticoagulant effect.
6. **Cyclosporin A:** Increased cyclosporin blood levels.
7. **PO hypoglycemic agents:** Increased hypoglycemic effect.
8. **Terfenadine:** concomitant use may result in ventricular arrhythmias.

Monitoring:

1. Liver function.
2. Adrenal function.

KETOROLAC

Trade Name: *Toradol.*

Drug Action:

1. Nonsteroidal anti-inflammatory.
2. Analgesic, antipyretic. Analgesic effect of 30–60 mg of ketorolac is similar to 12 mg morphine for acute surgical pain. Ceiling effect on analgesià at 30–60 mg dose. Higher doses prolong duration of analgesia without increasing analgesic efficacy.
3. Inhibits synthesis of prostaglandins.

Indications:

1. Pain.
2. Inflammation.

Pharmacokinetics:

1. **Absorption:** Give IM, IV, or PO. **Onset:** Pharmacologic effects after IM injection occur in 15 min with a peak analgesic effect in 2–3 hr.
2. **Metabolism:** Liver; <50% metabolized.
3. **Excretion:** Urine (clearance reduced in renal failure).
4. **Plasma-half life:** 4–6 hr.

Dosage:

1. **IM** 30–60 mg IM, then 15–30 mg q 6 hr for max. of 5 days. The lower recommended doses should be used for patients >60 yo or <50 kg weight.
2. **PO** 10 mg q 4–6 hr. Not recommended for chronic use.

Drug Preparations:

Preloaded syringes: 15 mg/mL, 30 mg/mL, 1–2 mL.
Tablets: 10 mg.

Adverse Effects:

1. **Respiratory:** Bronchospasm.
2. **GI:** Nausea, GI upset, ulcerations, gastritis, bleeding, perforations, hepatic injury, constipation, diarrhea, anorexia.
3. **Renal:** Nephrotoxicity, fluid retention.
4. **Hematologic:** Inhibits platelet aggregation (lasts 24–48 hr after drug discontinued), anemia, thrombocytopenia.
5. Headache, drowsiness, sweating, injection pain, seizures, vertigo, tremors, edema, hypertension, rash, pruritus.

Drug Interactions:

1. Should not be coadministered with aspirin or other NSAIDs. Side effects are additive.
2. Caution advised for use in patients on other anticoagulants; there is an increased risk of bleeding.
3. Diuretic response to furosemide reduced by 20% in healthy patients.
4. Excretion decreased by probenecid.
5. Inhibits renal excretion of lithium and clearance of methotrexate.

Monitoring:

1. Symptoms.
2. GI bleeding.
3. BUN, creatinine, liver function tests.

LABETALOL

Trade Names: *Normodyne, Trandate.*

Drug Action:

1. Selective α_1-adrenergic antagonist producing vasodilation.
2. Nonselective β-adrenergic antagonist with a potency of about one third to one quarter that of propranolol. Ratio of α-blockade to β-blockade is 1 : 3 to 1 : 7.

3. Membrane-stabilizing activity: not at clinically useful dosages.
4. Lacks intrinsic sympathomimetic activity (ISA).
5. Produces reduction in blood pressure while not affecting cardiac output and heart rate.

Indications:

1. Rapid control of acute hypertension.
2. Treatment of chronic hypertension.
3. Treatment of pheochromocytomia: Must be used with care, because paradoxical increases in blood pressure have been reported with this drug.

Pharmacokinetics:

1. **Absorption:** PO/IV.
2. **Metabolism:** Hepatic.
3. **Excretion:** 5% excreted unchanged in urine.
4. **Protein-binding:** 50%.
5. **Plasma half-life:** Approximately 5 hr.
6. **Onset of action:** Almost immediate.

Drug Preparations:

Vials: 100 mg/20 mL, 25 mg/5 mL, 200 mg/40 mL
Tablets: 100, 200, 300 mg.

Dosage:

1. **PO:** Begin with 100–200 mg bid; taper to effect. Usual maintenance dosage is 200–400 mg bid.
2. **IV:** For rapid control of blood pressure, IV bolus doses of 5–20 mg given slowly; can be repeated after 5 min. Dosage of 50–100 mg may be required.
3. **Continuous infusion** of 1 mg/mL can be started at 1–2 mg/min and titrated to effect.

Adverse Effects:

1. Worsening of congestive heart failure, bradycardia, dizziness.
2. Exacerbation of angina pectoris on withdrawal of drug.
3. May promote bronchospasm in patients with asthma or chronic obstructive pulmonary disease.
4. May block signs of hypoglycemia in diabetics.
5. Orthostatic hypotension.

Drug Interactions:

1. Cimetidine increases bioavailability of labetalol.
2. Labetalol blunts reflex tachycardia associated with concurrent nitroglycerin use.
3. Synergism with halothane to produce hypotension.
4. Potentiates antihypertensive effects of other antihypertensive agents.
5. Antagonizes bronchodilation from β-agonists.

Monitoring: Blood pressure, heart rate, respiratory status.

BIBLIOGRAPHY

Kates RA: Antianginal drug therapy. In Kaplan JA (ed): *Cardiac Anesthesia*, vol 1, New York, 1987, Grune & Stratton.

LAXATIVES/STOOL SOFTENERS

More than 120 laxative preparations are currently on the market. To cover them all would be exhaustive; therefore, selected products in each category are discussed.

Trade Names:

1. Bulking agents:
    Methylcellulose: *Citrucel.*
    Malt soup extract: *Maltsupex.*
    Polycarbophil: *Mitrolan.*
    Psyllium: *Metamucil, Naturacil, Konsyl, Perdiem* (contains stimulants).
    Plant gums: *Kondrem* (contains stimulants).
2. Emollients:
    Docusate sodium: *Colace, Peri-Colace* (contains stimulants), *Doxinate, Modane.*
    Docusate calcium: *Surfak, Doxidan* (contains stimulants).
    Docusate potassium: *Dialose.*
3. Lubricants:
    Mineral oils: *Fleet Enema Oil Retention, Haley's M-O* (contains saline solution), *Neo-Cultol*
4. Saline agents:

Magnesium citrate: *Citroma.*
Magnesium hydroxide: *Milk of Magnesia, Haley's M-O* (contains mineral oil).
Sodium phosphate: *Fleet Enema.*
5. Stimulants:
Bisacodyl: *Dulcolax, Carter's Little Pills.*
Cascara sagrada: *Caroid.*
Caster oil: *Neoloid.*
Casanthrol: *Peri-Colace* (contains emollients or mineral oil).
Danthron: *Doxidan.*
Phenophthalein: *Ex-Lax, Feen-A-Mint, Correctol* (contains emollients or mineral oil).
Senna: *Fletcher's Castoria, Senokot.*
6. Hyperosmotic agents:
Glycerin.
Lactulose: *Cephulac, Chronulac.*
Combination salts: *Go LYTELY.*

Drug Action:

1. Bulking agents swell, forming a gel that stimulates peristalsis.
2. Emollients are surfactants that facilitate stool mixing and softening.
3. Lubricants act by coating fecal contents and decreasing water absorption.
4. Saline agents are osmotically active products that increase intraluminal volume, thereby stimulating peristalsis.
5. Stimulants act by poorly understood mechanisms ranging from direct nerve stimulation to decreasing fluid, sodium, and glucose absorption.
6. Hyperosmotic agents increase intraluminal contents and stimulate peristalsis.

Indications:

1. Constipation.
2. Irritable bowel syndrome (bulking agents).
3. Acute bowel evacuation before procedures (e.g., barium enema, colonoscopy, surgery).
4. Hyperammonemia, acute and chronic therapy (lactulose).

Pharmacokinetics:

1. **Absorption:** All act locally with virtually no systemic absorption.

2. **Onset of action:**
   a. Bulking agents: 12–24 hr (up to 72 hr).
   b. Emollients: 24–48 hr (up to 3–5 days).
   c. Lubricants: 6–8 hr (12 hr if taken q hs).
   d. Saline solution: 30 min–3 hr.
   e. Stimulants: 6–8 hr, except castor oil, 2–6 hr.

Drug Preparations: *See* Table 16.

Dosage:

Drug	Daily Dosage
Bulk	
Methylcellulose	4–6 gm PO
Malt soup extract	12 gm PO
Polycarbophil	4–6 gm PO
Psyllium	Variable, generally 1 tablespoon bid/tid
Plant gums	Variable
Emollient	
Docusate sodium	50–360 mg PO
Docusate calcium	50–360 mg PO
Docusate potassium	100–300 mg PO
Saline solution	
Magnesium citrate	200 mL PO
Magnesium hydroxide	2.4–4.8 gm PO
Sodium phosphate	Variable, generally 10 oz PR
Lubricant	
Mineral oil	15–45 mL
Stimulant	
Bisacodyl	5–15 mg PO
Cascara	Variable
Castor oil	15–60 mg PO
Casanthrol	Variable
Danthron	75–150 mg PO
Phenophthalein	30–270 mg PO
Senna	Variable
Hyperosmotic	
Glycerin	3 gm suppository PR
Lactulose	15–60 mL PO

TABLE 16.

Drug Preparations

Drug	Tabs/Caps	Liquid	Powder
Bulk			
Methylcellulose	500 mg	450 mg/5 mL	Available
Malt soup extract	750 mg	5 g/5 mL	5 g/tsp
Polycarbophil	500 mg	—	—
Psyllium	1.7 g	—	3–5 g/tsp
Plant gums	—	Available	—
Emollient			
Docusate sodium	50–300 mg	10–50 mg/5 mL	—
Docusate calcium	50–240 mg	—	—
Docusate potassium	100–240 mg	—	—
Saline solution			
Magnesium citrate	—	2 g/dL	—
Magnesium hydroxide	325, 650 mg	400 mg/5 mL	—
Sodium phosphate	—	18–48 g/100 mL	2 g/10g

Lubricant		
Mineral oil	—	Available
Stimulant		
Bisacodyl	5 mg	—
Cascara	325 mg	Available
Castor oil	—	Available
Casanthrol	Combined with docusate in Peri-Colace	—
Danthron	37.5/75 mg	37.5 mg/5 mL
Phenophthalein	60, 90, 97.5 mg	65 mg/15 mL
Senna	187, 218 mg	325, 350, 400 mg/5 mL
Hyperosmotic		
Glycerin	Suppositories	3 gm
Lactulose	—	10 mg/15 mL
Combination agents	—	Available

Adverse Effects:

1. Bulk:
   a. GI impaction caused by insufficient fluid intake.
   b. Allergic rash, asthma occur rarely.
   c. In some patients, bulking agents cause abdominal bloating and flatus.
2. Emollient:
   a. Abdominal cramping.
   b. Rare skin rash.
3. Saline solution:
   a. Abdominal cramping.
   b. Confusion.
   c. Magnesium toxicity (e.g., weakness, dizziness, fatigue, decreased deep tendon reflexes), particularly in patients with chronic renal failure.
4. Lubricant:
   a. Rectal irritation.
   b. Lipoid pneumoconiosis can occur in chronic aspirators (elderly, neurologically impaired).
5. Stimulant:
   a. Abdominal cramping, diarrhea.
   b. Confusion.
   c. Electrolyte disorders.
   d. Cardiac complications.
6. Hyperosmotic: Abdominal cramping, diarrhea, increased gas formation.

Drug Interactions:

1. Bulk: Decreases absorption of digitalis, warfarin, tetracyclines.
2. Emollient: Enhances absorption of stimulant laxatives and phenothiazines. Decreases absorption of tetracycline.
3. Saline solution: Reduces effectiveness of warfarin, digitalis, phenothiazines. Decreases absorption of tetracycline.
4. Lubricant: Decreases absorption of warfarin, PO contraceptives, digitalis, fat-soluble vitamins (A, D, E, K).
5. Stimulant: Do not use concurrently with milk or antacids, because rapid tablet dissolution may result in gastric and duodenal irritation. Prolonged use can cause melanosis coli and "cathartic colon."

6. Hyperosmotic: Reduces effectiveness of warfarin, digitalis, phenothiazines. Decreases absorption of tetracycline.

Comments/Recommendations: Constipation, whether perceived or real, is common. The many prescription and over-the-counter laxatives available attest to the national concern about bowel habits. However, although confronting the problem almost daily, physicians receive little information about constipation and its treatment in medical school curriculums.

Normal bowel patterns range from one stool tid to one q 3 days. Convincing patients that moving the bowels once every 3 days is normal can be difficult, particularly if they perceive otherwise. Constipation is more common in the elderly, for multiple reasons, including low-residue diet, decreased abdominal muscle tone, sedentary life style, and medications (e.g., analgesics, diuretics, antidepressants, antacids).

Therapy for chronic constipation should begin with a trial of dietary changes coupled with increased exercise and elimination of unnecessary medications. Attempts should be made to increase dietary fiber to 30 g/day. Good food sources of fiber include bran cereals, sunflower seeds, various nuts, green peas, beans, squash, artichokes, dates, berries, pears, and raisins. A good rule of thumb that allows dietary flexibility and approaches the recommended 30 g/day is three slices of whole-wheat bread, one bowl of high-fiber cereal, and four products from the fruit and vegetable category, in any combination.

Bulk-forming laxatives should be the first drug therapy for patients with refractory chronic constipation. The most frequent dosing error is not encouraging adequate fluid intake. At least 8 oz water should be given with each dose, and daily fluid intake should be liberalized. Other than for short courses, stimulants should be avoided in patients with irritable bowel syndrome or diverticular disease. Bulking agents are recommended for bedridden or institutionalized patients. Additional agents are occasionally needed to prevent fecal impaction. Milk of magnesia, lactulose, and enemas are often effective. Mineral oil is to be avoided because of the risk of aspiration.

Stool softeners may be used in hospitalized patients in whom straining may be harmful (e.g., cardiac patients, postoperative patients).

For the outpatient with acute constipation, any product can be used for the short term. Patients who chronically use nonbulking laxatives, particularly stimulants, should be tapered off them and dietary or bulking substitutions made. Stimulants should be tapered, because the bowel becomes dependent with chronic use. Abrupt cessation may lead to ileus.

For bowel evacuation prior to radiographic, surgical, or endoscopic evaluation, it is best to consult the specialists performing the procedure.

BIBLIOGRAPHY

AMA Drug Evaluations, ed 6, Philadelphia, 1986, WB Saunders.
Drug Information for the Health Care Provider, ed 6, Rockville,
    1986, US Pharmacopeial Convention.
Tedesco F: Laxative use in constipation, *Am J Gastroenterol*
    1985, 80:303–309.

LIDOCAINE

Trade Name: *Xylocaine.*

Drug Action:

1. Local anesthetic effects by binding to and inhibiting sodium channels.
2. Depresses conduction velocity (phase 0) and slope of phase 4 of the action potential.
3. Prolongs refractoriness only in ventricular Purkinje fibers.
4. Slows conduction and prolongs refractoriness of accessory pathways.

Indications:

1. Local anesthetic.
2. Ventricular arrhythmias.
3. In patients with acute myocardial infarction:
   a. Treatment of premature ventricular contractions.
   b. Prevention of recurrent episodes of ventricular fibrillation in patients after resuscitation.

Pharmacokinetics:

1. **Metabolism:** Hepatic.
2. **Excretion:** Metabolites excreted in urine.
3. **Protein binding:** 50%–75%.
4. **Plasma half-life:** 100 min.

Drug Preparations:

Vials: 10, 20 mg/mL in 5, 30, 50 mL vials.

Dosage:

1. **Continuous infusion:** 1–4 mg/min; usually preceded by a bolus of 1.0–1.5 mg/kg given twice over 20 min.
2. **IM:** 200–300 mg.

Adverse Effects:

1. **Cardiac:** Toxic levels produce bradycardia, hypotension, myocardial depression.
2. **CNS:** High drug levels can produce anxiety, seizures, depression, lethargy, unconsciousness, respiratory arrest, confusion, tremor, paresthesias, slurred speech.
3. **Other:** Nausea/vomiting, rash, edema, bronchospasm, anaphylaxis.

Drug Interactions:

1. Reduced hepatic metabolism (elevated levels): Cimetadine, β-blockers.
2. Additive toxicity when used with other antiarrhythmic agents.

Drug Monitoring:

1. Drug levels, if available; therapeutic level 1.5–5 μg/mL.
2. Beware of lethargy, sedative effects; may be prodrome to seizure activity.

BIBLIOGRAPHY

Bigger JT Jr, Hoffman BF: Antiarrhythmic drugs. In Gilman AG, Goodman LS, Gilman A (eds): *The Pharmacological Basis of Therapeutics,* New York, 1980, Macmillan, pp 761–792.

Zipes DP: Management of cardiac arrhythmias: pharmacological, electrical, and surgical techniques. In Braunwald E (ed): *Heart Disease: A Textbook of Cardiovascular Medicine,* Philadelphia, 1988, WB Saunders, pp 621–657.

LITHIUM

Trade Names:

Lithium citrate: *Carbolith.*
Lithium carbonate: *Eskalith, Lithane, Lithonate, Lithotabs.*

Drug Action:

1. Antimanic, antidepressant.
2. Alters sodium transport in nerve and muscle.
3. Blocks antidiuretic hormone effect on renal collecting duct.
4. Stimulates granulopoiesis.
5. Blocks thyroid hormone release.

Indications:

1. Manic-depressive illness (bipolar disorders).
2. Depression (unipolar).
3. Syndrome of inappropriate antidiuresis (SIADH).
4. Cluster headache.
5. Hyperthyroidism.

Pharmacokinetics:

1. **Absorption:** PO; complete in 6–8 hr.
2. **Metabolism:** None.
3. **Distribution:** Total body water.
4. **Serum half-life:** 24 hr.
5. **Excretion:**
   a. 95% unchanged in urine; 80% reabsorbed in renal tubules.
   b. Competes with sodium for reabsorption; **decrease dose in patients with renal disease or advanced age.**
   c. Excreted in breast milk; crosses placenta.
6. **Therapeutic serum concentration for manic-depressive illness:** Acute: 1–1.5 mEq/L; maintenance 0.6–1.2 mEq/L.

Drug Preparations:

Lithium carbonate: *Capsules:* 300 mg; *Tablets:* 300 mg; *Controlled release tablets:* 450 mg.
Lithium citrate: *Syrup:* 8 mEq (300 mg)/5 mL.

Dosage:

1. Should be individualized using serum levels and clinical response.

2. **Acute mania:** 600 mg tid PO immediate release tablets; 900 mg bid controlled release tablets.
3. **Maintenance for bipolar disorder:** 300 mg tid–qid PO immediate release tablets; 450 mg bid controlled release tablets.
4. Immediate release tablets are given tid or qid; controlled release tablets are given bid.

Adverse Effects:

1. **Neurologic:** Drowsiness, stupor, coma, confusion, dysarthria, tremor, dizziness, ataxia, nystagmus, blurred vision, fasciculations, seizures, hyperactive reflexes, dry mouth, psychosis, choreoathetoid movements, rigidity, syncope, weakness, pseudotumor cerebri.
2. **Cardiovascular:** Arrhythmias, SA block, QRS widening, T-wave changes, bradycardia, hypotension, acute circulatory failure.
3. Nephrogenic diabetes insipidus, dehydration, thirst, polyuria, polydipsia. Approximately 60% of patients taking lithium exhibit a renal concentrating defect. Does not correlate with serum levels.
4. Hypothyroidism, goiter, hyperparathyroidism.
5. Diarrhea, anorexia, nausea/vomiting, abdominal pain.
6. Impaired renal function, leukopenia (rare), mild leukocytosis common, skin rashes, allergic reactions.

Drug Interactions:

1. Increased serum lithium levels and toxicity by decreased renal excretion: Antithyroid drugs, iodinated glycerol, potassium iodide, anti-inflammatory drugs, diuretics (cause increased proximal tubule reabsorption).
2. Decreased serum lithium levels by increased urinary excretion: Caffeine, xanthines.
3. Lithium prolongs effects of atracurium, pancuronium, succinylcholine.
4. Lithium decreases effects of phenothiazines, carbamazepine, desmopressin, lypressin, vasopressin.
5. Drugs that increase lithium effects include carbamazepine, haloperidol, methyldopa, phenothiazines, phenytoin, probenecid, spironolactone, tetracycline.
6. Drugs that decrease lithium effects include acetazolamide, osmotic diuretics, sodium chloride, sodium bicarbonate, verapamil.
7. Lithium and iodides have synergistic antithyroid effects.

8. Renal reabsorption of lithium is increased with volume depletion, decreased with sodium loading.

Monitoring:

1. Serum lithium level: 1.0–1.5 mEq/L during initial treatment;
0.6–1.2 mEq/L during maintenance therapy.
2. ECG.
3. Creatinine.
4. Serum sodium, potassium.
5. Thyroxine, thyroid-stimulating hormone.
6. Body weight.

BIBLIOGRAPHY

MacGregor DA, Baker AM. Hyperosmolar coma due to lithium-
induced nephrogenic diabetes insipidus, *Lancet* 1995,
346:413–417.
Lithium. In *AMA Drug Evaluations,* ed 6, Philadelphia, 1986, WB
Saunders, pp 148–150.
Lithium. In *Drug Facts and Comparisons,* Philadelphia, 1989, JB
Lippincott, pp 1111–1115.

LORAZEPAM

Trade Name: *Ativan.*

Drug Action: Anxiety reduction, sedation, anticonvulsant activity, muscle relaxation, amnesia.

Indications: Anxiety, insomnia, status epilepticus, alcohol withdrawal, anesthesia premedication.

Drug Preparations:

Tablets: 0.5, 1, 2 mg
Injection: 2, 4 mg/mL.

Dosage:

1. **Anxiety:** 2–10 mg/day in two to four divided doses PO/IV/IM.
2. **Other indications:** Premedication for anesthesia: 1–4 mg PO
or IM.
3. **Sedation:** 1–2 mg q 1–4 hr IV bolus; 1–4 mg/hr by IV infusion.

Pharmacokinetics:

1. **Metabolism:** Hepatic conjugation.
2. **Half-life:** 15 hr (mean).
3. **Excretion:** Renal excretion of inactive metabolites.
4. **Dialyzable?:** Limited.
5. **Renal failure:** Monitor for excess sedation.
6. **Hepatic failure:** Reduce dosage.

Adverse Effects: Sedation, psychomotor impairment, depression, amnesia, impaired concentration, weakness, impaired sexual function, paradoxical agitation, hypotension, respiratory depression.

Drug Interactions: Additive effect with other CNS depressants. Onset is slow (20–40 min) even when given by IV route.

Monitoring: Excess sedation vs. therapeutic effect.

BIBLIOGRAPHY

Drugs used for anxiety and sleep disorders. In *AMA Drug Evaluations,* ed 6, Philadelphia, 1986, WB Saunders, pp 81–110.
Sussman N: The benzodiazepines: selection and use in treating anxiety, insomnia, and other disorders, *Hosp Formul* 1985, 20:298–305.

MAGNESIUM

Trade Names:

Magnesium sulfate: Various.

Magnesium oxide: *Uro-Mag, Mag-Ox 400, Maox.*

Magnesium carbonate: (Primarily an antacid) *Gaviscon, Mylanta gelcaps.*

Magnesium gluconate: *Almora, Magonate.*

Magnesium hydroxide: (Primarily a laxative or antacid) *Milk of Magnesia, Maalox, Mylanta, Gelusil.*

Drug Action:

1. Coenzyme involved in many enzymatic reactions, including phosphatases, sodium potassium ATPases, protein and carbohydrate metabolism.

2. Important for muscle contraction and nerve conduction.
3. Regulates parathyroid gland function.
4. Calcium channel antagonist.
5. Important for maintenance of potassium and calcium homeostasis.
6. Stabilizes membranes.
7. Anticonvulsant action, inhibits neuromuscular transmission.
8. Inhibits uterine contractions.

Indications:

1. Hypomagnesemia.
2. Cellular magnesium depletion.
3. Cardiac arrhythmias.
4. Eclampsia/preeclampsia.

Pharmacokinetics:

1. **Absorption:** 15%–30% absorbed from GI tract (depends on form).
2. **Distribution:** Throughout body.
3. **Metabolism:** None.
4. **Excretion:** Renal. Reduce dose in patients with renal insufficiency.
5. **Duration:**
    a. IV: Immediately; effects last approximately 30 min (with normal renal function).
    b. IM: Peaks in 60 min; effects last 3–4 hr.
6. Crosses placenta; may cause respiratory and neuromuscular depression in newborn.
7. Excreted in breast milk.

Drug Preparations: (1 mEq = 12 mg elemental Mg):

1. Magnesium sulfate (1 g = 8.12 mEq Mg = 98 mg Mg):
    Solution: 10% (0.8 mEq/mL), 12.5% (1 mEq/mL), 25% (2 mEq/mL), 50% (4 mEq/mL), for injection. May give IV or IM. Granules: 40 mEq/5 G; Oral solution: 50% (500 mg/mL; 4 mEq/mL).
2. Magnesium gluconate (500 mg =27 mg Mg):
    Tablets: 500 mg.
3. Magnesium carbonate:
    Tablets: 250 mg.

4. Magnesium oxide:
   Capsules: 140 mg (84.5 mg Mg)
   Tablets: 400 mg (241 mg Mg).
5. Magnesium hydroxide (*Milk of Magnesia*): Primarily a laxative.
   Solution: 7.75% (405 mg Mg/5 mL).
   Tablets: 325 mg (311 mg Mg).

Dosage:

1. **Hypomagnesemic seizures/cardiac arrhythmias:** 1–2 g magnesium sulfate IV over 15 min, then 1–2 g IV q 4–6 hr.
2. **Eclampsia/preeclampsia:** Initial dose 4 g magnesium sulfate IV over 5–15 min, then 1–4 g IV per hr. Alternatively, 4 g IV over 15 min and 4 g IM as loading dose, then 4 g IM q 4 hr.
3. **Hypomagnesemia:**
   a. **Mild:** Adults, 1 g magnesium sulfate IV/IM q 6 hr (392 mg/day or 32 mEq/day) for 3–5 days, plus excess losses. Children, 3–6 mg/kg/day in divided doses three to four times/day.
   b. **Severe:** 5 g magnesium sulfate (40 mEq) over 4 hr, then 1 g q 4–6 hr for 3–5 days, plus excess losses.
   c. **PO:** May cause diarrhea.
4. **RDA:** Adult: 300–400 mg/day (4.5 mg/kg/day).
5. **Hyperalimentation:** Adult: 8–24 mEq/day.

Adverse Effects:

1. **Cardiovascular:** Vasodilation, flushing, sweating, hypotension, conduction abnormalities, heart block, asystole, ECG (increased PR interval, increased QRS complex, prolonged QT interval).
2. **Respiratory:** Weakness, paralysis, respiratory depression.
3. **Renal:** Magnesium accumulates in renal failure.
4. **Neuromuscular:** CNS depression, coma, drowsiness, depressed reflexes, muscle weakness, paralysis, hypothermia.
5. **GI:** Diarrhea (PO), abdominal cramps.
6. **Metabolic:** Hypocalcemia.

Drug Interactions:

1. Concomitant use with alcohol, narcotics, anxiolytics, barbiturates, antidepressants, hypnotics, antipsychotics, general anesthetics may increase CNS depressant effects.

2. Concomitant use with succinylcholine, tubocurarine, and other neuromuscular blockers potentiates and prolongs neuromuscular blockade.
3. Magnesium administration may potentiate heart block when used with digitalis; hypomagnesemia may potentiate arrhythmias in patients receiving digitalis.
4. Excretion increased by loop diuretics.
5. Ritodrine and magnesium sulfate have additive cardiac side effects.
6. Oral magnesium may decrease absorption of drugs (tetracyclines, digoxin, indomethacin, iron).

Overdose:

1. Respiratory depression and cardiac toxicity. Antagonized by IV calcium (5–10 mEq over 5 min).
2. Supportive.
3. Remove magnesium from body (e.g., diuresis, dialysis).

Monitoring:

1. Deep tendon reflexes, blood pressure, heart rate, respiratory rate, ECG.
2. **Serum magnesium level** (anticonvulsant serum levels range from 2.5–7.5 mEq/L).
   a. **Normal serum level:** 1.7–2.4 mEq/L.
   b. **Therapeutic level for eclampsia/preeclampsia:** 4–7 mEq/L.
   c. **Loss of deep tendon reflexes; hypotension:** 7–10 mEq/L.
   d. **Respiratory paralysis:** 12–15 mEq/L.
   e. **Heart block, cardiac arrest:** >15 mEq/L.
3. Renal Function.
4. Serum potassium, calcium.

BIBLIOGRAPHY

Zaloga GP, Chernow B: Divalent ions—calcium, magnesium, and phosphorus. In Chernow B (ed): *The Pharmacologic Approach to the Critically Ill Patient,* ed 3, Baltimore, 1994, Williams & Wilkins, pp 777–804.

MANNITOL

Trade Name: *Osmitrol.*

Drug Action:

1. **Cerebral dehydration:** Enhances movement of fluid across blood-brain barrier from brain tissue and CSF to intravascular compartment by elevating plasma osmolality. Could potentially worsen cerebral edema if blood-brain barrier is not intact. Free radical scavenging properties also are potentially beneficial in neurologic injury.
2. **Osmotic diuresis:** Mannitol is not absorbed by renal tubules; thus, increased osmolality of glomerular filtrate facilitates excretion of water and inhibits reabsorption of sodium, chloride, and other solutes.
3. **Antidote:** Induced diuresis facilitates excretion of solutes and promotes clearance of potentially nephrotoxic substances, thereby preventing accumulation in tubular fluid.
4. **Antiglaucoma action:** Enhances flow of fluid from the eye into the vascular compartment by osmotic action, with consequent reduction in intraocular pressure.

Indications:

1. **Acute oliguria:** Possible adjunct in therapy for oliguria when attempting to prevent acute renal failure in oliguric states. Other measures must also be taken to ensure adequate circulating blood volume and renal perfusion.
2. **Cerebral edema:** Reduces cerebral edema, thus decreasing intracranial pressure.
3. **Acute glaucoma:** Reduces acutely increased intraocular pressure.
4. **Toxin excretion:** Nonspecifically enhances renal excretion of potentially nephrotoxic substances, such as salicylates, barbiturates, bromides, lithium.

Pharmacokinetics:

1. **Absorption:** IV.
2. **Metabolism:** Slight hepatic metabolism to glycogen.
3. **Excretion:** Renal, 80% in 3 hr.

4. **Volume of distribution:** Extracellular fluid.
5. **Plasma half-life:** Approximately 100 min. May be increased in renal failure.
6. **Onset of action:** Diuresis in 1–3 hr, tissue osmotic effect approximately 15 min after start of infusion.
7. **Duration:** Reduction in intraocular and intracerebral pressure will persist for 3–8 hr.

Drug Preparations:

Solution: 5%, 10%, 15%, 20%, 25% concentrations.

Dosage:

1. **Adult:** Usual adult limit is up to 6 g/kg body weight/24 hr or until serum osmolality >310 mOsm/kg water.
   a. **Diuretic:** 50–100 g as 5%–25% solution IV over 1–2 hr.
   b. **Osmotic agent for cerebral edema:** IV infusion 0.15–2.0 g/kg as 15%–25% solution over 30–60 min.
   c. **Toxin excretion:** IV infusion 50–200 g as 5%–25% solution to maintain urinary flow at 100–500 mL/hr.
   d. **Glaucoma:** 1.5–2.0 g/kg as 20%–25% solution IV over 30–60 min.
2. **Pediatric:**
   a. **Diuretic:** 2.0 g/kg body weight as 15%–20% solution over 2–6 hr IV.
   b. **Osmotic agent for edema:** 0.15–2.0 g/kg body weight IV as 15%–20% solution over 30–60 min.
   c. **Toxin excretion:** Up to 2.0 g/kg body weight IV as 5%–10% solution.

Adverse Effects:

1. Common:
   a. Fluid/electrolyte imbalance:
      (1) Hypervolemia (particularly with large doses administered rapidly).
      (2) Hypovolemia (occasionally resulting in prerenal azotemia).
      (3) Dilutional hyponatremia (acutely or if renal excretion delayed).
      (4) Hypernatremia (loss of water in excess of sodium).
      (5) Hyperkalemia.

2. Uncommon:
    (1) Chills or fever.
    (2) Mental status changes, headache, confusion.
    (3) Chest pain (resembles angina).
    (4) Muscle cramps/pain.
    (5) Seizures.
    (6) Thrombophlebitis.
    (7) Acute renal failure.

Drug Interactions: Electrolyte-free mannitol solutions should not be given conjointly with blood; may enhance renal excretion of drugs (e.g., lithium).

Monitoring:

1. Follow serum osmolality.
2. Frequent blood pressure determinations.
3. Serum electrolyte determinations, including potassium and sodium.
4. Volume status.
5. Urinary output.

BIBLIOGRAPHY

Antianginal agents. In *AMA Drug Evaluations Annual,* 1995, American Medical Association, pp 841, 843, 2244.

Diuretics and cardiovasculars. In *Drug Facts and Comparisons,* Philadelphia, 1996, JB Lippincott, pp 669.

Mannitol. In *Drug Information for the Health Care Provider,* vol 1, ed 15, Rockville, 1995, US Pharmacopeial Convention, pp 1769.

MEPERIDINE

Trade Names: *Demerol, Mepergan* (in combination with promethazine); plus generic preparations.

Drug Action:

1. Similar to morphine (e.g., it acts at opiate receptors, producing analgesia and sedation), but morphine has about six to eight times the potency of meperidine.

2. Meperidine has some structural similarities with atropine and thus may produce less smooth muscle spasm.

Indications:

1. Moderate to severe pain; preoperative medication; adjunct to general, regional, or local anesthesia.
2. Not useful as an antitussive or antidiarrheal agent.
3. Effective in treating postoperative shivering.

Pharmacokinetics:

1. **Absorption:** Good PO absorption, although this route of administration is approximately half as effective as the parenteral route, owing to first-pass hepatic metabolism. Peak effects occur in 45 min with PO, 30 min with IM, 10 min with IV administration. Duration of action is 3–4 hr with PO/IM/IV administration.
2. **Metabolism:** Primarily in liver via hydrolysis or *N*-demethylation followed by hydrolysis. Glucuronide conjugation may then also occur after either of the previous steps.
3. **Excretion:** Predominantly urinary.
4. **Half-life:** Elimination t½ in plasma is 3–4 hr.

Drug Preparations:

Solution: 50 mg/5 mL PO.
Tablets: 50, 100 mg.
Vials: 25, 50, 75, 100 mg/mL IV/IM/SQ.

Dosage:

1. **Adult:**
   a. **PO/IM/SQ:** Usual dose 50–150 mg q 3–4 hr.
   b. **IV:** 20–40 mg given slowly over several minutes.
      (1) **Postoperative shivering:** 10–20 mg.
2. **Pediatric:**
   a. **PO/IM/SQ:** 1.1–1.5 mg/kg q 3–4 hr.
3. **Severe liver disease:** Decrease dosage and/or frequency of administration.

Adverse Effects:

1. Many adverse effects are similar to those of morphine, especially with equianalgesic doses. These include euphoria, drowsiness, confusion, respiratory depression, nausea/vomiting, constipation, urinary retention, hypotension, seizures.

2. Secondary to atropine-like effects, meperidine may produce mydriasis and dry mouth, and may increase ventricular response rate in patients with supraventricular tachycardia.
3. There may be less biliary spasm than with morphine.
4. Meperidine is the only narcotic that has a negative inotropic effect when used in high doses.
5. Normeperidine, a metabolite, has been reported to accumulate with prolonged administration in patients with renal disease and produce CNS excitation. A substitute narcotic should probably be used in these patients.

Drug Interactions:

1. Sedative and respiratory depressant actions may be augmented in patients receiving sedatives, hypnotics, tricyclic antidepressants, alcohol, phenothiazines, other CNS depressants.
2. Administration of meperidine in patients taking MAO inhibitors has been implicated in causing severe reactions, ranging from coma, hypotension, and respiratory depression to convulsions, hyperpyrexia, tachycardia, and hypertension.

Monitoring: Mental status; respiratory rate, blood pressure, heart rate.

BIBLIOGRAPHY

Gilman AG, Goodman LS, Rall TW, et al (eds): *Goodman and Gilman's The Pharmacological Basis of Therapeutics,* ed 7, New York, 1985, Macmillan.

McEvoy GK (ed): *AHFS Drug Information 89,* Bethesda, 1989, American Society of Hospital Pharmacists.

Physicians' Desk Reference, ed 42, Oradell, 1988, Medical Economics Co.

METHICILLIN

Trade Name: *Staphcillin.*

Drug Action:

1. Inhibits cell wall synthesis (penicillin).
2. Active against staphylococci.

Indications: Staphylococcal infections

Pharmacokinetics:

1. **Absorption:** Not appreciably absorbed PO.
2. **Excretion:** Renal.
3. **Serum half-life:** 30 min.
4. **Distribution:** CSF penetration enhanced by meningeal inflammation.

Drug Preparations:

Vials: 1, 4, 6 g for parenteral use.

Dosage:

1. **Normal renal function:** 1–2 g q 4–6 hr parenterally.
2. **Impaired renal function:**

Dose (g)	Creatinine Clearance	Interval (hr)
1–2	>80	4–6
	80–50	6
	50–10	8
	<10 (anuria)	12

3. **Hemodialysis:** Supplemental dose of 2 g after each dialysis.

Adverse Effects:

1. Similar to other penicillins, e.g., hypersensitivity reactions, cytopenias, positive Coombs test, neuropathy, seizures, cholestasis, diarrhea, hemolytic anemia.
2. **Methicillin nephritis:** Acute interstitial nephritis occurring 5 or more days after starting, and associated with:
   a. Abnormal urinalysis: Proteinuria, hematuria, eosinophiluria.
   b. Eosinophilia.
   c. Fever, rash; possibly arthralgias.
   d. Deteriorating renal function.
   e. 90% reversible.
   f. Also reported with other penicillins.

Monitoring: Urinalysis, neurologic status, periodic renal/hepatic/hematopoietic function, bacterial antibiotic sensitivity.

METHIMAZOLE

Trade Name: *Tapazole.*

Drug Action: Antithyroid drug; inhibits synthesis of thyroid hormones by interfering with incorporation of iodide into tyrosine.

Indication: Hyperthyroidism.

Pharmacokinetics:

1. **Absorption:** 70%–80% absorbed from GI tract.
2. **Distribution:** Concentrated in thyroid gland; crosses placenta; found in breast milk.
3. **Metabolism:** Hepatic.
4. **Excretion:** Renal; 7% unchanged.
5. **Half-life:** 3–9 hr.

Drug Preparations:

Tablets: 5, 10 mg.

Dosage:

1. **Adult:** Drug usually given q 8–24 hr.
   a. **Mild hyperthyroidism:** 15 mg/day PO.
   b. **Moderate hyperthyroidism:** 30–40 mg/day PO.
   c. **Severe hyperthyroidism:** 60 mg/day PO; max. 150 mg/day.
      (1) When patient is euthyroid, reduce dosage.
      (2) Average maintenance dose 5–15 mg/day.
2. **Pediatric:**
   a. 0.4 mg/kg/day, usually in divided doses q 8 hr.
   b. Usual maintenance dose 0.2 mg/kg/day, given divided q 8 hr.

Adverse Effects:

1. **CNS:** Headache, drowsiness, vertigo, depression, paresthesias, neuritis.
2. **Skin:** Rash, urticaria, pruritus, lupus-like syndrome, exfoliative dermatitis.
3. **GI:** Diarrhea, nausea/vomiting, anorexia, epigastric pain, sialadenopathy.
4. **Hematologic:** Agranulocytosis, leukopenia, thrombocytopenia, aplastic anemia.

5. **Hepatic:** Jaundice, hepatitis, hepatic necrosis, bleeding.
6. **Renal:** Nephritis.
7. **Other:** Arthralgia, myalgia, periarteritis, loss of taste, hair loss, fever, lymphadenopathy, toxic to fetus.
8. **Thyroid: Can cause hypothyroidism.** Hypertrophy of thyroid tissue. Thyroid and pituitary neoplasma may develop.

Drug Interactions:

1. May potentiate effects of other hepatotoxic or bone marrow depressant drugs.
2. Potentiates vitamin K anticoagulants.

Monitoring:

1. Thyroxine, triiodothyronine, thyroid-stimulating hormone.
2. Blood counts, ALT, AST, bilirubin, prothrombin time, partial thromboplastin time. Signs of infection, liver failure.

BIBLIOGRAPHY

Reasner CA, Isley WL: Thyrotoxicosis in the critically ill. In Zaloga GP (ed): Endocrine crisis, *Crit Care Clin* 1991, 7:57–74.
Burch HB, Wartofsky L: Life-threatening thyrotoxicosis—thyroid storm. In Ober KP (ed): Endocrine crisis, *Endocrinol Metab Clin North Am* 1993, 22:263–277.
Haynes RC: Thyroid and antithyroid drugs. In Gilman AG, et al (eds): *The Pharmacologic Basis of Therapeutics,* ed 8, New York, 1993, McGraw-Hill, pp 1361–1383.

METHYLDOPA

Trade Names: *Aldomet*; *methyldopa* (various).

Drug Action:

1. Its metabolite, α-methylnorepinephrine, stimulates central α-adrenergic receptors, which decrease blood pressure.
2. May act as a false neurotransmitter.
3. Reduces plasma renin.

Indication: Hypertension.

Pharmacokinetics:

1. **Absorption:** 50% absorbed from GI tract.
2. **Metabolism:** Liver, intestinal cells.
3. **Excretion:** Urine.
4. **Plasma half-life:** 2 hr.
5. **Onset of action:** 4–6 hr.
6. **Duration of action:** 16–24 hr.
7. **Max effect:** 2 days.

Drug Preparations:

Tablets: 125, 250, 500 mg.
PO suspension: 250 mg/5 mL.
Vials: 250 mg/5 mL (5 mL vials) for injection.

Dosage:

1. **Adult:**
   a. **PO:** Initial dose 250 mg bid–tid. Maintenance dose 500–2000 mg/day in two to four doses (max 3000 mg/day).
   b. **IV:** 250–500 mg over 30 min q 6 hr (max. 1 g q 6 hr).
2. **Pediatric:**
   a. **PO:** Initial dose 10 mg/kg/day in two to four doses (titrate to effect) (max. 65 mg/kg or 3 g/day).
   b. **IV:** 20–40 mg/kg/day in four divided doses.
3. **Renal failure:** Decrease dosage.

Adverse Effects:

1. **Cardiovascular:** Bradycardia, hypotension, angina, myocarditis, edema.
2. **GI:** Nausea/vomiting, diarrhea, pancreatitis, hepatic damage.
3. **Hematologic:** Hemolytic anemia, granulocytopenia, thrombocytopenia, positive Coombs test.
4. **CNS:** Sedation, headache, weakness, dizziness, depression, nightmares, paresthesias, memory impairment.
5. **Other:** Dry mouth, nasal stuffiness, gynecomastia, rash, fever, impotence, lactation, lupus-like syndrome.

Drug Interactions:

1. Potentiates other antihypertensives.
2. Antagonized by phenothiazines, tricyclic antidepressants.
3. Increased sedation and dementia with haloperidol.

4. Potentiated by verapamil.
5. Enhances hypoglycemic effect of tolbutamides.
6. Potentiates effects of anesthetics, sympathomimetic amines, levodopa.
7. Paradoxical hypertension with propranolol (rare).

Monitoring:

1. Blood pressure, heart rate.
2. Liver function tests, enzymes.

BIBLIOGRAPHY

Methyldopa. In *Drug Facts and Comparisons,* Philadelphia, 1989, JB Lippincott, p. 618.
Methyldopa. In *AMA Drug Evaluations,* ed 6, Philadelphia, 1986, WB Saunders, p 517.

METHYLPHENIDATE

Trade Name(s): *Ritalin, Ritalin-SR.*

Drug Actions: Similar to amphetamine, CNS stimulant, appetite suppressant. Blocks reuptake mechanism of dopaminergic neurons.

Indications: For children with attention deficit disorder. Also used rarely to treat narcolepsy in adults.

Pharmacokinetics:

1. **Absorption:** 67%–86% after PO dose.
2. **Onset of action:** 1–8 hr, depending on age; duration 3–6 hr (immediate-release tablet), 8 hr (sustained-release tablet).
3. **Metabolism:** Active metabolites, liver.
4. **Excretion:** Urinary excretion of metabolites.
5. **Half-life:** 2–4 hr.

Drug Preparations:

Tablets: 5, 10, 20 mg
SR tablets: 20 mg.

Dosage: Adults average dose is 20–30 mg daily in two or three doses.

Adverse Effects: Nervousness, anxiety, tachycardia, hypertension, hypotension, palpitations, arrhythmias, dizziness, stomach pain, insomnia, anorexia, toxic psychosis, fever, headache, seizures, rash, nausea, bone marrow depression.

Drug Interactions: Use cautiously with pressor agents and MAO inhibitors. May inhibit metabolism of drugs metabolized in the liver. May antagonize effects of guanethidine, bretylium; increases serum concentrations of tricyclic antidepressants, warfarin, phenytoin, phenobarbital, primidone. Potentiated by MAO inhibitors.

Monitoring: Tolerance may develop. Mental status, blood pressure, heart rate.

BIBLIOGRAPHY

Zarcone V: Narcolepsy, *N Engl J Med* 1973, 288:1156–1166.

METOLAZONE

Trade Names: *Zaroxolyn, Mykrox.*

Drug Action:

1. **Diuretic:** Increases excretion of sodium and water by inhibiting sodium reabsorption in the thick ascending limb of Henle's loop and distal convoluted tubule.
2. **Antihypertensive:** Direct vasodilation.

Indications:

1. Salt and water retention (e.g., edema).
2. Hypertension.
3. Cardiac and renal insufficiency.

Pharmacokinetics:

1. **Absorption:** 65% of PO dose in healthy individuals.
2. **Metabolism:** Insignificant.
3. **Excretion:** 70%–95% unchanged in urine.
4. **Plasma half-life:** 8 hr; prolonged in renal failure.
5. **Onset:** 1 hr.
6. **Duration:** 12–24 hr.

Drug Preparations:

Tablets: 0.5, 2.5, 5, 10 mg. Metolazone preparations are not bioequivalent or therapeutically equivalent at the same doses.

Dosage:

1. **Adult:** (Zaroxolyn, Diulo): 5–20 mg PO q day; (Mykrox) 0.5–1 mg PO q day.

Adverse Effects:

1. **Cardiovascular:** Volume depletion, hypotension, tachycardia, arrhythmias.
2. **GI:** Nausea/vomiting, anorexia, pancreatitis, hepatic encephalopathy.
3. **Dermatologic:** Dermatitis, photosensitivity.
4. **Hematologic:** Aplastic anemia, agranulocytosis, leukopenia, thrombocytopenia.
5. **Metabolic:** Hyperuricemia, hyperglycemia, hypokalemia, hypomagnesemia, metabolic alkalosis, hypercholesterolemia.
6. **Other:** Hypersensitivity, vasculitis, dizziness, headache, weakness, paresthesias, restlessness, fatigue, muscle spasms.

Drug Interactions:

1. Potentiates hypotensive effects of other antihypertensives.
2. Increases demand for insulin or oral hypoglycemics in diabetic patients
3. Decreases renal clearance of lithium, quinidine.
4. Absorption decreased by cholestyramine and colestipol.
5. Effect of nondepolarizing muscle relaxants may be prolonged.

Monitoring:

1. Blood pressure, heart rate.
2. Serum electrolytes (especially K^+, Mg^{++}).
3. Serum glucose.
4. BUN, creatinine.

BIBLIOGRAPHY

Metolazone. In *Drug Facts and Comparisons,* Philadelphia, 1996, JB Lippincott, pp 632–644.

Metolazone. In *AMA Drug Evaluations,* ed 6, Philadelphia, 1995, WB Saunders, p 847.

METRONIDAZOLE

Trade Names: *Flagyl, Metric 21, Protostat.*

Drug Action:

1. Mechanism of action not fully understood (?DNA strand-breaking effect).
2. Spectrum of activity selective for only protozoa and obligate anaerobes.

Indications:

1. Protozoal infections:
   a. Trichomoniasis.
   b. Amebiasis: Intestinal and hepatic infections.
   c. Giardiasis: Alternative to quinacrine.
   d. American mucocutaneous leishmaniasis.
2. Anaerobic infections:
   a. Multiple sites, including intraabdominal, pelvic, brain.
      (1) (?Inferior to penicillin or clindamycin in lung abscess).
   b. *Clostridium difficile*–associated pseudomembranous colitis; alternative to PO vancomycin or bacitracin.
   c. Bacterial vaginosis.

Pharmacokinetics:

1. **Absorption:** Almost complete after PO/PR use.
2. **Excretion:** Both natural compound and metabolites excreted in urine, with one third metabolized in liver.
3. **Penetration:** Excellent, including CSF.
4. **Serum half-life:** 6–14 hr.

Drug Preparations:

Tablets: 250, 500 mg.
Vials: 500 mg/100 mL, for parenteral use.

Dosage:

1. **Normal renal function:** 7.5 mg/kg q 6 hr PO/parenteral.
   a. **Trichomoniasis:** 2 g single dose for adult patients.
   b. **Bacterial vaginosis:** 500 mg bid for 7 days.
   c. **Pseudomembranous colitis:** 500 mg bid for 10 days.

  d. **Amebiasis:** 750 mg tid for 10 days.
  e. **Giardiasis:** 250 mg bid/tid for 5–7 days or 2 g/day for 3 days.
2. **Renal impairment/dialysis:** No change in dosage.
3. **Decompensated liver disease:** Approximately one-half dose.

Adverse Effects:

1. **Carcinogenic potential:** Tumorigenic in animals but no evidence in humans.
   a. Avoid in first trimester of pregnancy.
2. **Alcohol intolerance:** Disulfiram effect.
3. **Neurotoxicity:** Peripheral neuropathies (high doses), seizures (avoid use with history of seizure disorder), headache, incoordination, confusion, depression, weakness.
4. **GI:** Metallic, bitter taste; stomatitis, nausea/diarrhea.
5. **Transient leukopenia.**
6. **Dark urine,** common but harmless.
7. **Falsely depressed AST;** absorbed at same wavelength.
8. Pruritus, urticaria, edema, dysuria.

Drug Interactions:

1. **Alcohol:** Disulfiram reaction.
2. **PO anticoagulants:** Increased anticoagulant effect.
3. **Disulfiram:** Organic brain syndrome.
4. **Phenobarbital:** Decreased metronidazole effect.

MEZLOCILLIN

Trade Name: *Mezlin.*

Drug Action:

1. Inhibits cell wall synthesis (penicillin).
2. Spectrum of activity includes gram-positive aerobes (but not β-lactamase–producing staphylococci), most gram-negative aerobes (including *Pseudomonas aeruginosa*) and anaerobes (including *Bacteroides* family).

Indications:

1. Infections caused by susceptible organisms, most commonly with aminoglycosides to provide synergistic *P. aeruginosa* or mixed aerobic/anaerobic coverage.
   a. Multiple sites.

Pharmacokinetics:

1. **Excretion:** Renal.
2. **Monosodium salt:** 1.7 mEq/g.
3. **Serum half-life:** 1.1 hr.

Drug Preparations:

Vials: 1, 2, 3, 4 g for parenteral use.

Dosage:

1. **Normal renal function:** 3 g q 4 hr or 4 g q 6 hr IV/IM.
2. **Impaired renal function:**

Dose (g)	Creatinine Clearance	Interval (hr)
3–4	>80	4–6
	80–50	4–6
	50–10	6–8
	<10 (anuria)	8–12

3. **Hemodialysis:** Supplemental dose of 2–3 g after each dialysis.

Adverse Effects:

1. Similar to other penicillins, including hypersensitivity reactions, GI problems, cytopenias, neurotoxicity.
2. Sodium overload: Less with monosodium compounds.
3. Qualitative platelet defect.
4. Hypokalemia.

Drug Interactions:

1. Inactivation of aminoglycosides if administered in same IV line.

MICONAZOLE

Trade Name: *Monistat.*

Drug Actions:

1. An imidazole, miconazole inhibits sterol 14α-demethylase, a microsomal cytochrome P450–dependent enzyme system, resulting in accumulation of 14α-methyl sterols and reduced concentrations of ergosterol.
2. The spectrum of activity of the IV preparation is *Coccidioides immitis, Candida albicans, Cryptococcus neoformans, Pseudallescheria boydii,* and *Paracoccidioides brasiliensis.* Miconazole is important in the critical care setting owing to its role as drug of choice for treatment of *P. boydii* infections, which occur occasionally in immunocompromised patients (e.g., bone marrow transplant recipients).
3. Miconazole nitrate (topical form) inhibits the growth of *Trichophyton rubrum, T. mentagrophytes, Epidermophyton floccosum, C. albicans,* and *Malassezia furfur.*

Indications:

1. Pseudallescheriasis.
2. Miconazole (IV) may also be used to treat coccidioidomycosis in patients who do not respond to or have contraindications to amphotericin B and ketoconazole therapy.
3. Indications for topical use: candidal vulvavaginitis and skin infections, and dermatophytoses.

Pharmacokinetics:

1. **Absorption:** IV. Peak levels occur 5 min after a 1 hr infusion. There is no CNS penetration.
2. **Excretion:** 14%–22% in urine as inactive metabolites (<1% as active drug).
3. **Half-life:** 20–25 hr.

Drug Preparations:

Ampules: 20 mL (200 mg).
Topical: Numerous preparations.

Dosage: For treatment of pseudallescheriasis: 600–3000 mg/day (may be divided into three infusions). Administration of a 200 mg test dose should be considered. No dosage adjustment is necessary for patients with renal insufficiency or on dialysis.

Adverse Effects:

1. Phlebitis (29%), pruritus (21%), nausea (18%), fever and chills (10%), rash (9%), and emesis (7%).
2. Transient decreases of hematocrit and serum sodium values have been observed following infusion of miconazole.
3. Thrombocytopenia has been reported.
4. Anaphylaxis has occurred rarely.

Drug Interactions:

1. Anticoagulant effects of warfarin sodium may be enhanced.
2. Concomitantly administered rifampin reduces blood levels of miconazole.
3. A similar imidazole drug, ketoconazole, increases cyclosporine levels. Cyclosporine levels should be followed closely if miconazole and cyclosporine are to be given together.

BIBLIOGRAPHY

Miconazole. In *Drug Facts and Comparisons,* ed 49, St. Louis, MO, 1995, Facts and Comparisons, pp 2071–2072.
Physicians' Desk Reference, ed 50, Montvale, 1996, Medical Economics Co.

MIDAZOLAM

Trade Name: *Versed.*

Drug Action:

1. A water-soluble benzodiazepine.
2. Facilitates action of γ-aminobutyric acid at presynaptic nerve terminals to provide CNS depression.
3. Amnesia action, anxiolytic, hypnotic, sedative, anticonvulsant.

Indications:

1. Sedation.
2. Anxiety, agitation.
3. Alcohol withdrawal.
4. Seizures.

Pharmacokinetics:

1. **Absorption:** Give IV/IM. Oral dosing (of IV preparation) used as premedication in pediatric patients.
2. **Distribution:** Total body, crosses placenta.
3. **Metabolism:** Hepatic metabolism to 1-OH-midazolam (minimal activity).
4. **Excretion:** Conjugated metabolites in urine.
5. **Onset of action:** 15 min after IM; 1–5 min after IV.
6. **Half-life:** 2–6 hr.
7. **Duration of sedation:** 1–4 hr.

Drug Preparations:

Injection: 1 mg/mL in 2, 5, 10 mL vial.
5 mg/mL in 1, 2, 5, 10 mL vial.
5 mg/mL in 2 mL disposable syringe.

Dosage:

1. **Sedation:** Adults 1–4 mg IM/IV q 2–6 hr.
2. Continuous IV infusion of 1–4 mg/hr in ICU patients.
3. 0.5–0.75 mg/kg **PO** to premedicate pediatric patients.

Adverse Effects:

1. **CNS:** Amnesia, euphoria, confusion, slurred speech, ataxia, oversedation, stupor, coma, emergence delirium, agitation.
2. **Cardiovascular:** Hypotension, tachycardia.
3. **Dermatologic:** Rash, hives, pruritus, hypersensitivity.
4. **Respiratory:** Apnea, depression, bronchospasm.
5. **Miscellaneous:** Elevates intraocular pressure; blurred vision, diplopia, salivation, nausea/vomiting, phlebitis.

Drug Interactions:

1. Potentiates other CNS depressants.
2. Delayed metabolism in hepatic, renal, and congestive heart failure.
3. May be reversed with flumazenil.

Monitoring: Blood pressure, heart rate, mental alertness, respiratory rate.

MILRINONE

Trade Name: *Primacor.*

Drug Actions: Phosphodiesterase III inhibitor with positive inotropic and vasodilating properties. Much more potent than amrinone.

Indications:

1. Myocardial dysfunction, especially when accompanied by increased vascular (systemic and pulmonary) resistance.
2. Congestive heart failure.

Pharmacokinetics:

1. **Absorption:** Approved for IV use.
2. **Onset of action:** Almost immediate (<10 min).
3. **Metabolism:** Hepatic.
4. **Excretion:** 83% excreted unchanged in urine.
5. **Half-life:** Although 60% is excreted in first 2 hr after dosing, clinical effects may persist for up to 4–6 hr.

Drug Preparations:

IV injection solutions: 1 mg/mL.

Dosage:

50 µg/kg over 10–30 min (load) followed by infusion of 0.25–0.75 µg/kg/min.

Adverse Effects:

1. Hypotension (may be severe following loading dose). Ventricular arrhythmias may be potentiated by milrinone. Angina. Tachycardia.
2. Headache, hypokalemia, tremor.
3. Hypersensitivity reactions, thrombocytopenia.

Drug Interactions: May dramatically potentiate the effects of β-adrenergic agonists used for inotropic support. Also adds to hypotensive effects of other vasodilators.

Monitoring: Cardiac output, blood pressure, heart rate, serum potassium, clinical response.

BIBLIOGRAPHY

Prielipp RC, et al: Pharmacodynamics and pharmacokinetics of milrinone administration to increase oxygen delivery in critically ill patients, *Chest* 1996, 109:1291–1301.

Sherry KM, Locks IJ: Use of milrinone in cardiac surgical patients, *Cardiovasc Drugs Ther* 1993, 7:671–675.

Honerjager P, Nawrath H: Pharmacology of bipyridine phosphodiesterase III inhibitors, *Eur J Anaesthesiol* 1992, 5(suppl): 7–14.

MINOCYCLINE

Trade Names: *Minocin, Dynacin.*

Drug Actions:

1. Inhibits bacterial protein synthesis by binding to the 30S ribosomal subunit.
2. Spectrum of activity: Wide range of bacteria, including rickettsiae and mycoplasmas.

Indications:

1. Essentially the same as tetracycline, (*see* tetracycline indications), but has the additional advantage of not necessarily sharing cross-resistance with other tetracyclines, and thus is sometimes useful against tetracycline-resistant *Staphylococcus aureus* (including methicillin-resistant *S. aureus*) and *Haemophilus influenzae* strains.
2. Alternative to sulfonamides in treatment of actinomycosis and nocardiosis.

Pharmacokinetics:

1. **Absorption:** PO (may be taken without regard to food)/IV.
2. **Metabolism:** Enterohepatic circulation (minocycline is recoverable from urine and feces in lesser amounts than other tetracyclines, so it appears that it is metabolized to a greater extent).
3. **Half-life:** 11–17 hr PO, 15–23 hr IV.

Drug Preparations:

Capsules: 50, 100 mg.
Oral suspension: 50 mg/5 mL.
Vials: 100 mg.

Dosage:

100 mg PO bid or 50 mg PO q 6 hr.
100 mg IV q 12 hr or 200 mg IV q 24 hr.

Adverse Effects:

1. Pseudotumor cerebri (benign intracranial hypertension) in adults has been associated with the use of tetracyclines.
2. With complete absorption of oral minocycline, side effects involving the lower GI tract (i.e., diarrhea) are uncommon. Nausea/vomiting and, rarely, hepatitis can occur.
3. Lightheadedness, dizziness, and vertigo are fairly common.
4. Risk of esophageal irritation and ulceration with tetracycline-class drugs can be reduced through ingestion of adequate amounts of fluids with PO formulations.
5. Dark discoloration of the thyroid gland has occurred after prolonged use of tetracyclines.
6. Use of drugs in the tetracycline group during the latter half of pregnancy has resulted in permanent, yellow-gray-brown tooth discoloration and, more rarely, enamel hypoplasia (of the fetus).
7. Similarly, tetracycline drugs (including minocycline) should not be taken by children <8 yr of age owing to risk of tooth discoloration.
8. Decreased hearing has been rarely reported in patients taking minocycline capsules or tablets.

Drug Interactions:

1. Concurrent use of tetracyclines and oral contraceptives may render oral contraceptives less effective.
2. Tetracyclines may depress prothrombin activity; thus, anticoagulant dosages may need a downward adjustment.

BIBLIOGRAPHY

Physicians' Desk Reference, ed 50, Montvale, 1996, Medical Economics Co.

Sande MA, Mandell GL: Antimicrobial agents: tetracyclines, chloramphenicol, erythromycin, and miscellaneous antibacterial agents. In Gillman AG, Rall TW, Nies AS, et al (eds): *The Pharmacological Basis of Therapeutics,* ed 8, New York, 1990, McGraw-Hill, pp 1117–1145.

MISOPROSTOL

Trade Name: *Cytotec.*

Drug Actions: A synthetic prostaglandin E_1 analog; replaces gastric protective prostaglandins whose synthesis is inhibited by nonsteroidal anti-inflammatory drugs (NSAIDs).

Indications: Prevention of NSAID-induced gastric ulcers.

Pharmacokinetics:

1. **Absorption:** Rapid.
2. **Onset of action:** 15–30 min.
3. **Metabolism:** Deesterified to misoprostol acid.
4. **Excretion:** Urine (75%), feces (15%).
5. **Half-life:** 1.5 hr.

Drug Preparations:

   Tablets: 100, 200 µg.

Dosage: Adults: 200 µg qid PO (with food).

Adverse Effects:

1. GI: Diarrhea, abdominal pain, constipation, flatulence, nausea/vomiting.
2. CNS: Headache, sedation, tremor, seizures.
3. Uterine stimulation, vaginal bleeding.
4. Hypotension, bradycardia.

Drug Interactions: None reported.

Monitoring: Clinical response, signs of GI bleeding.

BIBLIOGRAPHY

Monk JP, Clissold SP: Misoprostol—a preliminary review of its pharmacodynamic and pharmacokinetic properties, and therapeutic efficacy in the treatment of peptic ulcer disease, *Drugs* 1987, 33:1–30.
Sontag SJ: Prostaglandins in peptic ulcer disease—an overview of current status and future directions, *Drugs* 1986, 32:445–457.

MORPHINE

Trade Names: *Astramorph, Duramorph, MS Contin, Roxanol SR.*

Drug Action:

1. Morphine has agonist actions at all opioid receptors, with a high affinity specifically at the μ and κ receptors. Thus, analgesia and sedation are the primary desired actions.
2. Peripheral vasodilation.

Indications:

1. Relief of moderate to severe pain.
2. Preoperative medication (sedation).
3. Analgesic supplementation with local or regional anesthesia.
4. As major/minor component of general anesthesia.
5. To relieve anxiety and produce vasodilation when treating cardiogenic pulmonary edema secondary to left ventricular dysfunction associated with myocardial infarction or ischemia.
6. Morphine is seldom used as an antitussive or antidiarrheal agent, although it is effective for both.

Pharmacokinetics:

1. **Absorption:** Good PO absorption. However, as much as 75%–80% of absorbed PO dose undergoes first-pass metabolism in the liver, decreasing the effectiveness of this route of administration.

a. Peak effect after IV/IM administration occurs at 15 and 40 min, respectively, with duration of action approximately 3–5 hr.

b. After intrathecal/epidural administration, onset of analgesia occurs at 15–60 min and lasts up to 24 hr.

2. **Metabolism:** Hepatic glucuronide conjugation is the predominant mode of metabolism. Less than 10% is excreted unchanged.

3. **Excretion:** 90% of metabolized drug is excreted via kidneys; remainder is excreted via biliary system.

4. **Plasma half-life:** 2–3 hr; 2–3 hr, longer in older patients.

a. Renal/hepatic dysfunction prolongs elimination half-life.

Drug Preparations:

Preservative-free solutions (Astramorph, Duramorph): 0.5 mg/mL, 1.0 mg/mL, intended primarily for intrathecal/epidural use but suitable for IV administration.

Solutions: 1, 2, 4, 5, 8, 10, 15 mg/mL for parenteral use.

Liquid: 10, 20, 100 mg/5 mL for PO use.

Tablets: 10, 15, 30 mg. 30 and 60 mg sustained release.

Suppositories: 5, 10, 20, 30 mg for PR use.

Dosage:

1. **IM/SQ**
   a. **Adult:** 2–10 mg/70 kg q 4–6 hr.
   b. **Pediatric:** 0.1–0.2 mg/kg q 4–6 hr.
2. **IV:**
   a. **Adult:** 1–5 mg q 3–4 hr.
   b. **Pediatric:** Approximately 0.1 mg/kg q 3–4 hr.
3. **Epidural:** 2–8 mg as bolus q 18–24 hr, depending on dermatomal level desired. Alternatively, continuous infusion of 0.01 mg/kg/hr after 0.1 mg/kg bolus.
4. **Intrathecal:** 0.1–0.3 mg q 12–24 hr.
5. **PO:** 10–30 mg q 4 hr.
6. **PR:** 10–20 mg q 4 hr.

Adverse Effects:

1. May produce euphoria, drowsiness, confusion, nausea/vomiting, respiratory depression, constipation, urinary retention.

2. If hemodynamic instability is present, morphine may exacerbate it. May cause hypotension, tachycardia.
3. May produce biliary spasm, even in patients with history of cholecystectomy, resulting in severe right upper quadrant pain.
4. Especially when given IV, can produce histamine release, with subsequent urticaria and pruritus.
5. In patients with closed head injury or other cause of increased intracranial pressure (ICP), may exacerbate elevated ICP, because narcotics can cause respiratory depression with resultant increases in $PaCO_2$ cerebral blood volume, and ICP.
6. Epidural and especially intrathecal administration of morphine can produce delayed respiratory depression, pruritus, urinary retention, nausea/vomiting.
   a. Intermittent IV boluses of 0.1–0.2 mg naloxone or continuous IV infusion at 5 μg/kg/hr reverse these adverse effects of intrathecal/epidural morphine without affecting quality of pain relief. This is in contrast to what may happen when naloxone is used to reverse undesired effects of systemically administered morphine (e.g., quality of analgesia may be diminished).

Drug Interactions: Sedative and respiratory effects of morphine may be augmented when patients are concomitantly receiving sedatives, hypnotics, tricyclic antidepressants, phenothiazines, MAO inhibitors, alcohol, other CNS depressants.

Monitoring:

1. Mental status, if possible.
2. Respiratory rate, blood pressure, heart rate.

BIBLIOGRAPHY

Chernow B (ed): *The Pharmacologic Approach to the Critically Ill Patient,* ed 2, Baltimore, 1988, Williams & Wilkins.

Gilman AG, Goodman LS, Rall TW, et al (eds): *Goodman and Gilman's The Pharmacological Basis of Therapeutics,* ed 7, New York, 1985, Macmillan.

McEvoy GK (ed): *AHFS Drug Information 89,* Bethesda, 1989, American Society of Hospital Pharmacists.

Physicians' Desk Reference, ed 42, Oradell, 1988, Medical Economics Co.

NAFCILLIN

Trade Names: *Nafcil, Unipen.*

Drug Action:

1. Inhibits cell wall synthesis (penicillin).
2. Antistaphylococcal activity.

Indications: Staphylococcal infections.

Pharmacokinetics:

1. **Absorption:** Erratic PO (not a preferred PO antistaphylococcal agent).
2. **Excretion:** Primary hepatic, with high biliary concentration.
3. **Serum half-life:** 30 min.
4. **Penetration:** Best of antistaphylococcal agents into CNS.
5. **Metabolism:** Liver, enterohepatic circulation.

Drug Preparations:

Capsules: 250 mg.
Tablets: 500 mg.
Solution: 250 mg/5 mL for PO use.
Vials: 0.5, 1, 2 g for parenteral use.

Dosage:

1. **Normal/impaired renal function:**
   a. **Adult:** Usual dose 4–9 g/day, depending on severity of infection (0.5–1.5 g q 4–6 hr) PO/IV/IM.
   b. **Pediatric:** 100–200 mg/kg/day in divided doses q 4–6 hr PO/IV/IM.
2. **Dialysis:** No modification.

Adverse Effects:

1. Similar to other penicillins, including hypersensitivity reactions, GI problems (asymptomatic liver enzyme elevation).
2. Neutropenia in 10% when given for >3 wk; occasionally severe.
3. Nephropathy rare.

Drug Interactions:

1. Incompatible when mixed with aminoglycosides.
2. Renal excretion inhibited by probenecid.

NALBUPHINE

Trade Name: *Nubain.*

Drug Action:

1. Exerts analgesic activity at κopioid receptors; has only minimal σopioid receptor activity; is an antagonist at μopioid receptors (where morphine is a potent agonist). On a mg/mg basis, nalbuphine is roughly equivalent to morphine in pain relief.
2. Nalbuphine and morphine have similar respiratory depressant activity, but nalbuphine effects do not significantly increase after a 10-mg dose in a healthy adult. There is a ceiling effect on pain relief.

Indications:

1. Indicated for relief of moderate to severe pain and as adjunct to local, regional, or general anesthesia.
2. In contrast to butorphanol (drug with similar actions), can also be used to treat pain related to myocardial ischemia and infarction, because it does not produce increases in heart rate or pulmonary artery, systemic, or left ventricular filling pressures.

Pharmacokinetics:

1. **Absorption:** After SQ/IM administration, onset of action occurs within 10–15 min, and usually within 3 min when drug is administered IV. Duration of action is usually 3–6 hr.
2. **Metabolism:** Hepatic.
3. **Excretion:** Metabolites are excreted predominantly via kidneys.
4. **Plasma half-life:** Approximately 5 hr.

Drug Preparations:

Vials: 10, 20 mg/mL.

Dosage:

1. IV/IM/SQ: 10–20 mg/70 kg adult (0.14 mg/kg) q 3–6 hr.

Adverse Effects:

1. Nausea/vomiting, sedation, dysphoria, dizziness, confusion, disorientation, vertigo; potential to increase intracranial pressure in susceptible patients.
2. "Ceiling effect" on respiratory depression, tachycardia, hypotension.
3. Nalbuphine may precipitate withdrawal symptoms in narcotic addicts.

Drug Interactions: Sedation is additive with other CNS depressants (e.g., phenothiazines, hypnotics, tranquilizers). However, nalbuphine has been used in doses of 10–20 mg to reverse narcotic-induced respiratory depression following surgery in which significant doses of narcotics were used as part of the anesthetic. This effect is a result of the μ receptor antagonism that nalbuphine exhibits.

Monitoring: Respiratory rate, blood pressure, heart rate; mental status.

BIBLIOGRAPHY

Gilman AG, Goodman LS, Rall TW, et al (eds): *Goodman and Gilman's The Pharmacological Basis of Therapeutics,* ed 7, New York, 1985, Macmillan.
McEvoy GK (ed): *AMA Drug Information 89,* Bethesda, 1989, American Society of Hospital Pharmacists.
Physicians' Desk Reference, ed 42, Oradell, 1988, Medical Economics Co.

NALOXONE

Trade Name: *Narcan;* generics.

Drug Action:

1. Pure opioid receptor antagonist with no agonist activity and no significant pharmacologic effects other than opioid receptor blockade.

2. Reverses effects of opioids, including analgesia, respiratory depression, sedation, dysphoria, pruritus, and urinary retention.

Indications:

1. To reverse adverse effects of all narcotics (most commonly respiratory depression).
2. Empiric therapy in coma of unknown origin to diagnose/rule out narcotic overdose as the cause.
3. Known overdose of narcotics.

Pharmacokinetics:

1. **Absorption:** Onset of action after IV administration within 2 min, and only slightly longer when administered IM/SQ. Can be administered endotracheally in a dose two and one half times its IV dose.
2. **Metabolism:** Predominantly glucuronidation in liver.
3. **Excretion:** Urinary.
4. **Serum half-life:** Approximately 60 min in adults, with a clinical duration of action 30–60 min (i.e., shorter than many narcotic agonists).

Drug Preparations:

Vials: 0.02 mg/mL (primarily for neonates), 0.4 mg/mL, 1.0 mg/mL. Available in both preservative and preservative-free formulations.

Adult Dosage: Varies depending on condition being treated.

1. **To reverse postoperative narcosis:** 0.5–1.0 µg/kg IV repeatedly administered q 2–3 min until desired clinical effects are achieved. Total dose of 0.2–0.3 mg is usually sufficient. If titrated carefully, naloxone can reverse respiratory depressant effects of narcotics without reversing analgesia. In treating postoperative respiratory depression, minimum amount of naloxone should be administered (*see* Adverse Effects).
2. **Suspected narcotic overdose:** Initial dose should be 2.0 mg IV and repeated q 2–5 hr PRN; as much as 10–20 mg may be necessary on occasion. If there is no effect after this dose has been administered, narcotic overdose is unlikely. Naloxone can be given IM, SQ, or via endotracheal tube if an IV route is not available. When given IM, duration of action is somewhat prolonged.

3. **For prolonged response:** (a) Continuous IV infusion at 4–5 µg/kg/hr may be used to reverse respiratory depression from epidural narcotics without reversing analgesia; (b) in overdose setting, an infusion administered at a rate of two thirds the initial reversal dose per hr may be used.

Adverse Effects/Drug Interactions:

Contraindications: Hypersensitivity; narcotic habituation (relative—use with caution).

1. Few, if any, significant adverse effects unless naloxone is given to postoperative patients (hemodynamic instability, pulmonary edema arrhythmias) or narcotic addicts (abstinence, syndrome, nausea, vomiting, abdominal pain, diaphoresis).
2. Severe hypertension, ventricular tachycardia and fibrillation, pulmonary edema, and cardiac arrest have occurred in patients, both healthy and ill, who have rapid reversal of narcotic analgesia with naloxone. Most commonly described in the immediate postoperative period, this occurs via an uncertain mechanism that apparently results in severe sympathetic discharge. Careful titration of small doses until achieval of adequate respiration is mandatory.
3. Can produce a withdrawal syndrome in patients addicted to narcotics.
4. Larger doses may be required for certain agonists (propoxyphene, pentazocine, buprenorphine, methadone).

Monitoring: Respiratory rate, heart rate, blood pressure; mental status. Resedation common owing to short duration of action relative to that of narcotic agonists.

BIBLIOGRAPHY

Physicians' Desk Reference, ed 49, Montvale 1995, Medical Economics Co., p 983.

Weisman RS: Naloxone. In Goldfrank LR, Flomenbaum NE, Lewin NA, et al (eds): *Toxicologic Emergencies,* ed 5, Norwalk, CT, 1994, Appleton & Lange, p 784.

Committee on Injury and Poison Prevention: *Handbook of Common Poisonings in Children,* ed 3, 1994, American Academy of Pediatrics, p 19.

Stoelting RK (ed): *Pharmacology and Physiology in Anesthetic Practice,* ed 2, Philadelphia, 1991, JB Lippincott, p 96.

NICARDIPINE

Trade Names: *Cardene, Cardene SR.*

Drug Actions: Slow calcium channel antagonist; dihydropyridine class, vascular selective (minimal myocardial depression in vivo), and conduction system depression in vivo.

Indications: Hypertension, angina pectoris (recent studies question long-term mortality with calcium blockers).

Pharmacokinetics:

1. **Absorption:** Well absorbed orally.
2. **Onset of action:** Max. plasma levels 30 min–2 hr after oral dose (peak effect), within minutes after IV administration.
3. **Metabolism:** (65% removed during first pass) saturable hepatic first-pass metabolism.
4. **Excretion:** <1% of intact drug in urine; 60% of metabolites excreted in urine, 35% in feces.
5. **Half-life:** Terminal half life 8–14 hr at steady state (3–4 hr after first dose).
6. **Offset of action:** Following IV administration: 50% decrease in 30–45 min; effect may last 50 hr.

Drug Preparations:

Capsules: 20, 30 mg.
Capsules, sustained action, oral: 30, 45, 60 mg.
Ampules, IV: 10 mL, 2.5 mg/mL.

Dosage: Titrate to effect: Begin 20–40 mg tid PO; IV: initiate at 5 mg/hr, increase by 2.5 mg/hr every 5–15 min until desired effect or max. dose of 15 mg/hr; IV—oral—equivalency 0.5 mg/hr ~20 mg q 8 hr, 1.2 mg/hr ~30 mg q 8 hr, 2.2 mg/hr ~40 mg q 8 hr; decrease dose in patients with hepatic disease and renal insufficiency.

Adverse Effects: Hypotension (esp. in patients with aortic outlet obstruction), tachycardia, palpitations, may worsen heart failure in patients with severe left ventricular dysfunction, may worsen angina pectoris in occasional patient, may reduce renal plasma flow and glomerular filtration rate, dizziness, headache, asthenia, flushing, nausea, syncope, tremor, pedal edema, overdose: hypotension, bradycardia, AV block.

Drug Interactions: Cimetidine increase plasma levels, may elevate digoxin levels, cyclosporin levels.

Monitoring: Blood pressure, heart rate (peak effect 1–2 hr after dose), clinical response.

BIBLIOGRAPHY

Tobias JD: Nicardipine—applications in anesthesia practice, *J Clin Anesth* 1995, 7:525–533.

Sabbatini M, Strocchi P, Amenta F: Nicardipine and treatment of cerebrovascular diseases with particular reference to hypertension-related disorders, *Clin Exp Hypertens* 1995, 17:719–750.

NIFEDIPINE

Trade Names: *Procardia, Adalat.*

Drug Action: Calcium antagonist; cardiovascular depression is limited by vasodilation and reflex sympathetic responses.

1. Slows conduction, depresses rate of spontaneous depolarization in AV and SA nodes. Has less effect than verapamil and diltiazem.
2. Myocardial depression, less than with verapamil and diltiazem.
3. Smooth muscle vasodilator; most pronounced of calcium antagonists.
4. Improves diastolic relaxation properties of ventricles.

Indications:

1. Myocardial ischemia secondary to coronary vasospasm.
2. Hypertension.

Pharmacokinetics:

1. **Absorption:** PO/SL.
2. **Metabolism:** Hepatic.
3. **Excretion:** 80% of metabolites by renal excretion.
4. **Protein binding:** 90%.
5. **Onset of action:** 5 min (SL), PO 20 min (intact capsule or tablet).
6. **Plasma half-life:** 2–5 hr.

Drug Preparations:

Soft capsules: 10, 20 mg. Liquid from capsule can be drawn with syringe for sublingual administration.

Extended-release tablets: 30, 60, 90 mg.

Dosage: Capsules 10 or 20 mg PO q 6–8 hr or 30 mg once daily (extended release). Soft capsules may be given SL if NPO. Taper drug to effect.

Adverse Effects:

1. Hypotension, dizziness, headache, flushing.
2. Reflex sympathetic effects (tachycardia) may precipitate myocardial ischemia, heart failure.
3. Edema, nasal congestion, nausea, diarrhea.

Drug Interactions:

1. Digoxin levels increase by 45%.
2. May result in myocardial depression in patients receiving β-blockers, which prevent sympathetic reflexes.

Monitoring: Blood pressure, heart rate.

BIBLIOGRAPHY

Antman EM, Stone P, Muller JE, et al: Calcium channel blocking agents in the treatment of cardiovascular disorders. I: Basic and clinical electrophysiologic effects, *Ann Intern Med* 1980, 93:875–885.

Braunwald E: Mechanism of action of calcium channel blocking agents, *N Engl J Med* 1982; 307:1618–1627.

Stone PH, Antman EM, Muller JE, et al: Calcium channel blocking drugs in the treatment of cardiovascular disorders. II: Hemodynamic and clinical applications, *Ann Intern Med* 1980; 93:886–904.

NIMODIPINE

Trade Name: *Nimotop.*

Drug Actions: Slow calcium channel blocker; greater vasodilatory effect on cerebral arteries than on other arteries.

Indications: Hypertension; cerebral vasospasm associated with subarachnoid hemorrhage.

Pharmacokinetics:

1. **Absorption:** Rapid with peak concentrations within 1 hr.
2. **Onset of action:** Rapid.
3. **Metabolism:** Liver.
4. **Excretion:** Urine, feces.
5. **Half-life:** Terminal t½ is 8–9 hr but effective t½ is only 1–2 hr.

Drug Preparations:

Capsules: 30 mg

Dosage: 60 mg (2 capsules) PO q 4 hr. May be switched to 30 mg q 2 hr if hypotension occurs.

Adverse Effects:

1. Hypotension, edema, ECG abnormalities, tachycardia, brady-cardia.
2. Headache, depression, confusion, stupor.
3. Rash, muscle cramps.
4. Diarrhea, nausea, hepatitis.

Drug Interactions:

1. Potentiates hypotensive effects of other antihypertensives, including diuretics.
2. Increased nimodipine effect: H_2 blockers, β-blockers.
3. Increased levels of carbamazepine, cyclosporin, digitalis, quinidine, theophylline.

Monitoring: Neurologic status must be observed closely in patients with subarachnoid hemorrhage; blood pressure, heart rate.

BIBLIOGRAPHY

Hongo K, Kobayashi S: Calcium antagonists for the treatment of vasospasm following subarachnoid haemorrhage, *Neurol Res* 1993, 15:218–224.

Wadworth AN, McTavish D: Nimodipine—a review of its pharmacological properties and therapeutic efficacy in cerebral disorders, *Drugs Aging* 1992, 2:262–286.

NITROGLYCERIN

Trade Names: *Nitrostat, Nitro-Bid, Nitro-Dur, Nitrodisc, Nitrocine, Nitrol, Nitrong, Transderm-Nitro, Nitrospan, Nitrolingual Spray.*

Drug Action: Organic nitrates produce direct smooth muscle relaxation. Nitrates must first be absorbed intracellularly and reduced by sulfhydryl compounds; reduced product then forms nitric oxide (NO). NO reacts with tissue thiols, which activate cGMP, which relaxes smooth muscles.

1. **Cardiac:**
   a. Venodilation and decreased pulmonary vascular resistance, producing decreased preload, decreased left ventricular end-diastolic pressure (LVEDP). This reduces ventricular wall tension and thus lowers myocardial oxygen demand. Because systematic arterial dilation occurs only at higher doses, decreased LVEDP and constant arterial pressure increase coronary perfusion pressure and subendocardial blood flow.
   b. Epicardial coronary vasodilation; increases myocardial oxygen supply; dose-dependent effect.
   c. Increased collateral blood flow to ischemic myocardium; dose-dependent effect.
   d. Redistribution of blood flow to subendocardial tissue.
2. **Noncardiac:** Relaxation of smooth muscle in bronchi, biliary tract, GI tract, ureters, uterus.

Indications:

1. **Myocardial ischemia:**
   a. Stable/unstable angina.
   b. Coronary vasospasm.
2. Congestive heart failure.
3. Esophageal spasm.
4. Systemic and pulmonary hypertension.

Pharmacokinetics:

1. **Absorption:** SL/IV/topical/PO.
2. **Metabolism:** Liver.

3. **Excretion:** Renal.
4. **Protein binding:** 60%.
5. **Onset of action:** Immediate for IV/sublingual; slight delay for PO.
6. **Plasma half-life:** IV 1–4 min; SL 20 min; PO 4 hr.

Drug Preparations:

Tablets: Sustained release: 2.6, 6.5, 9 mg; sublingual: 0.15, 0.3, 0.4, 0.6 mg.

IV: 0.5, 0.8, 5 mg/mL.

Topical: 2% ointment.

Transdermal: 2.5, 5, 7.5, 10, 15 mg per 24 hr patch.

Dosage:

1. 10–400 µg/min IV. Mean dose 75–100 µg/min required to relieve angina in CCU patients, although up to 400 µg/min is occasionally required.
2. Hypotension is a limiting factor at doses >150 µg/min when arteriolar vasodilation is seen.
3. In patients in whom volume status is unknown, initial dose is 10–25 µg/min.
4. One sustained-release capsule q 8–12 hr; 1/2–2 inches ointment q 8–12 hr; 2.5–15 mg transdermal patch q 24 hr; 1 sublingual tablet q 5–10 min.

Adverse Effects:

1. Tolerance with prolonged use; more common with sustained-release preparations. Higher IV doses may be required when managing these patients acutely.
2. Methemoglobinemia caused by nitrate metabolite. Can be treated with methylene blue. Clinically significant problems are extremely rare.
3. Blunting of hypoxic pulmonary vasoconstriction.
4. Headache, flushing, dizziness, nausea/vomiting, palpitations.
5. Postural hypotension.
6. Increased intracranial pressure.

Monitoring: Hemodynamic signs of hypotension with blood pressure cuff or arterial line. If hypotension develops, monitoring of cardiac filling pressures must be considered.

Drug Reversal: Hypotension may be reversed quickly with discontinuation of drug. If continued infusion or higher infusion rates are required for ongoing myocardial ischemia, pressure may be supported with volume replacement or use of vasopressors (e.g., phenylephrine, norepinephrine).

BIBLIOGRAPHY

Corwin S, Reiffel JA: Nitrate therapy for angina pectoris, *Arch Intern Med* 1985, 145:538–543.

Fung HL: Pharmacokinetics and pharmacodynamics of organic nitrates, *Am J Cardiol* 1987, 60:4H–9H.

NITROPRUSSIDE

Trade Names: *Nipride, Nitropress.*

Drug Action:

1. Vasodilation in arteries and veins. Binds to nitrate receptor, resulting in production of nitric oxide (NO). Production of NO results in formation of cGMP. cGMP activates a cascade system, with the end result relaxation of smooth muscles in precapillary resistance vessels and postcapillary capacitance vessels. These decreases may be accompanied by reflex increases in heart rate and renin release.
2. Coronary arteriolar vasodilation; may result in coronary steal and angina.
3. Increase in cerebral blood volume and cerebral blood flow, thus increasing intracranial pressure.
4. Blunting of hypoxic pulmonary vasoconstriction.

Indications:

1. Hypertension: Effects on arterial system greater than on venous system.
2. Production of deliberate hypotension during anesthesia.
3. Acute left ventricular failure.
4. Treatment of heart failure associated with mitral/aortic regurgitation and ventricular septal rupture.

Pharmacokinetics:

1. **Metabolism:** Rapidly broken down to cyanide by nonenzymatic reactions and is converted to thiocyanate in liver.
2. **Excretion:** Thiocyanate renally excreted.
3. **Plasma half-life:** Minutes.
4. **Thiocyanate half-life** approximately 4 days.
5. **Onset of action:** Immediate.

Drug Preparations:

Vials: 50 mg/5 mL.

Dosage: Mix 50 mg into 250 mg D_5W. Start at minimal effective dose (range 0.5–2 µg/kg/min), titrating to effect.

Adverse Effects:

1. **Toxicity:** Primarily related to production of thiocyanate and cyanide. Nausea/vomiting, sweating, restlessness, headache, coma, metabolic acidosis usually related to too high a dosage. Also more likely in renal/hepatic failure.
2. Tachycardia, hypotension, dizziness, hypoxia (pulmonary shunting).
3. Raised intracranial pressure.
4. Development of tachyphylaxis.
5. Rebound hypertension on discontinuation.
6. May cause qualitative platelet defect.

Drug Interactions: Hypotensive effects augmented by ganglionic blockers and other antihypertensives, volatile anesthetics.

Monitoring:

1. Thiocyanate levels (<10 mg/100 mL), if available, should be measured each day if therapy is required longer than 48 hr.
2. Observe blood pressure, heart rate, arterial pH.

Drug Reversal:

1. Toxicity related to abnormality in cyanide-thiocyanate pathway by low levels of rhodanese enzyme (liver), required in production of thiocyanate.
2. Toxicity may occur with doses >2 µg/kg/min or use in renal/hepatic failure.

3. Treat by administering amyl nitrite and sodium nitrite (converts hemoglobin to methemoglobin). Methemoglobin binds cyanide. Also administer sodium thiosulfate (converts cyanide to thiocyanate).
4. Addition of hydroxycobalamine can reduce serum cyanide levels.

BIBLIOGRAPHY

Tinker JH, Michenfelder JD: Sodium nitroprusside: pharmacology, toxicology and therapeutics, *Anesthesiology* 1976, 45:340–354.

Ivankovich AD, Miletich DJ, Tinker JH: Sodium nitroprusside—metabolism and general considerations, *Int Anesthesiol Clin* 1978, 16:1–29.

NONDEPOLARIZING MUSCLE RELAXANTS

Warning: Before using any neuromuscular relaxant, the clinician must be totally familiar with its action and be able to perform tracheal intubation and totally control ventilation in the patient.

Trade Names:
Long-acting: 25% recovery of motor function approximately 60 min after intubation doses:

  Doxacurium: *Nuromax.*
  Metocurine: *Metubine.*
  Pancuronium: *Pavulon.*
  Pipecuronium: *Arduan.*
  Tubocurarine: generics.

Intermediate-acting: 25% recovery of motor function approximately 30 min after intubation doses:

  Atracurium: *Tracrium.*
  Cisatracurium: *Nimbex.*
  Vecuronium: *Norcuron.*
  Rocuronium: *Zemuron.*

Short-acting: 25% recovery of motor function in less than 30 min after intubation doses.

  Mivacurium: *Mivacron.*

Drug Action: Primary site of action of each of these drugs is the postsynaptic cholinergic receptor of the neuromuscular junction. They competitively bind and block depolarization of the motor end plate produced by acetylcholine that is released from the presynaptic terminal membrane. None of these agents crosses the blood-brain barrier, and they do not produce sedation, amnesia, or anesthesia.

Indications:

1. Skeletal muscle relaxation for surgical procedures and tracheal intubation.
2. Skeletal muscle relaxation during mechanical ventilation and in various disease states, such as tetanus.

Pharmacokinetics:

1. All of these drugs are administered IV. *See* Table 17 for comparisons of distribution, metabolism, and excretion. Doxacurium, curare, metocurine, pipecuronium, and rocuronium are not metabolized. Doxacurium is excreted primarily by renal mechanisms, and while doxacurium can be recovered in the bile 35–90 min after administration, the extent of biliary excretion is unknown. Curare is excreted almost equally by renal and hepatic mechanisms; metocurine is predominantly excreted via the kidneys. 60%–80% of a dose of pancuronium and >75% of pipecuronium is excreted unchanged via the kidneys; 80% of a dose of vecuronium is excreted unchanged via the biliary system. Pancuronium and its analog, vecuronium, are metabolized similarly into three metabolites, with each metabolite having significantly less potency than the parent compound. Rocuronium and pipecuronium are not metabolized to any significant extent.
2. Both atracurium and cisatracurium undergo Hoffman degradation, a pH- and temperature-dependent process in which the molecule spontaneously breaks down. Atracurium also undergo hydrolysis by nonspecific plasma esterases. Cisatracurium, one of the ten sterioisomers comprising atracurium, does not undergo enzymatic ester hydrolysis. Renal and hepatic mechanisms and plasma cholinesterase are not involved in the metabolism of either atracurium or cisatracurium. Laudanosine (a metabolite of atracurium and its

sterioisomers, including cisatracurium), when exogenously administered in large quantities, causes CNS excitation and even seizures. In most patients this is not a problem. However, the potential for significant blood levels of laudanosine does exist in patients with renal failure who receive atracurium or cisatracurium infusions for several days.

3. In patients with renal failure, the preferred muscle relaxants would then be atracurium, cisatracurium, mivacurium, rocuronium, vecuronium (20% renal excretion), and curare (50% renal excretion). Independent of which muscle relaxant is chosen, the initial dose is the same for intubation, and subsequent doses are given on the basis of neuromuscular blockade monitoring and clinical assessment.

4. In patients with hepatic failure, the actions of pancuronium, rocuronium, and vecuronium are affected. The initial doses of these drugs may need to be increased because of increased volume of distribution. Once neuromuscular blockade is achieved, subsequent doses may need to be decreased because of delay in elimination.

5. In patients with combined renal-hepatic failure, the choice of muscle relaxant depends on the severity of the respective organ failure and the requirements for muscle relaxation. Short periods of paralysis can be safely achieved with atracurium, cisatracurium, and mivacurium. Prolonged relaxation can be achieved by administering any of the other relaxants, with subsequent doses titrated by neuromuscular blockade monitoring and clinical criteria.

Drug Preparations:

Arduan: 1 mg/mL, in 10 mL vials.

Metubine: 2 mg/mL, in 20 mL vials.

Mivacron: 0.5 mg/mL, in 50 and 100 mL vials. 2.0 mg/mL, in 5, 10, 20, and 50 mL vials.

Nimbex: (unknown)

Norcuron: 1 mg/mL, in 10 mL vials. 1 mg/mL in 10 mL prefilled syringes.

Nuromax: 1 mg/mL, in 5 mL vials.

Pavulon: 1 mg/mL, in 10 mL vials. 2 mg/mL, in 2, 5 mL ampules.

Tracrium: 10 mg/mL, in 5 mL and 10 mL vials.

Tubocurarine: 3 mg/mL, in 5, 10, and 20 mL vials.
Zemuron: 10 mg/mL, in 5 mL vials.

Dosage: *See* Table 17 for intubating doses of relaxants. Subsequent doses for relaxation must be individualized, depending on underlying disease, administration of other drugs, and organ dysfunction. In general, long-acting neuromuscular blocking drugs such as doxacurium, tubocurarine, metocurine, pipecuronium, and pancuronium need to be given q 1–2 hr at 25%–50% of the original dose. Intermediate-acting drugs such as atracurium, cisatracurium, rocuronium, and vecuronium need to be given q 30–60 min at 25%–50% of the original dose. The short-acting drug mivacurium requires frequent readministration (at 10–15 min intervals). For prolonged administration, (e.g., >1 hr) a continuous infusion, titrated to the desired effect, is more appropriate.

Adverse Effects:

1. Injection of intubating doses of curare over less than 60–90 sec frequently results in histamine release, with subsequent cutaneous flushing and possibly a drop in blood pressure. Rarely, bronchospasm occurs. Release of histamine also may occur infrequently with rapid bolus injection of an intubating dose of metocurine, atracurium, or mivacurium.
2. Tachycardia may occasionally result from administration of pancuronium as a result of its vagal blocking properties and possibly secondary to the increased release and decreased uptake of norepinephrine at the cardiac adrenergic nerve endings.
3. Ganglionic blockade as an adverse effect of curare resulting in hypotension has been reported. Only at doses 2–3 times the intubating dose does this effect become significant.
4. Inadequate airway protection can increase the risk of aspiration.

Problems Related to Altered Physiologic State:

1. Markedly prolonged neuromuscular blockade occurs after administration of nondepolarizing relaxants to patients with myasthenia gravis and myasthenic syndrome (Eaton-Lambert syndrome), especially when the long-acting agents are used. This occurs with as little as 1 mg pancuronium or 2–3 mg curare. Owing to its unique metabolism, atracurium seems to be

TABLE 17.

Pharmacokinetics of Nondepolarizing Muscle Relaxants

Agent	Intubating Dose (mg/kg)	Metabolism	Renal Excretion (%)	Elimination Half-Time (min)	Time from Administration to Intubation (min)	Histamine Release*	Cardiac Vagal Blockade	Infusion Rate (μg/kg/min)
Atracurium	0.4–0.5	Yes	<10	20	2–3	+	0	4–12
Cisatracurium	0.15–0.2	Yes	<10	20	1–2	0	0	2–3
Doxacurium	0.05–0.08	No	70	100	4–5	0+	0	—
Metocurine	0.3–0.4	No	80–90	300	3–5	0++	0	—
Mivacurium	0.2–0.3	Yes	<5	2–3	1–2	+++	0	3–15
Pancuronium	0.07–0.1	Yes	60–80	100–120	3–5	0	+++	—
Pipecuronium	0.08–0.14	No	>75	60–120	2–3	0	0	—
Rocuronium	0.6–1.0	No	<5	120–180	1–2	0	+	8–12
Tubocurarine	0.5–0.6	No	40–60	90–120	3–5	++++	0	—
Vecuronium	0.08–0.10	Yes	<25	70	2–3	0	0	.08–2.0

*Histamine release with intubating doses administered rapidly.
†With atropine being ++++.

the best agent in these patients, and with careful titration of reduced doses (approximately one fifth routine intubating dose
or less), the duration of blockade may not be significantly prolonged.
2. Other neurologic conditions (e.g., hemiplegia) alter the pharmacodynamics of neuromuscular relaxants, with decreased
sensitivity observed on the side affected by a cerebrovascular
accident.
3. Electrolyte alterations may affect the action of nondepolarizing
relaxants. Acute hypokalemia can increase the sensitivity; hyperkalemia can reduce the sensitivity. Usually, this is not a significant problem.
4. Respiratory acidosis, and to a lesser extent metabolic alkalosis,
will prolong the action of nondepolarizing agents.
5. Burn patients frequently require two or three times the dose to
obtain adequate relaxation.
6. Hypothermia prolongs neuromuscular blockade and increases
the sensitivity of the neuromuscular junction to nondepolarizing agents.
7. Prolonged atracurium infusions should be used with caution in
patients with renal failure, because of accumulation of potentially toxic metabolites.

Drug Interactions:

1. Certain antibiotics (e.g., the aminoglycosides, polymyxin B,
bacitracin, tetracycline, colistin, and others) may prolong the
duration of action of nondepolarizing relaxants. The penicillins
and cephalosporins have no effect on duration of action.
2. Administration of magnesium salts in eclamptic parturients or
of lithium in psychiatric patients increases the sensitivity to
nondepolarizing agents and prolongs paralysis.
3. Lidocaine and quinidine, used in treatment of cardiac dysrhythmias, may prolong and increase the sensitivity for neuromuscular blockade.
4. Various drugs, such as diuretics, steroids, and amphotericin B,
may result in hypokalemia, which increases sensitivity to nondepolarizing agents.

5. Various sedatives and narcotics may produce respiratory acidosis, which may potentiate or prolong neuromuscular relaxation.
6. Furosemide in relatively small doses (1 mg/kg IV) may enhance neuromuscular blockade by inhibition of cAMP production, leading to decreased prejunctional output of acetylcholine. Conversely, large doses may inhibit phosphodiesterase, making more cAMP available, leading to antagonism of neuromuscular blockade.
7. Cyclosporine has been shown to prolong the duration of neuromuscular blockade.

Monitoring:

1. Anesthesiologists frequently assess neuromuscular function with peripheral nerve stimulators. The ulnar nerve is most commonly stimulated, and the response produced by the adductor pollicis brevis is assessed.
2. Recovery of neuromuscular function can also be simply assessed in the ICU. A sustained head lift for 5 sec or inspiratory pressure (force) 30–40 cm H_2O indicates that sufficient motor function has returned to allow for extubation if neurologic status, oxygenation, and carbon dioxide elimination are adequate.

Reversal of Neuromuscular Relaxation:

1. If partial recovery of function has occurred, complete recovery can frequently be hastened by pharmacologic means. This involves use of a cholinesterase inhibitor to augment the amount of acetylcholine at the motor end plate and an anticholinergic agent to prevent the muscarinic effects, such as bradycardia and sialorrhea, which are not desired.
2. The following two regimens take advantage of onset of action of the various drugs:
   a. Atropine 7–9 μg/kg **plus** edrophonium 0.5–1.0 mg/kg.
   b. Glycopyrrolate 7.5 μg/kg or atropine 15 μg/kg **plus** neostigmine 40–70 μg/kg.

BIBLIOGRAPHY

Gilman AG, Rall TW, Nies AS, Taylor P (eds): *Goodman and Gilman's The Pharmacological Basis of Therapeutics,* ed 8, New York, 1990, Macmillan.

Miller RD (ed): *Anesthesia,* ed 4, New York, 1994, Churchill Livingstone.

Stoelting RK: *Pharmacology and Physiology in Anesthetic Practice,* ed 2, Philadelphia, 1987, JB Lippincott.

Denniston PL Jr (ed): 1995 *Physicians GenRx,* Riverside, 1995, Denniston Publishing.

Physicians' Desk Reference, ed 49, Montvale, 1995, Medical Economics Data Production.

NONSTEROIDAL ANTI-INFLAMMATORY DRUGS (NSAIDS)

Trade Names: *See* Table 18.

Aspirin: *see* Aspirin.
Ibuprofen: *see* Ibuprofen.
Ketorolac: *see* Ketorolac.

Drug Actions: Inhibits prostaglandin synthesis; inhibits hypothalamic heat-regulating center to reduce fever.

Indications:

1. Pain.
2. Fever.
3. Inflammation.
4. Antiplatelet agent (prevention of thrombosis).

Pharmacokinetics: *See* Table 18.

Drug Preparations: *See* Table 18.

Dosage: *See* Table 18.

Adverse Effects:

1. GI: Bleeding, gastritis, ulcer, nausea/vomiting, epigastric pain, perforation, heart burn, hepatic injury.

2. Bleeding (antiplatelet actions).
3. Renal dysfunction, renal failure, interstitial nephritis, cystitis.
4. Dizziness, tinnitus, blurred vision.
5. Confusion, agitation, hallucinations, weakness, tiredness, mental depression, coma, seizures, headache, peripheral neuropathy.
6. Rash, urticaria, hypersensitivity reactions.
7. Hemolytic anemia, iron deficiency anemia, bone marrow depression, leukopenia, thrombocytopenia.
8. Respiratory compromise, bronchospasm.
9. Metabolic acidosis, hypoglycemia, hyperkalemia.
10. Hypertension, tachycardia, angina, anaphylaxis, edema, heart failure, arrhythmias, flushing.

Drug Interactions:

1. There are many, and one should check the PDR for individual agents.
2. Increased risk of bleeding when used with other anticoagulants and antiplatelet agents.
3. May increase toxicity from digoxin, methotrexate, cyclosporin, lithium, insulin, sulfonylureas, potassium-sparing diuretics, phenytoin, sulfonamides, aminoglycosides, amphotericin B.
4. May decrease effect of antihypertensives, (diuretics, β-blockers, vasodilators).
5. Probenecid increases levels of NSAIDs.

Monitoring: Clinical response, signs of bleeding or peptic ulcer/gastritis, CBC, liver enzymes, BUN, creatinine.

BIBLIOGRAPHY

Williams RF: The selection of a nonsteroidal antiinflammatory drug—is there a difference?, *J Rheumatol* 1992, 19(suppl):9–12.

Insel PA: Analgesia-antipyretics and antiinflammatory agents—drugs employed in the treatment of rheumatoid arthritis and gout. In Gilman AG, et al (eds): *The Pharmacological Basis of Therapeutics,* ed 8, New York, 1993, Macmillan, pp 638–681.

TABLE 18.
Nonsteroidal Anti-inflammatory Drugs

DRUG	Trade Names	Dose	Metabolism	Half-Life	Preparations
Aspirin	Anacin Ascriptin Bayer aspirin Bufferin others	PO, rectal 325–650 mg q4–6h (max. 4 g/day)	Hepatic; hydrolyzed to salicylate	Parent drug 15–20 min Salicylate 3–5 hr	Tablets: 80, 325, 500 mg Suppositories: 120, 200, 300, 600 mg
Diclofenac	Cataflam Voltaren	PO: 25–75 50 mg tid	Hepatic	2 hr	Tablets 25, 50, 75 mg
Fenoprofen	Nalfon	PO: 200–600 mg q6–8h	Hepatic	2.5–3 hr	Tablet 600 mg Capsule 200, 300 mg
Ibuprofen	Motrin Advil Nupren Others	PO: 200–800 mg q6–8h	Hepatic	2–4 hr	Tablets: 200, 300, 400, 600, 800 mg Suspension 100 mg/5 mL
Indomethacin	Indocin	PO: 25–50 mg q8–12h (sustained release 75 mg daily) IV (patent ductus): Initial 0.2 mg/kg, followed by 0.1–0.25 mg/kg q12–24h	Hepatic	4.5 hr	Capsule 25, 50 mg Sustained release 75 mg Suppository 50 mg Oral suspension 25 mg/5 mL Injection 1 mg

Ketoprofen	Orudis	PO: 25–75 mg q6–8h (extended release 200 mg once daily)	Hepatic	1–4 hr	Capsule 25, 50 75 mg Extended release 200 mg
Ketorolac	Toradol Acular	PO: 10 mg q4–6h IM: Initial 30–60 mg, then 15–30 mg q6h IV: Initial 30 mg, then 15–30 mg q6h	Hepatic	2–8 hr	Tablet 10 mg Injection 15 and 30 mg/mL
Meclofenamate	Meclomen	PO: 50 mg q4–6h (max. 400 mg/day)	Hepatic	2–3 hr	Capsule 50, 100 mg
Naproxen	Aleve Naprosyn Anaprox	PO: 250 mg q6–8h	Hepatic	12–15 hr	Tablets 250, 375, 500 mg Suspension 125 mg/5 mL
Piroxicam	Feldene	PO: 10–20 mg/day	Hepatic	45–50 hr	Capsule 10, 20 mg
Salsalate	Argesic Salgesic Salflex Others	PO: 3 gm/day in 2–3 divided doses	Hepatic	7–8 hr	Tablets 500, 750 mg Tablets 150, 200 mg
Sulindac	Clinoril	PO: 150–200 mg bid	Hepatic (to active metabolite)	Parent drug 7 hr Active metabolite 18 hr	Tablets 150, 200 mg
Tolmetin	Tolectin	PO: 400 mg tid	Hepatic	5 hr	Capsule 400 mg Tablets 200, 600 mg

NOREPINEPHRINE

Trade Name: *Levophed.*

Drug Action:

1. Potent arterial and venous vasoconstriction (α-effect). Stimulates β_1 but not β_2 receptors.
2. Increases inotropic effects and blood pressure without increasing heart rate.

Indications:

1. Hypotension.
2. Refractory hypotension (sepsis; after removal of pheochromocytoma).
3. Cardiogenic shock.

Pharmacokinetics:

1. **Absorption:** IV.
2. **Metabolism:** Monoamine oxidase+catechol-*O*-methyl transferase in liver, kidney, GI tract. Reuptake into nerve terminals helps terminate biologic actions.
3. **Excretion:** Renal.
4. **Plasma half-life:** Minutes.
5. **Onset of action:** Almost immediate after IV administration.

Drug Preparations:

Ampules: 4 mg/4 mL.

Dosage:

1. **Decreased blood pressure:** 4–10 μg/min IV infusion.
2. **Higher doses** may be required in sepsis, cardiogenic shock, and in combination with vasodilator therapy.

Adverse Effects:

1. Decreased renal blood flow (dopamine may have protective effects).
2. Intense peripheral vasoconstriction making peripheral vascular disease worse, hypertension.
3. Venous extravasation causes skin necrosis.

4. Headache, anxiety, tremor, angina, bradycardia, dysrhythmias, myocardial infarction, stroke, nausea/vomiting, acidosis, seizures.

Drug Interactions:

1. Drugs that sensitize the heart to arrhythmias.
2. Potentiated by tricyclic antidepressants, MAO inhibitors, certain antihistamines.

Monitoring:

1. Heart rate, rhythm.
2. Blood pressure.
3. Urine output.
4. PA catheter when using contractility effects.

BIBLIOGRAPHY

Kaplan JA: Treatment of perioperative left ventricular failure. In Kaplan JA (ed): *Cardiac Anesthesia,* Orlando, 1987, Grune & Stratton, pp 963–994.

Weiner N: Norepinephrine, epinephrine, and the sympathomimetic amines. In Gilman AG, Goodman LS, Gilman A (eds): *The Pharmacological Basis of Therapeutics,* ed 6, New York, 1980, Macmillan, pp 138–175.

NORFLOXACIN

Trade Name: *Noroxin.*

Drug Action:

1. Inhibition of DNA gyrase.
2. Spectrum of activity includes gram-positive aerobes (better against staphylococci than against streptococci) and almost all clinically important gram-negative aerobes (including *Pseudomonas aeruginosa*).
   a. No anti-anaerobic activity.
   b. *P. maltophilia* and *P. cepacia* resistant.

Indications: Treatment of urinary tract infections caused by susceptible organisms in **adults.**

Pharmacokinetics:

1. **Absorption:** Variable but rapid from GI tract (presence of food and especially Mg- and Al-containing antacids interfere).
2. **Elimination:** Metabolism, hepatic and renal excretion.
3. **Serum half-life:** 3–4 hr (levels in tissues outside urinary tract not adequate for clinical use).

Drug Preparations:

Tablets: 400 mg.

Dosage:

1. **Normal renal function:** 400 mg bid PO.
2. **Impaired renal function:** 400 mg once daily with creatinine clearance <30.

Adverse Effects:

1. Cartilage damage in experimental animals.
   a. **Not approved** in patients younger than 18 yr or in pregnant or nursing women.
2. Generally well tolerated; most common side effects GI (e.g., nausea, abdominal pain, dyspepsia) and neurologic (e.g., headache, dizziness).

Drug Interactions:

1. **Antacids** decrease absorption of norfloxacin.

OCTREOTIDE

Trade Name: *Sandostatin.*

Drug Action:

1. Increases intestinal transit time.
2. Inhibits gastroenteropancreatic secretion.
3. Decreases fluid secretion in jejunum and ileum.
4. Increases water and electrolyte absorption by small intestine.

5. Suppresses secretion of vasoactive intestinal polypeptide (VIP), gastrin, glucagon, growth hormone, thyroid-stimulating hormone (TSH), insulin, pancreatic polypeptide, motilin, neurotensin, cholecystokinin, serotonin, gastric acid, pepsin, secretin, lipase, amylase, trypsin, bilirubin.
6. Decreases splanchnic blood flow.

Indications:

1. Neuroendocrine tumors of gut: metastatic carcinoids (controls flushing and diarrhea), VIP-secreting tumors (controls diarrhea).
2. Control of diarrhea and excess gut/pancreatic secretions (e.g., fistula).

Pharmacokinetics:

1. **Absorption:** Destroyed in GI tract; given parenterally; peak effect occurs 30 min after SQ injection.
2. **Metabolism:** Hepatic.
3. **Excretion:** Urine, 32% unchanged (clearance reduced with renal disease).
4. **Distribution:** Plasma, 65% protein bound.
5. **Serum half-life:** α: 0.2 hr; β: 1.4 hr.
6. **Duration of action:** Up to 12 hr.

Drug Preparations:

Ampules: 1 mL, containing 0.05, 0.1, 0.5 mg.

Dosage:

1. 50 μg SQ q day bid; taper to effect.
2. Average dose:
   a. **Carcinoid:** 100–600 μg/day.
   b. **VIPomas:** 150–750 μg/day.

Adverse Effects:

1. Pain at injection site.
2. (3%–10%): Nausea/vomiting, diarrhea, abdominal pain.
3. (1%–3%): Headache, fat malabsorption, dizziness, hyperglycemia, fatigue, flushing, hypoglycemia, edema, weakness, wheal/erythema.
4. (<1%): Constipation, flatulence, hepatitis, jaundice, GI bleeding, heartburn, cholelithiasis, hair loss, pruritus, rash, bruising, muscle pain, cramping, joint pain, chest pain, shortness of breath, hypertension, congestive heart failure, throm-

bophlebitis, anxiety, seizures, depression, drowsiness, insomnia, irritability, syncope, tremor, galactorrhea, rhinorrhea, oliguria, prostatitis.
5. (Possible): Hypothalamic pituitary dysfunction (e.g., hypothyroidism).

Drug Interactions:

1. Reduction in insulin requirements.
2. Decreased fat absorption.
3. May decrease absorption of nutrients and drugs.

Monitoring:

1. Glucose.
2. Thyroxine, TSH with long-term therapy.
3. Gallbladder ultrasound with long-term therapy.
4. 5-HIAA, serotonin, substance P (carcinoid tumors).
5. VIP (VIPoma).

BIBLIOGRAPHY

Paran H, Neufeld D, Kaplan O, et al: Oxtreotide for treatment of postoperative alimentary tract fistulas, *World J Surg* 1995, 19:430–433.

Harris AG, O'Dorisio TM, Woltering EA, et al: Consensus statement—octreotide dose titration in secretory diarrhea. Diarrhea Management Consensus Development Panel, *Diag Dis Sci* 1995, 40:1464–1473.

Gregor M: Therapeutic principles in the management of metastasising carcinoid tumors: drugs for symptomatic treatment, *Digestion* 1994, 55(suppl):60–63.

OFLOXACIN

Trade Name: *Floxin.*

Drug Actions:

1. Bactericidal through inhibition of bacterial DNA gyrase (topoisomerase II), an enzyme critical for duplication, transcription, and repair of bacterial DNA.

2. Spectrum of activity is broad and encompasses staphylococci and most gram-negative aerobes, including *Pseudomonas aeruginosa* (but not *P. cepacia* or *Stendtrophomonas* (formerly *Xanthomonas*) *maltophilia*), *Neisseria gonorrhoeae,* and *Chlamydia trachomatis.* Ofloxacin is moderately active against streptococci and anaerobes (not best choice for these). Many strains of enterococcus are resistant to ofloxacin.

3. Ofloxacin has some activity against *Mycobacterium tuberculosis.*

Indications:

1. Acute exacerbations of chronic bronchitis and community-acquired pneumonia.
2. Skin and skin structure infections.
3. Gonococcal cervicitis/urethritis.
4. Nongonococcal cervicitis/urethritis due to *C. trachomatis.*
5. Urinary tract infections.
6. Prostatitis due to *Escherichia coli.*
7. Second-line drug therapy for tuberculosis (mainly as treatment and prophylaxis for multidrug-resistant (MDR) tuberculosis)—not an FDA-approved indication.

Pharmacokinetics:

1. **Absorption:** PO/IV; good tissue penetration. Antacids, iron, or multivitamins containing zinc should not be taken within the 2 hr period before, or within the 2 hr period after ofloxacin administration.
2. **Excretion:** Mainly renal (65%–80%) with 4%–8% excreted in feces.
3. **Half-life:** Ofloxacin has biphasic elimination with half-lives of 4–5 hr and 20–25 hr (<5% of total at this half-life). Accumulation at steady state can be estimated using a half-life of 9 hr.

Drug Preparations:

Tablets: 200, 300, 400 mg.
Vials: 400 mg (10 mL of 40 mg/mL or 20 mL of 20 mg/mL).

Dosage:

1. Normal renal function:

Urinary tract infections: 200 mg q 12 hr.
Prostatitis, nongonococcal cervicitis/urethritis: 300 mg q 12 hr.
Exacerbation of chronic bronchitis, community-acquired pneumonia, skin and skin structure infections: 400 mg q 12 hr.
Uncomplicated gonorrhea: 400 mg PO once (note: Ofloxacin is not useful in chlamydial infections as a single dose).
Antituberculous therapy: 400 mg bid.

2. Impaired renal function:

Creatinine clearance (mL/min)	Dosage
10–50	Usual dose but q 24 hr.
<10	One half usual dose and give q 24 hr.

Adverse Effects:

1. The most commonly reported side effects are nausea (10%), headache (9%), insomnia (7%), external genital pruritus in women (6%), dizziness (5%), vaginitis (5%), diarrhea (4%), and vomiting (4%); numerous other events occur with lesser frequencies.
2. Osteochrondrosis in experimental animals. Ofloxacin is not approved for use in patients <18 yr of age, pregnant patients, or nursing women.

Drug Interactions:

1. Antacids, sucralfate, metal cations, and multivitamins interfere with absorption of quinolones (see above).
2. Cimetidine may increase half-lives of some quinolones.
3. May elevate levels of theophylline, cyclosporine, and other drugs metabolized by the cytochrome P-450 system.
4. Some quinolones have been reported to enhance the effects of warfarin.

BIBLIOGRAPHY

Physicians' Desk Reference, ed 50, Montvale, 1996, Medical Economics Co.

OMEPRAZOLE

Trade Name: *Prilosec.*

Drug Actions: Suppresses gastric acid secretion by inhibition of H^+-K^+-ATPase enzyme system in gastric parietal cell (proton pump)

Indications: Peptic ulcer disease, esophagitis, gastroesophageal reflux disease, hypersecretory conditions (e.g., Zollinger-Ellison syndrome)

Pharmacokinetics:

1. **Absorption:** Rapid PO: 30%–40% bioavailable, peak levels 0.5–3.5 hr.
2. **Onset of action:** 1 hr, max. effect 2 hr, duration 72 hr.
3. **Metabolism:** Hepatic.
4. **Excretion:** Metabolites in urine and bile.
5. **Half-life:** 0.5–1 hr.

Drug Preparations:

Delayed-release capsules: 20 mg.

Dosage: 20 mg PO daily (4–8 wk) before meals; do not open, chew, or crush (hypersecretory conditions—begin 60 mg daily and titrate to effect), do not adjust for renal/hepatic disease.

Adverse Effects: Hypergastronemia secondary to prolonged hypochlorhydria may lead to enterochromaffin cell hyperplasia and gastric carcinoid tumors; increase in gastric bacteria (similar to other agents that elevate pH), constipation, diarrhea, abdominal pain.

Drug Interactions: Prolongs elimination of diazepam, warfarin, phenytoin, carbamazepine, cyclosporin, and other P-450–metabolized drugs; interferes with absorption of drugs that require gastric acidity (ketoconazole, ampicillin esters, iron salts).

Monitoring: Gastric pH

BIBLIOGRAPHY

Eriksson S, Langstrom G, Rikner L, Carlsson R, Naesdal J: Omeprazole and H_2-receptor antagonists in the acute treatment of duodenal ulcer, gastric ulcer, and reflux oesophagitis: a meta-analysis, *Eur J Gastroenterol Hepatol* 1995, 7:467–475.

Schulman MI, Orlando RC: Treatment of gastroesophageal reflux: the role of proton pump inhibitors, *Adv Intern Med* 1995, 40:273–302.

ONDANSETRON

Trade Name: *Zofran.*

Drug Actions: Selective 5-HT$_3$ receptor antagonist.

Indications: Nausea and vomiting (cancer chemotherapy, postoperative).

Pharmacokinetics:

1. **Absorption:** PO or IV.
2. **Onset of action:** PO 1–2 hr, IV ~15–30 min.
3. **Metabolism:** Hepatic (cytochrome P-450 enzymes).
4. **Excretion:** 5% unchanged in urine.
5. **Half-life:** 3–6 hr.

Drug Preparations: Injection: 2 mg/mL in 2 and 20 mL vials; tablets: 4, 8 mg.

Dosage: Cancer chemotherapy: Dilute in 50 mL D$_5$W or 0.9% saline; give IV 8 mg PO tid (before, 4 and 8 hr after, chemotherapy), patients 4–12 yr old 4 mg PO tid. Alternate dosing: Administer 0.15 mg/kg IV dose (before, 4 and 8 hr after, chemotherapy) or single 32 mg IV dose before chemotherapy. Reduce dose in patients with impaired hepatic function (max. 8 mg daily). Postoperative nausea/vomiting: 4 mg undiluted IV over 2–5 min.

Adverse Effects: Constipation, diarrhea, abdominal cramps, liver injury, rash, hypersensitivity reactions, rare extrapyramidal CNS symptoms, transient dizziness and blurred vision, rare seizures, headache, bronchospasm, hypokalemia. Cardiovascular: Rare tachycardia, bradycardia, angina, hypotension, syncope, second-degree heart block.

Drug Interactions: Inducers (barbiturates, carbamazepine, rifampin, phenytoin, phenylbutazone or inhibitors (cimetidine, allopurinol, disulfiram) of cytochrome P-450 drug metabolizing enzyme in liver may alter clearance.

Monitoring: Clinical response, liver enzymes.

BIBLIOGRAPHY

Riola F, Del Favero A: Ondansetron clinical pharmacokinetics, *Clin Pharmacokinet* 1995, 29:95–109.
Claybon L: Single dose intravenous ondansetron for the 24 hour treatment of post-operative nausea and vomiting, *Anesthesia* 1994, 49(suppl):24–29.

OXACILLIN

Trade Names: *Bactocil, Prostaphlin.*

Drug Action:

1. Inhibition of cell wall synthesis (penicillin).
2. Antistaphylococcal activity.

Indications: Staphylococcal infections.

Pharmacokinetics:

1. **Absorption:** Variable from GI tract (best without food).
2. **Excretion:** Primarily renal.
3. **Metabolism:** Partial.
4. **Serum half-life:** 30 min.

Drug Preparations:

   Capsules: 250, 500 mg.
   PO suspension: 250 mg/5 mL.
   Vials: 500 mg, 1, 2, 4 g, for parenteral use.

Dosage: Normal/impaired renal function:

1. Adult:
   a. 2–4 g/day PO in divided doses q 6 hr.
   b. 0.5–2 g IV q 4–6 hr.
2. Pediatric:
   a. 50–100 mg/kg/day PO in four divided doses.
   b. 25–33.3 mg/kg IV q 4–6 hr.

Adverse Effects:

1. Similar to other penicillins (e.g., hypersensitivity reactions, GI problems, cytopenias).
2. Oxacillin hepatitis: Anicteric hepatic dysfunction with eosinophilia after high dose, long-term IV use.

Drug Interactions:

1. Incompatible with aminoglycosides.
2. Probenecid blocks renal excretion.

Monitoring: Serial liver/kidney function studies.

OXAZEPAM

Trade Name: *Serax.*

Drug Action: Anxiety reduction, sedation, anticonvulsant activity, muscle relaxation, amnesia.

Indications: Anxiety, insomnia, alcohol withdrawal.

Drug Preparations:

Tablets: 15 mg.
Capsules: 10, 15, 30 mg.

Dosage:

1. **Anxiety:** 30–120 mg/day PO in three to four doses.

Pharmacokinetics:

1. **Metabolism:** Hepatic conjugation.
2. **Half-life:** 5–15 hr.
3. **Excretion:** Renal excretion of inactive metabolites.
4. **Dialyzable?:** Limited.
5. **Renal failure:** Monitor sedation.
6. **Hepatic failure:** Reduce dose, monitor sedation.

Adverse Effects: Sedation, psychomotor impairment, depression, amnesia, impaired concentration, weakness, impaired sexual function, paradoxical agitation.

Drug Interactions: Additive effect with other CNS depressants.

Monitoring: Monitor for excess sedation vs. therapeutic effect.

BIBLIOGRAPHY

Drugs used for anxiety and sleep disorders. In *AMA Drug Evaluations,* ed 6, Philadelphia, 1986, WB Saunders, pp 81–110.
Sussman N: The benzodiazepines: selection and use in treating anxiety, insomnia, and other disorders, *Hosp Formul* 1985, 20:298–305.

OXYMORPHONE

Trade Name: *Numorphan.*

Drug Action:

1. Approximately 10 times more potent than morphine but causes more nausea/vomiting.
2. Produces mild sedation but has little antitussive activity.

Indications:

1. Treatment of moderate to severe pain.
2. Adjunct to general, regional, or local anesthesia.
3. Can be used for preoperative sedation.

Pharmacokinetics:

1. **Absorption:**
   a. **SQ/IM/PR:** Absorption good, with onset of action 10–20 min and duration 3–6 hr.
   b. **IV:** Onset within 5–10 min; similar duration of action as with other routes.
2. **Metabolism:** Glucuronide conjugation occurs in liver.
3. **Excretion:** Urinary.

Drug Preparations:

Parenteral: 1, 1.5 mg/mL.
PR suppositories: 5 mg.

Dosage:

1. IV: 0.5 mg q 4–6 hr.
2. IM/SQ: 1–1.5 mg q 4–6 hr.
3. PR: 5 mg q 4–6 hr.

Adverse Effects: Similar to those with morphine (e.g., dysphoria, lethargy, nausea/vomiting, urinary retention; potential for elevated intracranial pressure in patients at risk); sedation, drowsiness, respiratory depression, hypotension.

Drug Interactions: CNS depression may be augmented with concomitant administration of phenothiazines, tricyclic antidepressants, hypnotics, sedatives, alcohol, other CNS depressants.

Monitoring: Respiratory rate, blood pressure, heart rate, mental status.

BIBLIOGRAPHY

AMA Drug Evaluations, ed 6, Philadelphia, 1986, WB Saunders.
McEvoy GK (ed): *AHFS Drug Information 89,* Bethesda, 1989, American Society of Hospital Pharmacists.

PAMIDRONATE DISODIUM

Trade Name: *Aredia.*

Drug Actions: Bisphosphonate, inhibits bone resorption (but not formation); inhibits osteoclast activity

Indications:

1. Hypercalcemia of malignancy.
2. Paget's disease of bone.
3. Heterotopic ossification due to spinal cord injury or hip replacement.

Pharmacokinetics:

1. **Absorption:** Poorly absorbed after oral ingestion; give IV.
2. **Onset of action:** 24–48 hr; peak effect approximately 7 days.
3. **Metabolism:** Binds to bone.

4. **Excretion:** 51% unchanged in urine.
5. **Half-life:** 2.5 hr; elimination half-life in bone approximately 300 days.

Drug Preparations: 30, 60, 90 mg vials for IV administration (dilute dose in 1000 mL 0.45% or 0.9% NaCl or 5% dextrose).

Dosage: Moderate hypercalcemia (corrected Ca 12–14 mg/dL) 60–90 mg IV over 12–24 hr, severe hypercalcemia (corrected Ca >14 mg/dL) 90 mg IV over 12–24 hr (may repeat after 7 days); Paget's disease: 60 mg as single 12–24 hour infusion.

Adverse Effects: Hypophosphatemia, decreased Mg, decreased K, decreased Ca (may lead to symptoms such as paresthesias, spasm, tetany, seizures, hypotension), anemia, nephropathy, transient elevation in temperature, soft tissue symptoms at injection site, fluid overload, generalized pain, hypertension, tachycardia, bone pain, abdominal pain, anorexia, diarrhea, constipation, nausea/vomiting, vein irritation and thrombophlebitis with infusion, malaise, fever, seizures, hepatic dysfunction, skin rash, hypersensitivity reactions.

Drug Interactions: None reported.

Monitoring: Ca, PO_4, Mg, K, BUN, creatinine, CBC.

BIBLIOGRAPHY

Zaloga GP, Chernow B: Divalent ions—calcium, magnesium, and phosphorus. In Chernow B (ed): *The Pharmacologic Approach to the Critically Ill Patient,* ed 3, Baltimore, 1994, Williams & Wilkins, pp 777–804.

Purohit OP, Radstone CR, Anthony C, et al: A randomized double-blind comparison of intravenous pamidronate and clodronate in the hypercalcemia of malignancy, *Br J Cancer* 1995, 72:1289–1293.

Olson Y, Tomita A, Hasegawa H, et al: Pamidronate treatment in patients with tumor associated hypercalcemia: pharmacological effects and pharmacokinetics, *Endocrine J* 1994, 41:655–661.

PANCREATIC ENZYMES

Trade Names: *Ilozyme, Ku-Zyme HP, Cotazym, Pancrease, Viokase, Pancreatin 2400, Creon, Zymase, Entozyme.*

Drug Action:

1. Pancreatic extract: Contains multiple exogenous enzymes to enhance digestion of proteins, starches, and fats, primarily in the duodenum and upper jejunum. Activity is greatest in neutral or slightly alkaline environments.

Indications:

1. Pancreatic extract: Management of pancreatic insufficiency due to chronic pancreatitis, pancreatectomy, cystic fibrosis, bypass surgery (Billroth II), and neoplastic ductal obstruction usually characterized by steatorrhea or abdominal pain.
2. Occluded feeding tubes.

Pharmacokinetics: Pancreatic extract is not absorbed. It is degraded locally in the GI tract and inactivated by acid.

Drug Preparations: *See* Table 19. Only preparations with >600 U lipase/tablet or capsule are considered effective. Products with <600 U are not included. Do not chew capsules or tablets.

Dosage:

1. Actual dose depends on the digestive requirements of the patient.
2. Adults: 4000–16,000 units of lipase before or with meals and snacks (1–3 tablets/capsules). In severe deficiencies, patients may require 6–8 tablets/capsules with meals.
3. Relief of occluded feeding tubes: 1 tablet Viokase crushed with 325 mg tablet of sodium bicarbonate (to activate enzymes) in 5 mL of water instilled into feeding tube and left for 5–10 min, then flushed.

Adverse Effects:

1. Pancreatic extract:
   a. Can cause abdominal pain, nausea, diarrhea at high doses.
   b. At extremely high doses, hyperuricemia and gouty complications can occur.
   c. Hypersensitivity reactions.

TABLE 19.
Drug Preparations

Formulation	Protease (U)	Amylase (U)	Lipase (U)	Type
Pancreatic Extract Preparations:				
Ilozyme	30,000	30,000	11,000	T
Ku-Zyme HP	30,000	30,000	8000	C
Cotazym	30,000	30,000	8000	C
Pancrease	25,000	20,000	4000	E, C
Viokase	30,000	30,000	8000	T
Pancreatin 2400	60,000	60,000	12,000	T
Creon	13,000	30,000	8000	E

Lactase replacement:
Lactaid: 3,000 U lactase/tablet or 1,000 U lactase/5 drops solution
Lactrase: 125 mg lactase/capsule.

T—tablet; C—capsule; E—enteric coated.

Drug Interactions:

1. Pancreatic extract:
   a. Can decrease absorption of PO iron therapy.
   b. Because extracts are more effective in alkaline medium, antacids or sodium bicarbonate are occasionally given concurrently.
   c. Do not use antacids containing calcium carbonate or magnesium hydroxide, because they decrease extract effectiveness by forming insoluble soaps.

Comments/Recommendations: In most populations chronic pancreatitis is due to alcoholism. Chronic abdominal pain is common, and steatorrhea and/or diabetes can occur in patients with less than 10% pancreatic function. Steatorrhea is best documented by obtaining a 72 hr stool collection while on a diet containing 100 g fat/day (normal <6 g fat/day). If fat malabsorption is present, pancreatic extract replacement therapy should be instituted with 3–6 caps/tabs standard preparation just prior to meals. Pancreatic extracts are more effective at alkaline pH; hence, 325 mg sodium bicarbonate tablets, 2 before and 2 after meals, can enhance pancreatic replacement efficacy. In some patients with recurrent abdominal pain from chronic pancreatitis (usually women with nonalcoholic pancreatitis), enzyme replacement may also ease or relieve the pain.

BIBLIOGRAPHY

AMA Drug Evaluations, ed 6, Philadelphia, 1986, WB Saunders.
Drug Information for the Health Care Provider, ed 6, Rockville, 1986, US Pharmacopeial Convention.
Toskes P, Greenberger N: Acute and chronic pancreatitis, *Dis Mon* 1983, 24:69–81.

PARALDEHYDE

Trade Name: *Paraldehyde U.S.P.*

Drug Action: Rapidly acting sedative hypnotic. In high doses it is effective against all types of convulsions. It acts by depressing neuronal activity in the ascending reticular activating system. In therapeutic doses there is little effect on respiration and blood pressure. In higher doses respiratory depression and hypotension may develop.

Indications:

1. May be used as adjunctive therapy in treating seizures, delirium of the abstinence phenomenon.
2. May be used in emergency treatment of tetanus, eclampsia, status epilepticus, poisoning by convulsive drugs.
3. Sedative.

Pharmacokinetics:

1. **Absorption:** PO/PR/IV/IM.
2. **Metabolism:** 70%–80% metabolized in liver. Paraldehyde is depolymerized to acetaldehyde and oxidized to acetic acid. Metabolized to CO_2 and H_2O.
3. **Excretion:** Unmetabolized drug exhaled through the lungs; small amounts excreted by kidneys.
4. **Therapeutic levels:** Not available or established.
5. **Plasma half-life:** 7.5 hr (range 3.5–9.5 hr).
6. **Compatibilities:** Should be given using glass syringes or red rubber catheters. Paraldehyde reacts with most IV administration tubing. Unused portions of paraldehyde ampules should be disposed of within 24 hr, because of oxidation of paraldehyde when exposed to air.

Drug Preparations:

Capsules: 1 g.
PR/PO: 1 g/mL (30 mL).
IM/IV: 1 g/mL (5, 30 mL).

Anticonvulsant/Sedation Dosage:

1. **Adult:**
   a. **IM:** 5–10 mL.
   b. **IV:** 5 mL diluted in at least 100 mL 0.9% saline solution infused, not to exceed 1 mL/min.
   c. **PO/PR:** Up to 12 mL diluted to a 10% solution given via nasogastric tube, or total of 10–20 mL given as PO retention enema.
2. **Pediatric:**
   a. **IM:** 0.15 mL/kg or 6 mL/m^2 body surface area.
   b. **IV:** 0.1–0.15 mL/kg diluted with normal saline solution.
   c. **PO/PR:** 0.3 mL/kg.

Adverse Effects: Confusion, dizziness, sedation, circulatory collapse (IV), rash, nausea/vomiting, respiratory depression, hypotension.

Drug Interactions:

1. Additive sedation with other CNS depressants.
2. Incompatible with plastics.

Monitor: Mental status, respiratory rate.

BIBLIOGRAPHY

Cohen S, Armstrong M: *Drug Interactions: A Handbook for Clinical Use,* Baltimore, 1974, Williams & Wilkins.

Drug Information for the Health Care Professional, ed 8, Rockville, 1988, US Pharmacopeial Convention.

Evans WE, Oellerich M: *Therapeutic Drug Monitoring Clinical Guide,* ed 2, Irving, 1984, Abbott Laboratories Publications.

Gilman A, Goodman L, Rall T, et al (eds): *The Pharmacological Basis of Therapeutics,* ed 7, New York, 1985, Macmillan.

Johnson G: *Blue Book of Pharmacologic Therapeutics,* Philadelphia, 1985, WB Saunders.

McEvoy GK: *Drug Information 88,* Bethesda, 1988, American Society of Hospital Pharmacists.

PENICILLIN

Trade Names: *Penicillin G, Benzathine: Bicillin C-R, Bicillin L-A, Penicillin G, Potassium: Pfizerpen. Penicillin G, Procaine: Pfizerpen-AS, Wycillin, Bicillin C-R, Penicillin V, Potassium: Betapen-VK, Pen-Vee K, Veetids.*

Drug Action:

1. Inhibition of cell wall synthesis.
2. Narrow spectrum of activity increases with higher doses.
   a. Highly effective against gram-positive aerobic cocci (streptococci, pneumococci).
      (1) Most staphylococci resistant via penicillinase production.
      (2) Effective against enterococci with aminoglycoside.
   b. Excellent antianaerobic activity against all anaerobes except *Bacteroides fragilis* family.
      (1) Drug of choice against *Actinomyces*.
   c. Excellent against spirochetes (e.g., treponemes, *Borrelia*).
   d. Excellent against meningococci.
   e. Effective against many other organisms, including *Neisseria* spp. (increasing resistance among gonococci), *Pasteurella multocida*, agents of rat-bite fever (*Spirillum minus, Streptobacillus moniliformis*), and others.

Indications: Drug of first choice.

1. Streptococcal infections (including pneumococci).
2. Enterococcal infections (with aminoglycoside).
3. Non–penicillinase-producing staphylococcal infections.
4. Meningococcal infections (*Neisseria meningitidis*).
5. Anthrax (*Bacillus anthracis*).
6. Clostridial infections (except *Clostridium difficile*).
   a. Tetanus.
   b. Gangrene.
7. *P. multocida* infections.
8. Rat-bite fevers.
9. Actinomycosis.
10. Treponemal infections.
    a. Syphilis.
11. *Leptospira* infections.

Pharmacokinetics:

1. **PO absorption:** Penicillin V resists gastric acid breakdown better than penicillin G, providing two to five times higher blood levels.
2. **Excretion:** Renal.
3. **Electrolyte content:** Aqueous crystalline potassium (1.7 mEq K/million units) and sodium (2 mEq Na/million units).
4. **Serum half-life:** Dependent on drug form:
   a. **PO/IV penicillin G or V:** 30 min.
   b. **Procaine penicillin:** Blood levels for 8–24 hr.
   c. **Benzathine penicillin:** Blood levels for 3–4 wk.

Drug Preparations:

1. **Penicillin G potassium:**

   Tablets: 125 mg (200,000 U), 250 mg (400,000 U), 500 mg (800,000 U).

   Vials: 1, 5, 10, 20 million U.

   PO suspension: 200,000; 250,000; 400,000 U/5 mL.
2. **Penicillin V:**

   Tablets: 125 mg (200,000 U), 250 mg (400,000 U), 500 mg (800,000 U).

   PO suspension: 125, 250 mg/5mL.
3. **Procaine penicillin:**

   Injection: 300,000; 500,000; 600,000 U/mL.

Benzathine penicillin:

   Injection:
   a. L-A (long-acting): 600,000 U/1 mL in 1, 2, 4 mL sizes.
   b. C-R: 300,000 U each benzathine and procaine penicillin G/1 mL in 1, 2, 4 mL sizes.
   c. C-R 900/300: 900,000 U benzathine and 300,000 U procaine penicillin G/2 mL.

Dosage:

1. **Penicillin G:**
   a. **Adult:** 0.5–1 g PO q 6 hr.
   b. **Pediatric:** 6.25–12.5 mg/kg PO q 6 hr.
2. **Penicillin V:**
   a. **Adult:** 0.25–0.5 g PO q 6 hr.
   b. **Pediatric:** 6.25–12.5 mg/kg PO q 6 hr.

3. **Aqueous penicillin G potassium (or sodium):**
   a. **High dose:** 18–24 million U/day IM/IV in divided doses q 4 hr.
      (1) Used in serious infections such as endocarditis or meningitis.
   b. **Intermediate dose:** 8–12 million U/day IM/IV in divided doses q 4 hr.
      (1) Used in anaerobic lung infections (aspiration pneumonia or abscess), with an aminoglycoside for synergy (e.g., enterococci or resistant streptococci) or in moderate to severe group A streptococcal skin and soft tissue infections.
   c. **With renal impairment:** One half–one third max. daily dose when creatinine clearance drops below 10 or in anuric patients.
4. **Procaine penicillin:**
   a. 300,000–4.8 million U/day IM divided q 6–24 hr.
5. **Benzathine penicillin:**
   a. 2.4 million U IM as single dose or weekly × 3 doses (depending on severity).
      (1) Reserved for syphilis treatment.

Adverse Effects:

1. **Hypersensitivity reactions:** Rashes, fever, anaphylaxis.
2. **Neurotoxicity:** Metabolic encephalopathy (usually associated with high doses, renal insufficiency, intrathecal/intraventricular use) seizures.
3. **Autoimmune phenomenon:** Coombs-positive reaction with rare hemolytic anemia, vasculitis.
4. **Nephrotoxicity:** Most often reported with methicillin (acute interstitial nephritis), hypersthenuria, pseudoproteinuria.
5. **Hematologic:** Cytopenias; qualitative platelet defect, usually with antipseudomonal penicillins.
6. **Jarisch-Herxheimer reaction:** Acute, systemic febrile reaction; occurs 12–24 hr after first dose in treatment of syphilis, other spirochetal infections.
   a. Temperature rise, then fall, associated with aggravation of signs and symptoms of illness.
   b. Duration usually less than 6–12 hr.
   c. Not a contraindication to continued treatment.

7. **Procaine reaction:** After large dose or inadvertent IV dose of procaine penicillin:
   a. Immediate reaction manifested predominantly by mental disturbances, including anxiety, confusion, agitation, depression, weakness, hallucinations, "fear of impending death," combativeness, and even seizures.
   b. Transient, lasting 15–30 min.
   c. Secondary to procaine toxicity (increased in patients with decreased levels of pseudocholinesterase), not hypersensitivity.
8. **GI:** Nausea/vomiting, diarrhea, hepatic dysfunction.
9. **Electrolyte disturbances:**
   a. **Hyperkalemia:** With high doses of aqueous penicillin G potassium.
   b. **Hypokalemia:** penicillin acting as nonreabsorbable anion.

Drug Interactions:

1. Incompatible with aminoglycosides.
2. Probenecid blocks renal tubular secretion (higher serum levels).
3. Delays renal excretion of methotrexate.
4. Prolonged half-life with NSAIDs, sulfinpyrazone.
5. Increased hyperkalemia with potassium-sparing diuretics.

Monitor:

1. Serum potassium, renal functions.
2. Blood cell counts.

PENTAMIDINE

Trade Name: *Pentam 300, Pentacarinat, NebuPent (for inhalation.*

Drug Action: Antiprotozoal action, inhibits nucleic acid and protein synthesis.

Indications:

1. Pneumonia caused by *Pneumocystis carinii.*
2. Active against *P. carinii* and *Trypanosoma* organisms.

3. Prophylaxis for prevention of Pneumocystis carinii pneumonia (via inhalation route).

Pharmacokinetics:

1. **Absorption:** Give IV.
2. **Metabolism:** Unknown.
3. **Excretion:** Urine (mostly unchanged); accumulates in renal failure.
4. **Penetration:** Extensively tissue bound; CNS penetration poor.

Drug Preparations:

Vials: 300 mg for injection.
Inhalation: (NebuPent) 300 mg/vial.

Dosage:

1. 4 mg/kg IV or deep IM once daily for 14 days.
2. Prophylaxis for prevention of Pneumocystis carinii pneumonia: inhalation (NebuPent) 300 mg once q 4 wk via Respirgard II nebulizer.
3. **Renal failure:** Reduce dosage.

Adverse Effects:

1. **Cardiovascular:** Hypotension, arrhythmias.
2. **GI:** Nausea/vomiting, diarrhea, anorexia, metallic taste, pancreatitis, islet cell necrosis, hepatic toxicity.
3. **GU:** Elevated BUN and creatinine; renal toxicity.
4. **Dermatologic:** Rash, pruritus, toxic epidermal necrosis, Stevens-Johnson syndrome.
5. **Hematologic:** Leukopenia, thrombocytopenia, anemia, megaloblastic changes.
6. **Endocrine:** Hypoglycemia, late hyperglycemia (months after therapy), hypocalcemia, hyperkalemia.
7. **Other:** Sterile abscess, local injection pain, phlebitis, fever, anaphylaxis, confusion, hallucinations.

Drug Interactions: Increased nephrotoxicity when used with vancomycin, polymyxin B, methoxyflurane, cisplatin, colistin, aminoglycosides, amphotericin B, capreomycin.

Monitoring:

1. Blood pressure, heart rate, ECG.
2. BUN, creatinine; liver function tests.

3. Blood cell counts.
4. Glucose, calcium.

BIBLIOGRAPHY

Pentamidine isethionate. In *Drug Facts and Comparisons,* Philadelphia, 1989, JB Lippincott, p 1637.
Pentamidine isethionate. In *AMA Drug Evaluations,* ed 6, Philadelphia, 1986, WB Saunders, p 1581.

PHENOBARBITAL

Trade Names: *Solfoton, Luminal,* generics.

Drug Action:

1. **Anticonvulsant:** Enhances effects of GABA, decreases neuronal excitability, raises seizure threshold.
2. **Sedative-hypnotic:** Depresses reticular activating system, cortex, cerebellum.

Indications: Seizures, sedation.

Pharmacokinetics:

1. **Absorption:** PO/PR/IM.
2. **Metabolism:** Liver.
3. **Excretion:** 25%–50% unchanged in urine.
4. **Onset:** IV: 5 min; PO: 20–60 min.
5. **Plasma half-life:** 53–118 hr.
6. **Sedative dosage:** 30–120 mg PO.
7. **Hypnotic dosage: range:** 100–320 mg PO:

Drug Preparations:

PO solution: 15, 20 mg/5 mL.
Elixir: 20 mg/5 mL.
Capsules: 16 mg.
Tablets: 8, 15, 16, 30, 32, 60, 65, 100 mg.
Injection: 30, 60, 65, 130 mg/mL.
Powder for injection: 120 mg/ampule.

Dosage:

1. **Anticonvulsant:**
   a. **Adult:** 50–100 mg bid/tid PO/IV/IM.
      (1) IV rate should not exceed 50 mg/min.
   b. **Pediatric:** 4–6 mg/kg/day in one to three doses.
2. **Status epilepticus:**
   a. **Adult:** 10 mg/kg IV at 50 mg/min; may give up to 20 mg/kg total.
   b. **Pediatric:** 5–10 mg/kg IV at 50 mg/min; may give up to 20 mg/kg total.
3. **Sedation:**
   a. **Adult:** 30–120 mg/day PO/IM/IV in two to three doses.
   b. **Pediatric:** 6 mg/kg/day PO/IM in three doses.
4. **Sleep induction:**
   a. **Adult:** 100–320 mg PO/IM/IV.

Adverse Effects:

1. **Respiratory:** Depression, laryngospasm, bronchospasm.
2. **Cardiovascular:** Hypotension, bradycardia, circulatory collapse.
3. **GI:** Nausea/vomiting, diarrhea, constipation.
4. **Dermatologic:** Urticaria, rash, dermatitis, Stevens-Johnson syndrome.
5. **CNS:** Drowsiness, coma, lethargy, vertigo, paradoxical excitement, confusion.
6. **Other:** Vitamin K deficiency and bleeding in newborns of mothers treated during pregnancy, thrombophlebitis, pain at injection site.

Drug Interactions:

1. CNS and respiratory depression potentiated by other sedative drugs.
2. Increases hepatic metabolism (decreases effect of PO anticoagulants, digitoxin, corticosteroids, estrogens, theophylline, doxycycline, tricyclic antidepressants, β-blockers, quinidine, metronidazole, vitamin D).
3. Phenobarbital metabolism decreased by valproic acid, phenytoin, disulfiram, MAO inhibitors, chloramphenicol.
4. Phenobarbital metabolism increased by rifampin.
5. Increased risk of acetaminophen toxicity.

6. Effect of phenobarbital on phenytoin metabolism unpredictable; monitor serum levels of both drugs.

Monitoring:

1. **Serum levels:** 10–25 μg/mL (for seizure control).
2. Blood pressure, heart rate.
3. CNS and respiratory status.

BIBLIOGRAPHY

Phenobarbital. In *Drug Facts and Comparisons,* Philadelphia,
1989, JB Lippincott, p 1153.
Phenobarbital. In *AMA Drug Evaluations,* ed 6, Philadelphia,
1986, WB Saunders, pp 104, 187.

PHENOXYBENZAMINE

Trade Name: *Dibenzyline.*

Drug Action:

1. Noncompetitive blocker of α-adrenergic receptors.
2. Causes vascular smooth muscle relaxation (chemical sympa-
thectomy).

Indications:

1. Antihypertensive (especially caused by pheochromocytoma).
2. Peripheral vasodilation.

Pharmacokinetics:

1. **Absorption:** PO (20%–30%).
2. **Metabolism:** Hepatic.
3. **Excretion:** Urine and bile.
4. **Half-life:** Lipid soluble; effects may last up to 7 days after discontinuation of therapy.

Drug Preparations:

Capsules: 10 mg.

Dosage:

1. **Adult:**
   a. Initial dose 10 mg PO bid; increase every other day until desired effect.
   b. Maintenance dose usually 20–40 mg PO bid/tid.
2. **Pediatric:**
   a. Initial dose 0.2 mg/kg PO once a day; increase to desired effect.
   b. Maintenance dose usually 0.4–1.2 mg/kg/day.

Adverse Effects:

1. **Cardiovascular:** Hypotension, orthostatic hypotension, tachycardia.
2. **GI:** Nausea/vomiting, abdominal distress.
3. **CNS:** Drowsiness, lethargy, dizziness.
4. **Other:** Dry mouth, miosis, nasal congestion, impotence, inhibition of ejaculation.

Drug Interactions:

1. Antagonizes α-adrenergic agonists.
2. Increased vasodilation (i.e., hypotension) and tachycardia with vasodilator drugs and β-adrenergic agonists.

Monitoring: Blood pressure, heart rate.

BIBLIOGRAPHY

Phenoxybenzamine. In *Drug Facts and Comparisons,* Philadelphia, 1989, JB Lippincott, p 664.
Phenoxybenzamine. In *AMA Drug Evaluations,* ed 6, Philadelphia, 1986, WB Saunders, p 529.

PHENTOLAMINE

Trade Name: *Regitine.*

Drug Action:

1. α-Adrenergic receptor blocker (competitive); blocks both α_1 and α_2 receptors.
2. Vasodilator.

Indications:

1. Antihypertensive (especially caused by pheochromocytoma, clonidine withdrawal, MAO inhibitors).
2. Vasodilator.

Pharmacokinetics:

1. **Absorption:** Give IV.
2. **Metabolism:** Liver.
3. **Excretion:** 10% unchanged in urine.
4. **Plasma half-life:** 19 min (after IV administration).

Drug Preparations:

Vials: 5 mg/mL in 1 mL vials.

Dosage:

1. **Adult:** 5 mg IV/IM prn; taper to effect.
2. **Pediatric:** 0.1 mg/kg IV prn; taper to effect.

Adverse Effects:

1. **Cardiovascular:** Hypotension, tachycardia, palpitations, arrhythmias.
2. **GI:** Nausea/vomiting, diarrhea, hyperperistalsis, abdominal pain.
3. **CNS:** Dizziness, lethargy, weakness.
4. **Other:** Nasal congestion, hypoglycemia, flushing.

Drug Interactions:

1. Antagonizes action of α-adrenergic agonists.
2. Additive hypotensive effect when given with other vasodilators.

Monitoring: Blood pressure, heart rate.

BIBLIOGRAPHY

Phentolamine. In *Drug Facts and Comparisons,* Philadelphia, 1989, JB Lippincott, pp 662–663.
Phentolamine. In *AMA Drug Evaluations,* ed 6, Philadelphia, 1986, WB Saunders, p 529.

PHENYLEPHRINE

Trade Name: *Neo-Synephrine injection 1%.*

Drug Action:

1. α_1-Adrenergic agonist; produces peripheral arteriolar and venous constriction.
2. α_1-Adrenergic receptors on myocardial cells when activated lead to influx of Ca^{++}ions. This action is thought to be mediated by the phosphoinositol system. The result is a slow-to-develop increase in inotropy.
3. Rise in systolic and diastolic blood pressure, with accompanying reflex decrease in heart rate.

Indications:

1. Hypotension (to maintain diastolic blood pressure and coronary perfusion pressure).
2. Postcardiopulmonary bypass with hyperdynamic state of high cardiac output and low systemic vascular resistance.
3. To convert some supraventricular tachycardias.
4. As nasal decongestant when applied topically or taken PO.
5. As a mydriatic when applied topically.

Pharmacokinetics:

1. **Metabolism:** Liver, intestine, MAO.
2. **Excretion:** Renal.
3. **Plasma half-life:** Minutes. Cardiovascular responses may last 20 min after IV administration.
4. **Onset of action:** Immediate.

Drug Preparations:

Ampules: 10 mg/mL.

Dosage: 15 mg dissolved in 250 mL D_5W = 60 μg/mL. Begin at 20–30 μg/min, titrate to desired blood pressure.

Adverse Effects:

1. Headache.
2. Severe hypertension.
3. Reflex bradycardia.

4. Excitability.
5. Myocardial depression.
6. Myocardial ischemia.
7. Decreased organ blood flow.

Drug Interactions:

1. MAO inhibitors may markedly potentiate vasopressor effects.
2. Tricyclic antidepressants may potentiate vasopressor effects.

Monitoring: Blood pressure, heart rate, ECG, urine output.

BIBLIOGRAPHY

Colucci WS, Wright RF, Braunwald E: New positive inotropic agents in the treatment of congestive heart failure, *N Engl J Med* 1986, 314:290–297.
Weiner W: Norepinephrine, epinephrine, and the sympathomimetic amines. In Gilman AG, Goodman LS, Gilman A (eds): *The Pharmacologic Basis of Therapeutics,* New York, 1980, Macmillan, pp 158–175.

PHENYTOIN

Trade Name: *Dilantin.*

Many hydantoin derivatives have been and still are used in the treatment of epilepsy. By far the most commonly used member of this class of drugs is phenytoin. For the purpose and intent of this publication, phenytoin is considered the primary choice.

Drug Action:

1. Limits the propagation of seizures by reduction of posttetanic potentiation.
2. May increase efficiency of the cell membrane sodium pump and prevent passive influx of sodium.
3. Decreasing posttetanic potentials prevents cortical seizure foci from spreading to adjacent brain tissue.

Indications:

1. Used mainly in prophylactic treatment of tonic-clonic (grand mal) seizures and selected varieties of partial seizures, and in the treatment of status epilepticus.
2. Not recommended as a primary agent for treatment of absence seizures, but may be used in conjunction with other agents in cases of complex absence seizures combined with tonic-clonic seizures.
3. Ventricular arrhythmia (especially tricyclic overdose).

Pharmacokinetics:

1. **Absorption:** PO/IV.
2. **Metabolism:** Accomplished through oxidation in the liver to inactive metabolite 5-(*p*-hydroxyphenyl)-5-phenylhydantoin (HPPH). This is a saturable enzyme system; small increases in dosage may result in marked elevation of circulating drug level and toxic side effects.
3. **Excretion:** HPPH is excreted in the urine but undergoes enterohepatic circulation. 60%–75% of the daily dose is excreted in this form; 1% is excreted unchanged.
4. **Volume of distribution:** 95% of the dose is bound to plasma proteins. Protein binding decreases in renal or hepatic disease.
5. **Basal circulation:** Therapeutic plasma levels range from 10–20 µg/mL. The free fraction is the active agent for passage into the CNS.
6. **Plasma half-life:** On average, 22 hr; range 7–42 hr.

Compatibilities:

1. With IV administration, phenytoin precipitates from solution in the presence of glucose.
2. Should not be administered IM because the drug precipitates in muscle tissue and is erratically resorbed.

Drug Preparations:

Capsules: 100 mg.
Chewable tablets: 50 mg.
Suspension: 30, 125 mg/5 mL.
Ampules/prepackaged syringes: 50 mg/mL for IV.

Dosage:

1. **Initial PO dose** 100 mg tid, 5–10 days required to reach steady state. A 1000 mg or loading dose may be given in three divided doses over 24 hr to achieve higher blood levels more rapidly. Warning: Phenytoin demonstrates zero order kinetics; care must be taken when increasing dose since small increases in dosage can result in dramatic increases in serum levels.
2. **Maintenance dose** 300 mg q day or divided tid. Taper to desired blood level.
3. **Status epilepticus:**
   a. **IV loading dose** 10–15 mg/kg, not to exceed 50 mg/min, to avoid cardiac arrhythmias.
   b. **Maintenance dose** 300 mg IV q day or divided tid. Taper to desired blood level.

Adverse Effects: Adverse effects from Dilantin administration are numerous and are often related to dose and blood level.

1. **GI:** May occur with PO administration and include nausea/vomiting, constipation, epigastric pain, dysphagia, loss of taste, anorexia, weight loss.
2. **CNS:** Mental confusion, nystagmus, ataxia, blurred vision, diplopia, toxic amblyopia, dizziness, insomnia, nervousness, muscle twitching, headache. Drowsiness and lethargy, especially when serum levels exceed 20 μg/mL. Rarely, involuntary movements.
3. Long-term administration of phenytoin may be associated with gingival hyperplasia, which can result in significant peridontal disease.
4. Phenytoin produces hypertrichosis in some patients. Coarsening of facial features may also occur.
5. **Allergic reactions:** Skin eruptions; in more severe cases, Stevens-Johnson syndrome.
6. Rarely, phenytoin will produce a clinical picture of systemic lupus erythematosus.
7. May rarely be associated with lymphadenopathy.
8. Toxic hepatitis and liver enzyme elevations may occur.
9. Rarely, severe bone marrow suppression may occur.
10. Macrocytosis and megaloblastic anemia, responsive to folic acid therapy.

11. Too rapid IV administration may result in circulatory collapse and ventricular arrhythmias.

Drug Interactions:

1. Multiple drug interactions with phenytoin and other medications, especially other anticonvulsants, have been reported.
2. **Increased phenytoin effects:** Allopurinol, chloramphenicol, cimetidine, diazepam, ethanol, phenylbutazone, trimethoprim, NSAIDs, imipramine.
3. **Decreased phenytoin effects:** Barbiturates, folic acid, carbamazepine, theophylline, calcium.
4. **Phenytoin decreases effects of** corticosteroids, cyclosporin, dicumarol, disopyramide, haloperidol, quinidine, dopamine, sulfonylureas.

Monitoring: Phenytoin blood levels are readily available in most hospital laboratories.

1. For routine monitoring, a morning trough level prior to the first medication dosage of the day should be obtained.
2. After IV loading doses, a representative blood level may be obtained after 2 hr.
3. Therapeutic level: 10–20 μg/mL.

BIBLIOGRAPHY

Cohen S, Armstrong M: *Drug Interactions: A Handbook for Clinical Use,* Baltimore, 1974, Williams & Wilkins.

Drug Information for the Health Care Professional, ed 8, Rockville, MD, 1988, US Pharmacopeial Convention.

Evans WE, Oellerich M: *Therapeutic Drug Monitoring Clinical Guide,* ed 2, Irving, 1984, Abbott Laboratories Publications.

Gilman A, Goodman L, Rall T, et al (eds): *Goodman and Gilman's The Pharmacological Basis of Therapeutics,* ed 7, New York, 1985, Macmillan.

Johnson G: *Blue Book of Pharmacologic Therapeutics,* Philadelphia, 1985, WB Saunders.

McEvoy GK: *Drug Information 88,* Bethesda, 1988, American Society of Hospital Pharmacists.

PHOSPHORUS

Trade Names:

1. Potassium phosphate: *Neutra-Phos-K, potassium phosphate injection.*
2. Potassium phosphate and sodium phosphate: *K-Phos Neutral, Neutra-Phos, Uro-KP-Neutral.*
3. Sodium phosphate: *Fleet Phospho-Soda, sodium phosphate injection.*

Drug Action:

1. Component of high-energy phosphates (e.g., ATP, creatine phosphate), membrane phospholipids, intracellular messengers (e.g., cAMP, cGMP, phosphoinositides), nucleic acids, 2,3-DPG, bone.
2. Supplies energy for normal cell function.
3. Renal buffering of acids.

Drug Indications:

1. Phosphorus depletion.
2. Hypophosphatemia.

Pharmacokinetics:

1. **Metabolism:** None.
2. **Absorption:** Gut.
3. **Excretion:** Predominantly renal, some GI. Reduce dose in patients with renal insufficiency.
4. **RDA:** 800 mg or 26 mmol (adults); normal requirements (oral): 0–6 mo 240 mg, 6–12 mo 360 mg, 1–10 yr 800 mg, >10 yr 1200 mg.
5. **Normal serum level:**
   a. **Adult:** 3–4.5 mg/dL.
   b. **Pediatric:** 4–7 mg/dL.
6. 31 mg phosphorus =1 mmol.

Drug Preparations:

1. **PO:**

   Neutra-Phos: 250 mg capsule or powder (8 mmol); 7 mEq K, 7 mEq Na.

Neutra-Phos-K: 250 mg capsule or powder (8 mmol); 14 mEq K.

K-Phos Neutral Tabs: 250 mg (8 mmol); 1.1 mEq K, 13 mEq Na.

Uro-KP-Neutral Tabs: 250 mg (8 mmol); 1.3 mEq K, 11 mEq Na.

Fleet Phospho-Soda: 4.15 mmol/mL, 4.8 mEq Na/mL.

2. **IV:**

Potassium phosphate injection: 3 mmol PO_4 and 4.4 mEq K/mL.

Sodium phosphate injection: 3 mmol PO_4 and 4 mEq Na/mL.

Dosage:

1. It is difficult to predict the extent of total body deficits and response to therapy of this intracellular anion.
2. **Maintenance:**
    a. **PO:** Adults 1000–2000 mg/day in divided doses q 6 hr; children 250–1000 mg/day in divided doses q 6 hr.
    b. **IV:** Adults 10–30 mmol/day (310–930 mg elemental phosphorus); children 0.5–1.5 mmol/kg/24 hr.
3. PO_4 depletion:
    a. Adults: If depletion is recent and uncomplicated, 0.6 mg (0.02 mmol)/kg/hr IV.
    b. Adults: If depletion is chronic and multifactorial, 0.9 mg (0.03 mmol)/kg/hr IV.
    c. Children: 1–2 mmol/kg/24 hr IV.
4. Repletion of severe hypophosphatemia (<1 mg/dL) is best done IV because large doses of oral phosphate may cause diarrhea.

Adverse Effects:

1. Hyperphosphatemia.
2. **GI:** Diarrhea, nausea/vomiting, abdominal pain.
3. Renal damage. Phosphorous/potassium excretion is reduced in patients with renal insufficiency.
4. Hyperkalemia with potassium compounds.
5. Hypocalcemia, calcium precipitation.
6. Uncommon: Headache, dizziness, mental confusion, seizures, weakness, muscle cramps, numbness, tingling, tachycardia, shortness of breath, edema, paresthesias, flaccid paralysis, confusion, hypotension, cardiac arrhythmias, heart block.

Drug Interactions:

1. Sucralfate and antacids containing magnesium, aluminum, or calcium bind PO_4 and decrease in absorption.
2. PO_4 lowers circulating calcium levels and may cause calcium precipitation.
3. Potassium phosphate and potassium-sparing diuretics may cause hyperkalemia (*see* Potassium salts).

Monitoring:

1. Serum phosphate and calcium.
2. Serum BUN and creatinine.
3. Serum sodium and potassium (and ECG).

BIBLIOGRAPHY

Zaloga GP, Chernow B: Divalent ions: calcium, magnesium and phosphorus. In Chernow B (ed): *The Pharmacologic Approach to the Critically Ill Patient,* ed 3, Baltimore, 1993, Williams & Wilkins, pp 777–804.

Kovach KL, Hruska KA: Hypophosphatemia. In Jacobson HR, et al (ed): *The Principles and Practice of Nephrology,* St. Louis, 1995, Mosby–Year Book, pp 993–999.

PIPERACILLIN

Trade Name: *Pipracil.*

Drug Action:

1. Inhibition of cell wall synthesis (penicillin).
2. Spectrum of activity includes non–β-lactamase-producing gram-positive aerobes (streptococci but not staphylococci), most gram-negative aerobes (including *Pseudomonas aeruginosa*), and anaerobes (including *Bacteroides fragilis* family).

Indications: Infections caused by susceptible organisms usually involving *P. aeruginosa* (with synergistic combination of an aminoglycoside) or mixed aerobes/anaerobes (e.g., intra-abdominal infection).

Pharmacokinetics:

1. **Absorption:** IV/IM.
2. **Excretion:** Renal.
3. **Monosodium salt:** 1.98 mEq sodium/g.
4. **Serum half-life:** 1.3–1.5 hr.

Drug Preparations:

Vials: 2, 3, 4, g for parenteral use.

Dosage:

1. **Normal renal function:** 3–4 g q 4–6 hr parenterally.
3. **Impaired renal function:**

Dose (g)	Creatinine Clearance	Interval (hr)
3–4	>80	4–6
	80–50	4–6
2–3	50–10	6–12
2	<10 (anuria)	12

3. Hemodialysis: Use 2 g q 8 hr +1 g after each dialysis.

Adverse Effects:

1. Similar to those with penicillin, including hypersensitivity reactions, GI problems, cytopenias, phlebitis, headache, seizures.
2. Sodium overload or hypokalemia.
3. Qualitative platelet defect (? less than with carbenicillin or ticarcillin).

Drug Interactions:

1. Incompatible with aminoglycosides.
2. Excretion blocked by probenecid.
3. Elevates serum concentration of methotrexate.

Monitor: Electrolytes, blood cell counts, renal function, neurologic status.

PIPERACILLIN/TAZOBACTAM

Trade Name: *Zosyn.*

Drug Actions:

1. Piperacillin inhibits bacterial cell wall synthesis; tazobactam acts as a β-lactamase inhibitor.
2. Spectrum of activity includes gram-positive aerobes (including staphylococci due to the tazobactam- but not methicillin-oxacillin-resistant strains), most gram-negative aerobes, and anaerobes including *Bacteroides fragilis.*

Indications: Infections caused by susceptible organisms. Piperacillin/tazobactam as monotherapy is *not* adequate for treatment of complicated urinary tract infections or nosocomial pneumonias.

Pharmacokinetics:

1. **Absorption:** IV.
2. **Excretion:** Renal.
3. **Half-life:** 0.7–1.2 hr.

Drug Preparations: *Vials:* 2.25 g (2 g piperacillin sodium equivalent and 0.25 g tazobactam sodium equivalent), 3.375 g (3 g piperacillin sodium equivalent and 0.375 g tazobactam sodium equivalent), and 4.5 g (4 g piperacillin sodium equivalent and 0.5 g tazobactam sodium equivalent), for parenteral use.

Dosage:

1. **Normal renal function:** 3.375 g q 6 hr.
2. **Impaired renal function:**

Creatinine Clearance (mL/min)	Dosage
>40	3.375 g q 6 hr.
20–40	2.25 g q 6 hr.
<20	2.25 g q 8 hr.

Adverse Effects:

1. Similar to those with penicillin, including hypersensitivity reactions, GI problems, cytopenias, phlebitis, headache, seizures.

2. Sodium overload or hypokalemia.
3. Qualitative platelet defect (? less than with carbenicillin or ticarcillin).

Drug Interactions:

1. Incompatible with aminoglycosides (i.e., should be reconstituted and administered separately).
2. Excretion blocked by probenecid.
3. Piperacillin may prolong the neuromuscular blockade produced by nondepolarizing muscle relaxants.

Monitoring: Electrolytes, blood cell counts, renal function, neurologic status.

BIBLIOGRAPHY

Physicians' Desk Reference, ed 50, Montvale, 1996, Medical Economics Co.

PLICAMYCIN (MITHRAMYCIN)

Trade Name: *Mithracin.*

Drug Action:

1. Hypocalcemic agent.
2. Decreases release of calcium from bone. Inhibits action of PTH and vitamin D on osteoclasts.
3. Antineoplastic agent (binds to DNA).

Indications:

1. Hypercalcemia of malignancy.
2. Testicular cancer.

Pharmacokinetics:

1. **Absorption:** Must be given IV.
2. **Distribution:** Distributed in most cells of the body, including Kupffer cells of liver, renal tubular cells, bone, CSF. Not detected in brain.
3. **Metabolism:** Primarily liver; most drug metabolized.

4. **Excretion:** Less than 10% of active drug excreted in urine or bile.
5. **Half life:** 1 hr.

Drug Preparations:

Vials: 2.5 mg for injection.

Dosage:

1. **Hypercalcemia:** 15–25 µg/kg/day IV over 4–6 hr for 3–4 days; repeat at intervals of 1 wk if necessary.
2. **Testicular cancer:** 25–30 µg/kg/day IV over 4–6 hr for up to 10 days.
3. **Dilute** daily dose in 1 L saline solution or D_5W; administer over 4–6 hr.

Adverse Effects:

1. **CNS:** Headache, lethargy, depression.
2. **Skin:** Periorbital pallor, facial flushing, irritation with extravasation.
3. **GI:** Nausea/vomiting, anorexia, diarrhea, stomatitis, metallic taste, liver damage, depression of clotting factors.
4. **GU:** Proteinuria, renal impairment.
5. **Hematologic:** Bone marrow depression, leukopenia, anemia, thrombocytopenia, hemorrhagic syndrome.
6. **Hypocalcemia, hypophosphatemia, hypokalemia.**
7. Contradicted during pregnancy.
8. Fever, weakness, phlebitis.

Drug Interactions: Potentiates cardiotoxicity of doxorubicin.

Monitoring:

1. Serum ionized calcium, phosphate, potassium.
2. Blood cell counts, temperature, signs of infection.
3. BUN, creatinine.
4. ALT, AST, bilirubin, PT/PTT, signs of bleeding.

BIBLIOGRAPHY

Attie MF: Treatment of hypercalcemia, *Endocrinol Metab Clin North Am* 1989, 18:807–828.

Plicamycin. In *Drug Facts and Comparisons,* Philadelphia, 1989, JB Lippincott, pp 2111–2112.

Zaloga GP, Chernow B: Divalent ions: calcium, magnesium and phosphorus. In Chernow B (ed): *The Pharmacologic Approach to the Critically Ill Patient,* ed 3, Baltimore, 1994, Williams & Wilkins, pp 777–804.

POTASSIUM SALTS

Trade Names:

Potassium chloride: *Cena-K, Kaochlor, Kaochlor S-F, Kaon-Cl, Kato, Kay Ciel, K-Dur, K-Lor, Klor-Con, Klor-Con/25, Klorvess, Klotrix, K-Lyte/Cl, K-Tab, Micro-K, Potasalan, Rum-K, Slow-K, Ten-K*

Potassium bicarbonate and potassium citrate, effervescent: *Klor-Con/EF, K-Lyte, Effer-K,* and others.

Potassium acetate (1 mEq acetate = alkalinizing effect of 1 mEq bicarbonate).

Potassium gluconate: *Kaon, Kaylixer, K-G elixir.*

Potassium phosphate: *Neutra-Phos-K. See* Phosphorus.

Drug Action:

1. Major intracellular cation.
2. Responsible for maintenance of membrane potentials.
3. Required for transmission of nerve impulse.
4. Required for cardiac action potential, muscle contraction.
5. Important for cellular metabolism, acid-base balance, maintenance of intracellular tonicity.
6. Required for protein synthesis.

Indication: Hypokalemia.

Pharmacokinetics:

1. **Absorption:** Well absorbed from GI tract.
2. **Distribution:** Primarily intracellular fluid.
3. **Serum level:** 3.5–5.0 mEq/L.
4. **Metabolism:** None.
5. **Excretion:** Renal, some in stool. Reduce dose in patients with renal failure.
6. **Normal daily requirements:** Adults 40–80 mEq/day, children 2–3 mEq/kg/day, infants 1–2 mEq/kg/day.

Drug Preparations:

1. *Sustained-release tablets* (potassium chloride): 10, 20 mEq.
2. *Extended release capsules* (potassium bicarbonate and potassium citrate, potassium chloride): 8, 10 mEq.
3. *Powder:* (potassium citrate and potassium bicarbonates, potassium chloride*): 15, 20, 25 mEq/package.*
4. *Liquid* (chloride and gluconate): 10, 15, 20, 30, 40, 45 mEq/15 mL.
5. *Effervescent tablets* (potassium bicarbonate and potassium citrate, potassium chloride): 20, 25, 50 mEq.
6. *Vials for injection* (potassium chloride, potassium acetate): 1.5–4.0 mEq/mL.

Dosage:

1. **Life-threatening hypokalemia:** Adults, may give up to 40 mEq/hr IV; best to keep rate 10–20 mEq/hr. Children, 1–2 mEq/kg over 1–2 hr (repeat as needed).
2. **Maintenance:** Consider ongoing losses and renal function. Most adult patients require 60–100 mEq/day, children 2–5 mEq/kg/day; may give as IV infusion or in divided doses PO q 4–6 hr.
3. **Administration:** Max. concentration (peripheral line) 10 mEq/dL; max. concentration (central line) 30 mEq/dL; do not give by IV push—infuse over 1–2 hr; PO liquid supplements should be diluted into water or juice prior to administration.

Adverse Effects:

1. **Hyperkalemia**
2. **Renal failure:** Use with caution because of impaired ability to excrete potassium.
3. **Cardiovascular:** Arrhythmias, heart block, bradycardia, cardiac arrest, hypotension.
4. **ECG:** Prolonged PR, peaked T waves, wide QRS, ST depression.
5. **Neurologic:** Paresthesias, headache, lethargy, confusion, weakness, paralysis, respiratory failure.
6. **GI:** Nausea/vomiting, diarrhea, abdominal pain, ulcerations, perforation, stricture, hemorrhage.
7. **Phlebitis.** Tissue necrosis with extravasation.

Drug Interactions:

1. Potassium-sparing diuretics, aldosterone-inhibiting agents and angiotensin converting enzyme inhibitors (e.g., captopril, enalapril) decrease renal excretion.
2. Succinylcholine may raise serum level.
3. Thiazide and loop diuretics increase renal potassium excretion.
4. Hypokalemia predisposes to digitalis toxicity.
5. Insulin (and dextrose), bicarbonate, and β-adrenergic agonists may lower serum potassium by shifting it intracellularly.
6. Anticholinergics decrease GI motility and increase risk of GI ulceration.
7. Potassium citrate, a urinary alkalinizer, may affect the following:
    a. Decreased excretion (increased pharmacologic effect): Flecainide, mecamylamine, quinidine, quinine, sympathomimetics.
    b. Increased excretion (decreased pharmacologic effect): Chlorpropamide, lithium, methotrexate, salicylates, tetracycline.

Treatment of Overdose:

1. Discontinue agent.
2. Lavage GI tract.
3. Give calcium, fluids, diuretics (furosemide), sodium bicarbonate, dextrose plus insulin, sodium polystyrene resin (Kayexalate).
4. Dialysis.

Monitoring:

1. Serum potassium.
2. ECG.

BIBLIOGRAPHY

Oh MS, Carroll HJ: Electrolyte and acid-base disorders. In Chernow B (ed): *The Pharmacologic Approach to the Critically Ill Patient,* ed 3, Baltimore, 1994, Williams & Wilkins, pp 957–968.
Mudge GH, Weiner IM: Agents affecting volume and composition of body fluids. In Gilman AG, et al (eds): *The Pharmaco-*

logical Basis of Therapeutics, ed 8, New York, 1993, McGraw-Hill, pp 697–704.

Linas SL, Singh H: Hypokalemia. In Jacobson HR, et al (eds): *The Principles and Practice of Nephrology,* ed 2, St. Louis, 1995, Mosby–Year Book, pp 903–910.

PRALIDOXIME

Trade Name: *Protopam.*

Drug Actions: Cholinesterase reactivator: usually reserved for use as an antidote for organophosphates that have anticholinesterase activity.

Indications: Organophosphate poisoning with paralysis of respiratory muscles, or with respiratory compromise. May also be used to control overdose of anticholinesterase drugs used in the treatment of myasthenia gravis.

Pharmacokinetics:

1. **Absorption:** IV or IM routes only.
2. **Onset of action:** Minimum therapeutic level of 4 μg/mL is reached in about 16 min after a single injection of 600 mg.
3. **Metabolism:** Hepatic.
4. **Excretion:** Urinary.
5. **Half-life:** Approximately 75 min.

Drug Preparations: 50 mg/mL in 20 mL ampules.

Dosage: Infusion of 1–2 g over 15–60 min generally reverses symptoms of muscular weakness. A second dose may be indicated. Intermittent infusions have been used for up to 2 days.

Adverse Effects: Tachycardia, laryngospasm, and muscle rigidity may occur with too rapid IV administration. May induce a myasthenic crisis if used to correct anticholinesterase overdose. Blurred vision, diplopia, dizziness, tachycardia, hypertension, and GI distress are all common.

Drug Interactions: Frequently combined with atropine to reduce depression of CNS respiratory center.

Monitoring: Close monitoring of neuromuscular function is necessary.

BIBLIOGRAPHY

Wilson IB, Ginsburg S: A powerful reactivator of alkyl phosphate–inhibited acelylcholinesterase, *Biochim Biophys Acta* 1955, 18:168–170.

Sidell FR: Clinical effects of organophosphorus cholinesterase inhibitors, *J Appl Toxicol* 1994, 14:111–113.

Marrs TC: Organophosphate poisoning, *Pharmacol Ther* 1993, 58:51–66.

PRAZOSIN

Trade Name: *Minipress.*

Drug Action:

1. Inhibits α_1-adrenergic receptors.
2. Vasodilator (arterial, venous).

Indications:

1. Hypertension.
2. Afterload reduction in congestive heart failure.

Pharmacokinetics:

1. **Absorption:** PO (50%).
2. **Metabolism:** Liver.
3. **Excretion:** Feces (90%), urine.
4. **Plasma half-life:** 2–4 hr.
5. **Onset after PO administration:** 2 hr.
6. **Peak effect after PO administration:** 2–4 hr.
7. **Duration:** 18–24 hr.

Drug Preparations:

Capsules: 1, 2, 5 mg.

Dosage:

1. **Adult:** Initial dose 1 mg PO bid/tid; titrate to effect (max. dose 20 mg/day in divided doses). First dose best given at bedtime.

Adverse Effects:

1. **Cardiovascular:** Postural hypotension, palpitations, tachycardia, angina, fluid retention, edema.
2. **GI:** Nausea/vomiting, diarrhea, constipation, abdominal cramps.
3. **CNS:** Headache, dizziness, drowsiness, weakness, syncope, depression.
4. **Other:** Impotence, blurred vision, dry mouth.

Drug Interactions: Potentiated by diuretics and other antihypertensives.

Monitoring: Blood pressure, heart rate.

BIBLIOGRAPHY

Prazosin. In *Drug Facts and Comparisons,* Philadelphia, 1989, JB Lippincott, p 644.
Prazosin. In *AMA Drug Evaluations,* ed 6, Philadelphia, 1986, WB Saunders, p 528.

PRIMAQUINE

Trade Name: *Primaquine.*

Drug Actions:

1. Interferes with mitochondrial function.
2. Spectrum of activity includes exoerythrocytic (tissue) forms of *Plasmodium vivax* and *P. ovale,* and *Pneumocystic carinii.*

Indications:

1. *P. vivax* malaria (cure and prevention of relapse).
2. Terminal prophylaxis after chloroquine phosphate suppressive therapy in an area endemic for *P. vivax* malaria.
3. Alternative (used with clindamycin) to trimethoprim/sulfamethoxazole for treatment of *P. carinii* pneumonia.

Pharmacokinetics:

1. **Absorption:** PO.

2. **Metabolism:** Rapidly metabolized to metabolites that are also active. Primaquine is found in relatively low concentrations in tissues.
3. **Excretion:** 1% is excreted unchanged in urine.
4. **Half-life:** 4–6 hr.

Drug Preparations:

Tablets: 26.3 mg primaquine phosphate (=15 mg primaquine base).

Dosage: Dosage of primaquine is usually expressed in terms of the *base.*

Malaria (treatment, or prophylaxis after chloroquine): 15 mg PO q day for 14 days.

P. carinii pneumonia: 15–30 mg PO q day for 21 days (and is used with clindamycin).

Adverse Effects:

1. Hemolytic reactions in patients with G6PD or NADH methemoglobin reductase deficiencies.
2. Anemia, methemoglobinemia, and leukopenia have occurred following large doses.
3. Abdominal cramps, epigastric distress, nausea/vomiting. GI symptoms may be lessened by taking primaquine at mealtime.
4. Hypertension, arrhythmias, CNS symptoms (rare).

Drug Interactions: Quinacrine may potentiate the toxicities of antimalarial compounds and should not be given with primaquine.

Monitoring: Periodic CBCs.

BIBLIOGRAPHY

Primaquine. In *Drug Facts and Comparisons,* ed 49, New York, 1995, JB Lippincott, pp 2108–2109.

Webster LT Jr: Drugs used in the chemotherapy of protozoal infections: malaria. In Gillman AG, Rall TW, Nies AS, et al (eds): *The Pharmacological Basis of Therapeutics,* ed 8, New York, 1990, McGraw-Hill, pp 1117–1145.

PRIMIDONE

Trade Names: *Myidone, Mysoline.*

Drug Action: Anticonvulsant activity of this agent is unknown, but effects are thought to be due to parent compound primidone and its two active metabolites, phenobarbital and phenylethyl-malonamide (PEMA), whose actions may be synergistic. Much of primidone's anticonvulsant properties must come from the pheno-barbital-induced depression of cortical activity.

Indications: Use either alone or in conjunction with other anti-convulsants, as indicated in control of tonic-clonic, complex par-tial, and simple partial epileptic seizures.

Pharmacokinetics:

1. **Metabolism:** Primidone is slowly metabolized by the liver to PEMA, phenobarbital and *p*-hydroxyphenobarbital. Phenobar-bital is further metabolized by the liver. Resultant compounds are then slowly excreted by kidneys.
2. **Excretion:** Approximately 15%–25% of PO dose is excreted unchanged in urine. 15%–25% is metabolized to phenobarbi-tal, and 50%–70% excreted as PEMA. Primidone is removed by hemodialysis.
3. **Volume of distribution:** Protein binding is 0%–19% for prim-idone, negligible for PEMA, and 50% for phenobarbital. 92% $\pm 18\%$ of drug available after PO administration. Volume of distribution 0.59 ± 0.47 L/kg. Clearance for primidone is 0.94 ± 0.35 mL/min/kg.
4. **Plasma half-life:** Primidone 3–24 hr.
   Phenobarbital 72–144 hr.
   PEMA 24–48 hr.
5. **Compatibilities:** No major compatibility considerations. Drug is available for PO administration only.

Drug Preparations:

Suspension: 250 mg/5 mL.
Tablets: 50, 250 mg.

Dosage: *Mysoline:* Usual maintenance dose in adults and chil-dren >8 yr is 250 mg PO tid/qid, depending on blood levels. For children <8 yr the usual dose is 125–250 mg PO tid or 10–25 mg/kg/day. Alternatively, 1.25 gm/m^2 PO in two to four divided doses daily may be used in the pediatric population. In all patients, dosage should be increased in small increments over 10–14 days to maintenance levels.

Adverse Reactions:

1. Sedation, ataxia, vertigo, lethargy, anorexia, nausea/vomiting are common side effects of Primidone.
2. Occasional hyperexcitability in children.
3. Others: Diplopia, rash, alopecia, edema, leukopenia, impotence, eosinophilia, systemic lupus erythematosus–like syndrome, megaloblastic anemia, malignant lymphoma–like syndrome.
4. Safety of the drug in pregnancy is not established.

Drug Interactions:

1. Multiple drug interactions stem mostly from enzyme induction in competition with phenobarbital.
2. Increased sedation when used with other CNS depressants.
3. Carbamazepine and phenytoin increase metabolism.

Monitoring: Primidone, phenobarbital, and PEMA levels are readily available at most medical centers. Therapeutic level for primidone is 5–10 μg/mL; for phenobarbital, 10–25 μg/mL; for PEMA, not established.

BIBLIOGRAPHY

Cohen S, Armstrong M: *Drug Interactions: A Handbook for Clinical Use,* Baltimore, 1974, Williams & Wilkins.

Drug Information for the Health Care Professional, ed 8, Rockville, 1988, US Pharmacopeial Convention.

Evans WE, Oellerich M: *Therapeutic Drug Monitoring Clinical Guide,* ed 2, Irving, 1984, Abbott Laboratories Publications.

Gilman A, Goodman L, Rall T, et al (eds): *The Pharmacological Basis of Therapeutics,* ed 7, New York, 1985, Macmillan.

Johnson G: *Blue Book of Pharmacologic Therapeutics,* Philadelphia, 1985, WB Saunders.

McEvoy GK: *Drug Information 88,* Bethesda, 1988, American Society of Hospital Pharmacists.

PROCAINAMIDE

Trade Name: *Procan SR, Procan.*

Drug Action:

1. Antiarrhythmic effects similar to those of quinidine (class 1A).
2. Prolongs effective refractory period of atria and ventricles.
3. Depresses conduction velocity (phase 0) and slope of phase 4 of the action potential. Suppresses automaticity.
4. Slows conduction and refractoriness of accessory pathways.
5. Mild anticholinergic and no α-blocker properties.
6. Shortens effective refractory period of AV node. Increases AV nodal conduction.
7. Prolongs PR and QT intervals.
8. Vasodilation when given IV.

Indications:

1. Treatment of supraventricular arrhythmias.
2. Treatment of ventricular arrhythmias.
3. Prevent recurrences of atrial fibrillation/flutter.

Pharmacokinetics:

1. **Absorption:** PO/IV/IM.
2. **Metabolism:** Hepatic into metabolites, including *N*-acetyl derivative (NAPA), which has antiarrhythmic effects.
3. **Excretion:** Renal excretion of unchanged procainamide and metabolites.
4. **Protein-binding:** 20%.
5. **Plasma half-life:** 3–5 hr.

Drug Preparations:

Tablets: 250, 500 mg.
Extended-release tablets: 250, 500, 750, 1000 mg.
Capsules: 250, 375, 500 mg.
Vials: 1 g/2 mL, 1 g/10 mL.

Dosage:

1. **PO:** Total daily dose 2–6 g. Give in divided doses q 4–6 hr.
2. **IV:** 100 mg/min to effect or to total dose of 1000 mg, followed by infusion of 2–5 mg/min.

Adverse Effects:

1. **Cardiac:** Conduction disturbances, including AV block, prolongation of QT interval, leading to development of torsades de pointes, junctional tachycardia.
2. Hypotension, myocardial depression.
3. Nausea/vomiting, diarrhea, confusion, seizures, depression.
4. Lupus-like syndrome, cytopenia.

Drug Interactions:

1. Enhances anticholinergic effects of other anticholinergic drugs.
2. Antagonizes anticholinesterases in myasthenia gravis.
3. Tagamet increases serum levels and serum half-life.
4. Potentiates neuromuscular blockade.
5. Additive hypotension when used with antihypertensive agents.

Monitoring:

1. Plasma levels: Therapeutic 4–12 µg/mL.
2. NAPA levels should be measured in renal failure and congestive heart failure. Therapeutic: 10–30 µg/mL for combined levels of 10–30 µg/mL (procainamide plus NAPA) of procainamide and NAPA, although controversial.
3. Monitor for lupus-like reaction, ANA titers, blood cell counts.
4. Monitor heart rate, ECG, blood pressure.

BIBLIOGRAPHY

Bigger JT Jr, Hoffman BF: Antiarrhythmic drugs. In Gilman AG, Goodman LS, Gilman A (eds): *The Pharmacological Basis of Therapeutics,* New York, 1980, Macmillan, pp 761–792.

Davis RF: Etiology and treatment of perioperative cardiac dysrhythmias. In Kaplan JA (ed): *Cardiac Anesthesia,* Orlando, FL, 1987, Grune & Stratton, pp 411–450.

Zipes DP: Management of cardiac arrhythmias: pharmacological, electrical, and surgical techniques. In Braunwald E (ed): *Heart Disease: A Textbook of Cardiovascular Medicine,* Philadelphia, 1988, WB Saunders, pp 621–657.

PROCHLORPERAZINE

Trade Name: *Compazine,* generics.

Drug Action:

1. **Antipsychotic:** Postsynaptic blockade of CNS dopamine receptors.
2. **Antiemetic:** Blocks dopamine receptors in chemoreceptor trigger zone of CNS.
3. Anticholinergic and α-adrenergic blocking properties.
4. Depresses reticular activating system.

Indications: Nausea/vomiting.

Pharmacokinetics:

1. **Absorption:** PO/IM/IV.
2. **Metabolism:** Liver.
3. **Excretion:** Urine, feces (enterohepatic circulation).
4. **Duration of effect:** 4–6 hr.

Drug Preparations:

Tablets: 5, 10, 25 mg.
Spansules (time-release): 10, 15, 30 mg.
Syrup: 1 mg/mL.
Injection: 5 mg/mL.
Suppositories: 2.5, 5, 25 mg.

Dosage:

1. **Adult:**
   a. **PO:** 5–10 mg tid/qid. Sustained release, 10–30 mg q day bid.
   b. **IM/IV:** 5–10 mg q 3–4 hr; max. 40 mg/day.
   c. **PR:** 25 mg bid.
2. **Pediatric:**
   a. **PO/PR:** 2.5–5 mg bid/tid.
   b. **IM:** 0.132 mg/kg qd/bid.

Adverse Effects:

1. **Cardiovascular:** Arrhythmias, hypotension, hypertension, tachycardia/bradycardia, ECG changes, pulmonary edema, heart failure, circulatory collapse, syncope.

2. **GI:** Dry mouth, ileus, constipation, nausea/vomiting, diarrhea, anorexia, hepatic damage.
3. **GU:** Urinary retention, gynecomastia, hypermenorrhea.
4. **Hematologic:** Leukopenia/leukocytosis, agranulocytosis, thrombocytopenia, anemia.
5. **CNS:** Sedation, extrapyramidal symptoms/signs, torticollis, tardive dyskinesia, pseudoparkinsonism, neuroleptic malignant syndrome, headache, dizziness, sedation, tremors, psychosis, insomnia, seizures, weakness, ataxia.
6. **Other:** Blurred vision, tinnitus, mydriasis, dermatitis, muscle necrosis (with injection), hyperprolactinemia, photosensitivity, urticaria, fever, edema.

Drug Interactions:

1. May decrease α-adrenergic and dopaminergic effects of sympathomimetics; potentiates β-adrenergic effects.
2. Additive sedation when used with other CNS depressants.
3. Increased incidence of arrhythmias when used with quinidine, disopyramide, procainamide.
4. Oversedation, ileus, constipation, visual changes when used with anticholinergics.
5. Metabolism inhibited by β-blockers.
6. Increased risk of agranulocytosis when used with propylithiouracil.
7. Increased risk of toxicity when used with lithium.
8. Antagonizes effects of dopamine, bromocriptine.
9. Inhibits metabolism of phenytoin (increases risk of toxicity).
10. Increased risk of seizures with metrizamide.
11. Inhibits guanethidine.
12. Enhances effects of nitrates (e.g., hypotension).

Monitoring:

1. Symptoms.
2. BUN, creatinine; liver function tests.
3. Blood cell counts.

BIBLIOGRAPHY

Prochlorperazine. In *Drug Facts and Comparisons,* Philadelphia, 1989, JB Lippincott, pp 1004, 1080.
Prochlorperazine. In *AMA Drug Evaluations,* ed 6, Philadelphia, 1986, WB Saunders, p 267.

PROMOTILITY/PROKINETIC AGENTS

Trade Names:

Metoclopramide: *Reglan*.
Bethanechol: *Urecholine, Myotonachol, Duvoid*.
Cisapride (Propulsed): *See* Cisapride.

Drug Action: Metoclopramide is a dopamine antagonist; bethanechol is a muscarinic cholinergic agonist.

1. Increases lower esophageal sphincter pressure.
2. Increases esophageal acid clearance.
3. Improves delayed gastric emptying and peristalsis.
4. Raises threshold of chemoreceptor trigger zone or vomiting center (metoclopramide).

Indications:

1. Augment H_2 blockers to control gastroesophageal reflux disease (GERD).
2. Delayed gastric emptying due to diabetic gastroparesis (metoclopramide).
3. Peristaltic stimulant: Facilitates migration of nasoduodenal tubes from stomach into duodenum; improves gastric emptying.
4. Antiemetic in high doses (metoclopramide).

Pharmacokinetics: *See* Table 20.

Drug Preparations:

1. **Metoclopramide:**

    Tablets: 5, 10 mg.
    Syrup: 5 mg/mL.
    Vials: 5 mg/mL for IM/IV use.

2. **Bethanechol:**

    Tablets: 5, 10, 25, 50 mg.
    Vials: 5 mg/mL for SQ use.

Dosage:

1. **Metoclopramide:**
    a. **GERD:** 10–20 mg PO 30 min ac and qhs.

TABLE 20.
Pharmacokinetics

Drug	Absorption	Metabolism	t½ (hr)	Duration of Action (hr)	Excretion
Metoclopramide	100% PO	Hepatic	4–6	1–2	85% Renal
Bethanechol	Poor	None	—	1–2	Renal

b. **Gastroparesis;** 10 mg PO 30 min ac and qhs. May also be given IV q 6 hr.

c. **Antiemetic:** 1–2 mg/kg IV 30 min prior to chemotherapy; may repeat q 2–4 hr.

d. Properistaltic: 10 mg IV as single dose or q 6 hr.

2. **Bethanechol:**

a. **GERD:** 10–25 mg PO pc and qhs.

(1) 5 mg tid/qid SQ if NPO.

Adverse Side Effects:

1. **Metoclopramide:** Extrapyramidal signs (including acute dystonic reactions), drowsiness, fatigue, restlessness.

a. NOTE: Acute extrapyramidal/dystonic reactions are best treated with diphenhydramine (Benadryl) 50 mg IM/IV and discontinuation of metoclopramide. Rarely, these reactions have not been reversible.

2. **Bethanechol:** Bronchoconstriction (particularly in patients with underlying reactive airways), blurred vision, diarrhea, abdominal cramps, nausea/vomiting, dizziness, urinary frequency, flushing, bradycardia, hypotension, heart block, urinary retention, miosis.

Drug Interactions:

1. **Metoclopramide:**

a. May be additive with other CNS depressants (e.g., alcohol).

b. Accelerates gastric emptying of medications; long-acting preparations may not dissolve adequately.

2. **Bethanechol:**

a. Effects antagonized by procainamide or quinidine.

b. Ganglionic blockers may cause marked hypotension.

Comments/Recommendations: Metoclopramide and bethanechol are primarily used in conjunction with H_2 blockers in patients with reflux symptoms not controlled by H_2 blockers alone. They are generally not used as monotherapy for GERD, although bethanechol alone has been shown to improve reflux esophagitis. Widespread use of these agents has been limited because of the frequency of troubling side effects and patient intolerance. Metoclopramide has been shown to improve gastric emptying in patients with diabetic gastroparesis, and its properistaltic activity facilitates migration of nasoduodenal tubes from the stomach into the duodenum. At high doses (1–2 mg/kg) metoclopramide also raises the threshold of the chemoreceptor trigger zone, giving it antiemetic properties. This use is generally limited to oncology, and the drug is given before and during chemotherapy. Extrapyramidal side effects must be monitored carefully.

BIBLIOGRAPHY

Lux G, Katschinski M, Ludwig S, et al: The effect of cisapride and metoclopramide on human digestive and interdigestive antroduodenal motility, *Scand J Gastroenterol* 1994, 29:1105–1110.

Orihata M, Sarna SK: Contractile mechanisms of action of gastroprokinetic agents—cisapride, metoclopramide, and domperidone, *Am J Physiol* 1994, 266:G665–676.

McHugh S, Lico S, Diamant NE: Cisapride vs metoclopramide—an acute study in diabetic gastroparesis, *Dig Dis Sci* 1992, 37:997–1001.

PROPOFOL

Trade Name: *Diprivan.*

Drug Actions: Short-acting, rapidly metabolized, IV sedative hypnotic.

Indications: Induction of anesthesia; sedation of adult ICU patients.

Pharmacokinetics:

1. **Absorption:** IV formulation of propofol emulsified in Intralipid.
2. **Onset of action:** 1–2 min.
3. **Metabolism:** Hepatic conjugation to inactive metabolites.
4. **Excretion:** Metabolites excreted by kidneys.
5. **Half-life:** Distribution 1.8–8 min; slow 34–64 min; terminal 300–700 min (termination of biologic effect due largely to redistribution from CNS to peripheral tissues).
6. **Therapeutic level:** 1 μg/mL (sedation) to 5 μg/mL (light general anesthesia).

Drug Preparations: 1% propofol emulsion containing soybean oil (100 mg/mL), glycerol 22.5 mg/mL, and egg lecithin (12 mg/mL), single-dose vial for injection, no preservatives. 20 mL ampules and 50 and 100 mL infusion vials.

Dosage: Titrate to desired effect; induction of anesthesia: 2–2.5 mg/kg as slow IV bolus. ICU sedation: 0.5–1.0 mg/kg/hr in surgical patients, up to 2.5 mg/kg/hr in medical ICU patients.

Adverse Effects: The vehicle is capable of supporting rapid growth of microorganisms. *Strict aseptic techniques* must be followed when handling propofol. Use within 6 hr of preparation. Anesthesia induction: Pain on injection, hypotension, respiratory depression, allergic reactions, bradycardia. ICU sedation: Significant hypotension; cardiovascular depression. Reduce doses in elderly or other compromised patients.

Drug Interactions: Increased effect; with other CNS depressants (and narcotics).

Monitoring: Blood pressure, heart rate, respiratory status, airway, level of sedation/anesthesia, oxygenation.

BIBLIOGRAPHY

Fulton B, Sorkin EM: Propofol—an overview of its pharmacology and a review of its clinical efficacy in intensive care sedation, *Drugs* 1994, 50:636–657.

Lund N, Papadakos PJ: Barbiturates, neuroleptics, and propofol for sedation, *Crit Care Clin* 1995, 11:875–886.

PROPOXYPHENE

Trade Names: *Darvon (hydrochloride), Darvon-N (napsylate), Dolene.*

Drug Actions: Binds to opiate receptors in CNS, causing analgesia (one half to two thirds as potent as codeine).

Indications:

1. Management of mild to moderate pain.

Pharmacokinetics:

1. **Absorption:** PO (30%–70% bioavailable).
2. **Onset of action:** 0.5–1 hr, duration 4–5 hr.
3. **Metabolism:** Liver, metabolized to active metabolite (norpropoxyphene) and inactive metabolites.
4. **Excretion:** Urine.
5. **Half-life:** Parent drug 8–24 hr, norpropoxyphene 34 hr.

Drug Preparations:

Hydrochloride:
  Capsules: 32, 65 mg.
Napsylate:
  Tablets: 100 mg.
  Suspension: 50 mg/5 mL.

Dosage: Adults, 65 mg hydrochloride PO q 3–4 hr as needed for pain; 100 mg napsylate q 4 hr prn for pain; reduce dose in hepatic and renal failure.

Adverse Effects:

1. Hypersensitivity reactions, histamine release, rash, hives.
2. Hypotension.
3. CNS: dizziness, weakness, sedation, drowsiness, paradoxical excitement, nervousness, headache, confusion, hallucinations.
4. GI: Nausea/vomiting, constipation, anorexia, stomach cramps, dry mouth, biliary spasm, increased liver enzymes, ileus.
5. Decreased urination, ureteral spasms, shortness of breath, psychological and physical dependence, respiratory depression (overdose).

Drug Interactions:

1. Synergistic with other CNS depressants.
2. Decreased effect: Charcoal, smoking.
3. Increased serum levels of carbamazepine, phenobarbital, MAO inhibitors, tricyclics, warfarin.

Monitoring: Clinical response, mental status, respiratory status, blood pressure.

BIBLIOGRAPHY

Zieglar K: Opiate and opioid use in patients with refractory
  headache, *Cephalagia* 1994, 14:5–10.

PROPRANOLOL

Trade Name: *Inderal.*

Drug Action:

1. β_1 and β_2 blockade, leading to decreased heart rate and decreased inotropic effects.
2. Electrophysiologic effects, antiarrhythmic action.
3. Antihypertensive; blocks adrenergic receptors, decreases CNS
   sympathetic outflow, suppresses renin release.

Indications:

1. Antiarrhythmic:
   a. Supraventricular tachyarrhythmias.
   b. Sinus tachycardia.
   c. Slows ventricular response in atrial fibrillation/flutter.
   d. Treatment of digitalis-induced arrhythmias.
   e. Treatment of certain ventricular arrhythmias.
   f. Mitral valve prolapse.
   g. Thyrotoxicosis/pheochromocytoma.
2. Antianginal.
3. Antihypertensive.
4. Idiopathic hypertrophic subaortic stenosis.
5. Acute myocardial infarction.

Pharmacokinetics:

1. **Absorption:** PO/IV; peak concentrations occur 60–90 min after PO intake.
2. **Distribution:** Most tissues, 90% protein bound.
3. **Metabolism:** Hepatic.
4. **Excretion:** Urine.
5. **Biologic half-life:** 4 hr.

Drug Preparations:

Tablets: 10, 20, 40, 60, 80, 90 mg.
Extended-release capsules: 80, 120, 160 mg.
Injection: 1 mg/mL.

Dosage:

1. Titrate 0.5–1.0 mg IV q 5 min to effect.
2. Typical dose required in patients not on β-blockers is 0.075–0.15 mg/kg.
3. 20–120 mg tablet q 6–8 hr PO or one 80 mg sustained-release tablet daily; taper to effect.

Adverse Effects:

1. Cardiovascular: Bradycardia, hypotension, congestive heart failure.
2. Exacerbation of asthma or chronic obstructive pulmonary disease.
3. Mental depression, fatigue/weakness.
4. Increased risk of hypoglycemia.

Drug Interactions:

1. Usage with verapamil or digoxin may produce heart block or heart failure.
2. Aluminum hydroxide and ethanol reduce intestinal absorption.
3. Dilantin and phenobarbital accelerate propranolol clearance.
4. Tegretol when used concurrently with propranolol results in increased clearance of both drugs.
5. Lidocaine clearance is reduced.
6. Cimetidine delays clearance of propranolol and increases plasma half-life.
7. Theophylline clearance is reduced by propranolol.
8. Potentiates hypotensive effects of other antihypertensive agents.
9. Antagonizes β-adrenergic agonists, MAO inhibitors.
10. Usage with epinephrine can cause vasoconstriction.

Monitoring: Heart rate, blood pressure.

BIBLIOGRAPHY

Bigger JT Jr, Hoffman BF: Antiarrhythmic drugs. In Gilman AG, Goodman LS, Gilman A (eds): *The Pharmacological Basis of Therapeutics,* New York, 1980, Macmillan, pp 761–792.

Davis RF: Etiology and treatment of perioperative cardiac dysrhythmias. In Kaplan JA (ed): *Cardiac Anesthesia,* Orlando, 1987, Grune & Stratton, pp 411–450.

Zipes DP: Management of cardiac arrhythmias: pharmacological, electrical, and surgical techniques. In Braunwald E (ed): *Heart Disease: A Textbook of Cardiovascular Medicine,* Philadelphia, 1988, WB Saunders, pp 621–657.

PROPYLITHIOURACIL

Trade Name: generics.

Drug Action: Antithyroid drug. Inhibits synthesis of thyroid hormones by blocking iodination of tyrosine to form thyroxine (T_4); inhibits peripheral conversion of T_4 to triiodothyronine T_3.

Indication: Treatment of hyperthyroidism.

Pharmacokinetics:

1. **Absorption:** 80% from GI tract; peak levels 1–1.5 hr.
2. **Distribution:** Concentrated in thyroid gland; crosses placenta; distributed in breast milk.
3. **Metabolism:** Liver.
4. **Excretion:** 35% excreted in urine.
5. **Half-life:** 1–2 hr in patients with normal renal function; 8.5 hr in anuric patients.

Drug Preparations:

Tablets: 50 mg.

Dosage:

1. **Adults:** 100 mg PO tid up to 300 mg q 6 hr until patient is euthyroid; maintenance dose 100–300 mg/day in divided doses q 8–12 hr. Reduce dose in patients with renal insufficiency.
2. **Pediatric:**
   a. 6–10 yr: 15–50 mg q 8 hr.
   b. >10 yr: 100 mg tid; maintenance dose 75–200 mg/day.

Adverse Effects:

1. **CNS:** Headache, drowsiness, dizziness, vertigo, depression, paresthesias, neuritis.
2. **Skin:** Rash, urticaria, pruritus, lupus-like syndrome, exfoliative dermatitis, cutaneous vasculitis, hair loss.
3. **GI:** Diarrhea, loss of taste, nausea/vomiting, epigastric pain, sialadenopathy, constipation.
4. **Hematologic:** Aplastic anemia, agranulocytosis, leukopenia, thrombocytopenia.
5. **Hepatic:** Jaundice, hepatitis, hepatic necrosis, hypoprothrombinemia.
6. **Renal:** Nephritis.
7. **Other:** Arthralgia, myalgia, loss of taste, fever, lymphadenopathy, hypersensitivity reactions, bleeding, lupus-like syndrome.
8. Can cause hypothyroidism and goiter.

Drug Interactions:

1. May potentiate effect of other hepatotoxic or bone marrow depressant drugs.
2. Potentiates vitamin K anticoagulants.

Monitoring:

1. T_4, T_3 thyroid-stimulating hormone.
2. Blood cell counts, alanine aminotransferase (SGPT), aspartate aminotransferase (SGOT), bilirubin, PT, PTT.

BIBLIOGRAPHY

Burman KD: Thyroid hormones. In Chernow B (ed): *The Pharmacologic Approach to the Critically Ill Patient,* Baltimore, 1994, Williams & Wilkins, pp 741–757.

Cooper DS, Saxe VC, Maloff F, et al: Studies of propylthiouracil using a newly developed radioimmunoassay, *J Clin Endocrinol Metab* 1981, 52:204–213.

McMurry JF, Gilliland PF, Ratliff CR, Bourland PO: Pharmacodynamics of propylthiouracil in normal and hyperthyroid subjects after a single dose, *J Clin Endocrinol Metab* 1975, 41:362–364.

Haynes RC: Thyroid and antithyroid drugs. In Gilman AG, et al (eds): *The Pharmacological Basis of Therapeutics,* ed 8, New York, 1994, McGraw-Hill, pp 1361–1383.

PROTAMINE

Trade Name: *Protamine sulfate* (various).

Drug Action: Heparin antagonist (forms salt with heparin).

Indications: Reverse heparin effect.

Pharmacokinetics:

1. **Absorption:** Give IV.
2. **Metabolism:** Unknown; heparin-protamine complex may be attacked by fibrinolysin, freeing heparin.
3. **Onset of action:** Within 5 min.
4. **Duration of action:** 2 hr.

Drug Preparations:

  Vials: 50, 250 mg/vial for injection.

Dosage:

1. Give 1 mg for each 90 U lung heparin or 1 mg for each 115 U intestinal heparin, by slow IV injection over 1–3 min; max. dose 50 mg in any 10 min.
2. Protamine requirements decrease with time after heparin (because of metabolism of heparin); give half dose when taken 30 min after heparin.

Adverse Effects:

1. **Respiratory:** Dyspnea.
2. **Cardiovascular:** Hypotension, bradycardia.
3. **Other:** Flushing, hypersensitivity, anaphylaxis, heparin rebound, nausea/vomiting.
4. **Bleeding:** Protamine has anticoagulant effect; large doses may cause bleeding.

Drug Interactions: Incompatible with several cephalosporins and penicillins.

Monitoring: Clotting times (PT, PTT, activated clotting time).

BIBLIOGRAPHY

Protamine sulfate. In *Drug Facts and Comparisons,* Philadelphia, 1989, JB Lippincott, p 220.

PYRAZINAMIDE

Trade Name: generics.

Drug Actions: Pyrazinamide is a synthetic pyrazine analog of nicotinamide. It inhibits the growth of *Mycobacterium tuberculosis,* but the exact mechanism of this is unknown.

Indications:

1. Treatment of tuberculosis (as part of a four drug regimen that includes also isoniazid, rifampin, and ethambutol).
2. Pyrazinamide may be indicated in combination with another antituberculous drug (e.g., rifampin, ethambutol, ciprofloxacin, ofloxacin) for prophylaxis of a positive tuberculin test without disease when exposure was likely to have been by isoniazid-resistant organisms.

Pharmacokinetics:

1. **Absorption:** PO; well absorbed from GI tract.
2. **Metabolism:** Hydrolyzed in liver to its major active metabolite pyrazinoic acid (which is hydroxylated to the main excretory product, 5-hydroxypyrazinoic acid).
3. **Excretion:** 70% in urine.
4. **Half-life:** 9–10 hr.

Drug Preparations:

Tablets: 500 mg.

Dosage: 25 mg/kg/day with max. daily dosage of 2 g.

Adverse Effects:

1. Hepatic damage (<2%).
2. Hyperuricemia and gout (pyrazinamide inhibits urate excretion).
3. Arthralgias, anorexia, nausea/vomiting, dysuria, malaise, and fever have also been observed.

Drug Interactions: None found.

Monitoring: Consider baseline uric acid and liver function determinations. In patients with preexisting liver disease or at risk for drug-related hepatitis (e.g., alcohol abusers), liver function should be monitored periodically.

BIBLIOGRAPHY

Mandell GL, Sande MA: Antimicrobial agents: drugs used in the chemotherapy of tuberculosis and leprosy. In Gillman AG, Rall TW, Nies AS, et al (eds): *The Pharmacological Basis of Therapeutics,* ed 8, New York, 1990, McGraw-Hill, pp 1146–1164.

Physicians' Desk Reference, ed 50, Montvale, 1996, Medical Economics Co.

PYRIMETHAMINE

Trade Names: *Daraprim, Fansidar.*

Drug Action:

1. Folic acid antagonist.
2. Highly selective activity against *Plasmodium* spp. and *Toxoplasma gondii.*

Indications:

1. Malaria chemoprophylaxis.
2. Treatment of toxoplasmosis.

Pharmacokinetics:

1. **Absorption:** Good PO.
2. Penetrates well into all tissues, including CNS.
3. **Excretion:** Urine.
4. **Half-life:** 2–6 days.

Drug Preparations:

1. *Tablets:*
   Daraprim: 25 mg.
   Fansidar: Combination: Pyrimethamine 25 mg, sulfadoxine 500 mg.

Dosage:

1. **Chemoprophylaxis of malaria:**
   a. **Adult:** 25 mg/wk PO.

b. **Pediatric:** >10 yr: 25 mg/wk PO. 4–10 yr: 12.5 mg/wk (½ tablet) PO. <4 yr: 6.25 mg/wk (one-quarter tablet) PO.
2. Toxoplasmosis (in combination with a sulfonamide):
   a. **Adult:** Initial dose 50–100 mg/day PO, then lower (approximately one half initial dose) as treatment continuation (usually 4–5 wk) or as life-long prophylaxis (e.g., in AIDS patients).
   b. **Pediatric:** Initial dose 1 mg/kg/day divided in 2 doses; after 2–4 days, decrease by one half and continue for about 1 mo.

Adverse Effects:

1. Decreased hematopoiesis secondary to folate deficiency, leading to megaloblastic anemia, leukopenia, thrombocytopenia, pancytopenia.
   a. **Folinic acid (leucovorin) should be given 5–15 mg/day PO/IV/IM.**
2. Nausea/vomiting, diarrhea, anorexia; decreased by giving medication with meals.
3. Neurotoxicity including seizures with overdose, ataxia, tremor.
4. Rash, erythema multiforme, hemolytic anemia in patients with G6PD deficiency.

Drug Interactions:

1. Folic acid reduces drug effects.
2. Additive effect with sulfonamides.

Monitoring:

1. Blood cell counts.
2. Monitor for bleeding.
3. Signs of folate deficiency.

QUINIDINE

Trade Names:

Quinidex Extentabs.
Quinidine sulfate: *Quinora.*
Quinidine gluconate sustained action: *Dura-Tab.*
Quinidine gluconate: *Quinaglute, Quinalan.*

Drug Action:

1. Increases sinus rate and AV nodal conduction by anticholinergic effect.
2. Prolongs effective refractory period and action potential duration of atrial and ventricular muscle fibers.
3. Depresses conduction velocity (phase 0) and slope of phase 4 of the action potential.
4. Slows conduction and prolongs refractoriness of accessory pathways.
5. α-Blocking properties may decrease blood pressure.

Indications:

1. Acute/chronic treatment of ventricular arrhythmias, supraventricular arrhythmias.
2. Paroxysmal supraventricular tachycardia including Wolff-Parkinson-White syndrome.
3. Atrial fibrillation/flutter.

Pharmacokinetics:

1. **Absorption:** PO/IM.
2. **Metabolism:** Hepatic.
3. **Excretion:** Renal.
4. **Plasma half-life:** 6 hr.
5. **Protein binding:** 70%–80%.

Drug Preparations:

Tablets: 100, 200, 300, 324 mg. Also available as extended-release sulfate tablets.

Vials: 800 mg/10 mL (gluconate); 200 mg/mL (sulfate) for IV/IM use.

Dosage:

1. Quinidine sulfate: Usual dose 300–600 mg PO qid; or 600 mg extended-release form q 8–12 hr.
2. Quinidine gluconate: 200–300 mg IM q 2–6 hr or PO 324 mg q 8–12 hr.

Adverse Effects:

1. **Cardiac:** SA and AV block, asystole, prolongation of QT interval may result in torsades des pointes, increased ventricular re-

sponse in atrial fibrillation, hypotension, worsening CHF, may result in dysrhythmias.
2. **GI:** Nausea/vomiting, diarrhea, hepatotoxicity.
3. **HEENT:** Tinnitus, loss of hearing, blurred vision.
4. **Hematologic:** Thrombocytopenia, hemolytic anemia, cytopenias.
5. **CNS:** Headache, light-headedness, confusion, rash, pruritus, seizures.

Drug Interactions:

1. Anticholinergics, increased vagolytic effects; antagonism of cholinergic drugs.
2. Potentiates coumarin anticoagulant effect.
3. Neuromuscular blockers, potentiation of neuromuscular blockade.
4. Phenobarbital or phenytoin (Dilantin), decreased plasma half-life of quinidine.
5. Increases serum concentration of digoxin.
6. Tagamet prolongs quinidine plasma half-life and serum level.
7. Verapamil increases quinidine plasma half-life and plasma level.
8. Additive hypotensive effects when used with hypotensive agents.

Monitoring:

1. QT intervals (ECG).
2. Serum levels (therapeutic): 2–8 μg/mL.
3. Blood cell counts, liver/kidney function.

BIBLIOGRAPHY

Bigger JT Jr, Hoffman BF: Antiarrhythmic drugs. In Gilman AG, Goodman LS, Gilman A (eds): *The Pharmacological Basis of Therapeutics,* New York, 1980, Macmillan, pp 761–792.
Davis RF: Etiology and treatment of perioperative cardiac dysrhythmias. In Kaplan JA (ed): *Cardiac Anesthesia,* Orlando, 1987, Grune & Stratton, pp 411–450.
Zipes DP: Management of cardiac arrhythmias: pharmacological, electrical, and surgical techniques. In Braunwald E (ed): *Heart Disease: A Textbook of Cardiovascular Medicine,* Philadelphia, 1988, WB Saunders, pp 621–657.

RIBAVIRIN

Trade Name: *Virazole.*

Drug Action:

1. Antiviral activity against respiratory syncytial virus (RSV), influenza virus, and herpes simplex virus.
2. Inhibits RNA and DNA synthesis, RNA polymerase, synthesis of viral protein coat.

Indications: RSV infection in infants and young children.

Pharmacokinetics:

1. **Absorption:** Give by inhalation.
2. **Excretion:** Urine.
3. **Half-life:** First phase 9.5 hr; second phase 40 hr.
4. Concentrated in bronchial secretions.

Drug Preparations:

   Powder to be reconstituted for inhalation: 6 g in 100 mL vial.

Dosage: Administer concentrated solution of 20 mg/mL via Viratek Small Particle Aerosol Generator (SPAG-2); mist produced has a concentration of 190 µg/L. Use flow rate 12.5 L/min mist; treat for 12–18 hr/day for 3–7 days.

Adverse Reactions:

1. **Respiratory:** Respiratory failure, apnea, pneumonia, pneumothorax.
2. **Cardiovascular:** Cardiac arrest, hypotension.
3. **Hematologic:** Reticulocytosis, anemia.
4. **Other:** Rash, conjunctivitis.

Drug Interactions: Digitalis toxicity.

Monitoring:

1. Respiratory status.
2. Blood pressure, heart rate.

BIBLIOGRAPHY

Ribavirin. In *Drug Facts and Comparisons,* Philadelphia, 1989, JB Lippincott, p 1615.

Ribavirin. In *AMA Drug Evaluations,* ed 6, Philadelphia, 1986, WB Saunders, p 1620.

RIFABUTIN

Trade Name: *Mycobutin.*

Drug Actions: Inhibits bacterial DNA-dependent RNA polymerase in *Escherichia coli* and *Bacillus subtilis* (not known whether this is the mechanism of antimycobacterial action against *Mycobacterium avium* and *M. intracellulare*).

Indications: Prevention (prophylaxis) of disseminated *M. avium* complex (MAC) disease in patients with AIDS (recommended by Infectious Diseases Society of America to be begun when CD4 count is <75/mm³). Patients with HIV infection taking rifabutin are one third–one half as likely to develop MAC bacteremia as those not taking rifabutin.

Pharmacokinetics:

1. **Absorption:** PO; readily absorbed from GI tract.
2. **Metabolism:** High lipophilicity.
3. **Excretion:** 53% in urine; 30% in feces.
4. **Half-life:** 45 ($\pm$17) hr.

Drug Preparations:

   Capsules: 150 mg.

Dosage: 300 mg PO q day (may be given 150 mg PO bid with food to patients with propensity to nausea/vomiting).

Adverse Effects: Generally well tolerated, but rash (4%), GI intolerance (3%), and neutropenia (2%) can occur.

Drug Interactions:

1. Rifabutin has liver enzyme-inducing properties, but probably less so than the related drug rifampin. Numerous medications, including dapsone, narcotics, anticoagulants, corticosteroids, cyclosporine, cardiac glycoside preparations, quinidine, oral contraceptives, oral hypoglycemic agents (sulfonylureas), and analgesics, may have reduced activity when given concurrently

with rifabutin (based on known interactions of these drugs with rifampin). Additionally, ketoconazole, barbiturates, diazepam, verapamil, β-adrenergic blockers, clofibrate, progestins, disopyramide, mexiletine, theophylline, chloramphenicol, and anticonvulsants may have lessened effects in patients taking rifabutin (also based on experiences with rifampin).
2. Rifabutin should not be used with protease inhibitors owing to profound drug interactions.

BIBLIOGRAPHY

Kaplan JE, Masur H, Holmes KK, et al: USPHS/IDSA guidelines for the prevention of opportunistic infections in persons infected with human immunodeficiency virus: an overview, *Clin Infect Dis* 1995, 21(suppl 1):S12–S31.

Physicians' Desk Reference, ed 50, Montvale, 1996, Medical Economics Co.

RIFAMPIN

Trade Names: *Rifadin, Rifamate, Rimactane.*

Drug Action:

1. Bactericidal effect in inhibition of DNA-dependent RNA polymerase.
2. Spectrum of activity includes wide range of organisms:
   a. Mycobacteria.
   b. Gram-positive (esp. staphylococci) and gram-negative (esp. *Neisseria* spp. and *Haemophilus influenzae*) organisms.
   c. *Legionella* spp.
   d. Others, including *Chlamydia, Clostridium difficile.*

Indications:

1. Tuberculosis.
2. Meningococcal carriers and close contacts.
3. *H. influenzae B* meningitis contacts.
4. Synergistic addition to other antibiotic regimens (e.g., foreign body infections, endocarditis, legionellosis, osteomyelitis, brucellosis).

Pharmacokinetics:

1. **Absorption:** Well absorbed PO.
2. **Metabolism:** Penetrates well into all tissues, including CNS.
3. **Excretion:** Deacetylated by liver. Excreted in bile.
4. **Serum half-life:** 1.5–5 hr; prolonged in hepatic disease.

Drug Preparations:

Capsules: 150, 300 mg. In combination with isoniazid (INH): 300 mg rifampin/150 mg INH; 600 mg rifampin/300 mg INH.

Dosage: Tuberculosis:

1. **Adult:** 600 mg/day PO, single dose.
2. **Pediatric:** 10–20 mg/kg/day PO, single dose.

Adverse Effects:

1. **Hepatoxicity:** Worse with underlying liver disease, concurrent use of other hepatotoxins.
2. **Immunologic reactions:**
   a. Hypersensitivity/allergic reactions: Fever, rash, eosinophilia.
   b. Flulike syndrome, with fever, malaise, headache, particularly with irregular use.
3. **Immunosuppression:** Demonstrated in animals but of unknown clinical importance.
4. Red-orange discoloration of urine, tears, sweat.
   a. "Red lobster" syndrome with overdose and liver damage.
   b. Stains contact lenses orange-brown.
5. **Other:** Nephrotoxicity, thrombocytopenia, exudative conjunctivitis, hemolysis, headache, fatigue, dizziness, confusion, nausea/vomiting, anorexia, diarrhea, pseudomembranous colitis.

Drug Interactions:

1. PO anticoagulants: Decreased anticoagulant effect.
2. PO contraceptives: Decreased contraceptive effect.
3. Barbiturates: Decreased barbiturate effect.
4. β-adrenergic blockers: Decreased β-blocker effect.
5. Clofibrate: Decreased pharmacologic effect of clofibrate.
6. Corticosteroids: Decreased corticosteroid effect.

7. Diazepam: Decreased IV diazepam effect.
8. Digitoxin: Decreased digitoxin effect.
9. Disopyramide: Decreased disopyramide effect.
10. PO hypoglycemics, sulfonylurea: Decreased hypoglycemic effect.
11. INH: Possible increased hepatotoxicity.
12. Ketoconazole: Decreased fungistatic activity.
13. Methadone: Methadone withdrawal symptoms.
14. Mexiletine: Decreased antiarrhythmic effect.
15. Progestins: Decreased plasma levels.
16. Quinidine: Decreased quinidine effect.
17. Dapsone: Decreased dapsone effect.
18. Theophylline: Decreased theophylline level.

Monitoring: Serial liver function studies, renal function studies, hematologic status.

BIBLIOGRAPHY

Baciewicz AM, Self TH: Rifampin drug interactions, *Arch Intern Med* 1984, 144:1667.

RIMANTADINE

Trade Name: *Flumadine*.

Drug Actions:

1. Not fully understood, but probably exerts viral inhibitory effect by inhibiting uncoating of the virus.
2. Active against influenza A virus (little or no activity against influenza B virus). Small studies have shown that upon treatment with rimantadine, 10%–30% of patients with initially sensitive virus shed resistant virus (clinical response slower but not significantly different from those not shedding resistant virus).

Indications:

1. Prophylaxis and treatment of influenza A in adults.
2. Prophylaxis of influenza A in children.

Pharmacokinetics:

1. **Absorption:** PO.
2. **Metabolism:** Hepatic; three hydroxylated metabolites and parent drug found in plasma.
3. **Excretion:** <25% of dose excreted in urine as unchanged drug.
4. **Half-life:** 25.4 hr (32 hr in 71–79-year-old subjects).

Drug Preparations:

Tablets: 100 mg.
Syrup: 50 mg/5 mL.

Dosage:

1. Prophylaxis and treatment in adults: 100 mg PO bid. (A dose reduction to 100 mg PO q day is recommended for patients with severe hepatic or renal insufficiency, and elderly nursing home patients.) Rimantadine administration for treatment of influenza A should begin within 48 hr of onset of symptoms and signs of influenza A infection; recommended duration of therapy is 7 days.
2. Prophylaxis in children.

   10 yr of age or older: Adult dosage
   <10 yr of age: 5 mg/kg PO q day but not exceeding 150 mg.

Adverse Effects:

1. CNS side effects are less with rimantadine than with amantadine.
2. Nausea (2.8%), insomnia (2.1%), dizziness (1.9%), vomiting (1.7%), and others, including impaired concentration.

Drug Interactions:

1. Cimetidine decreases rimantadine clearance by 18%.
2. Coadministration of rimantadine with acetaminophen or aspirin mildly reduces rimantadine concentrations.

BIBLIOGRAPHY

Physicians' Desk Reference, ed 50, Montvale, 1996, Medical Economics Co.

Sanford JP, Gilbert DN, Sande MA (eds): *The Sanford Guide to Antimicrobial Therapy,* ed 26, Dallas, TX, 1996, Antimicrobial Therapy, Inc.

RITODRINE HYDROCHLORIDE

Trade Name: *Yutopar.*

Drug Action:

1. Tocolytic agent; β_2 agonist; inhibits contractility of uterus.
2. β-adrenergic receptor agonist (preferentially β_2).

Indication: Management of premature labor.

Pharmacokinetics:

1. **Absorption:** 30% PO.
2. **Metabolism:** Liver.
3. **Excretion:** 70%–90% in urine; removed by hemodialysis.
4. Crosses placenta.
5. **Time to peak level** after PO administration: 20–60 min.
6. **Plasma half-life:**
   a. Initial phase: 1.3–2.6 hr.
   b. Elimination phase 12–20 hr.
   c. Distribution phase (IV) 6–9 min.

Drug Preparations:

Vials: 10 mg/mL (5 mL vial), and 15 mg/ml (10 ml vial) for injection.
Tablets: 10 mg.

Dosage:

1. **Initial dose:** 50–100 µg/min by IV infusion; increase q 10 min by increments of 50 µg/min to reach effective dose (usual effective dose 150–350 µg/min).
2. **Maintenance:** 10 mg PO before stopping IV therapy, then 10 mg PO q 2 hr for 24 hr; thereafter, 10–20 mg q 4–6 hr.

Adverse Effects:

1. **Cardiovascular:** Hypertension, hypotension, chest pain, myocardial ischemia, palpitations, pulmonary edema, arrhythmias, tachycardia, ECG changes, altered maternal and fetal heart rate.
2. **GI:** Nausea/vomiting, diarrhea, constipation, epigastric pain, bloating, hepatotoxicity.
3. **CNS:** Nervousness, anxiety, headache, malaise, emotional lability.
4. **Other:** Hyperglycemia, hypokalemia, anaphylaxis, erythema, sweating, chills, ketoacidosis, hypersensitivity, tremor.

Drug Interactions:

1. Increased risk of pulmonary edema when used with corticosteroids.
2. Effects additive when used with sympathomimetic drugs.
3. Inhibited by β-blockers.
4. Increased effects when used with magnesium sulfate, diazoxide, meperidine, general anesthetics, potassium-sparing diuretics.
5. Hypertension exaggerated with parasympatholytics (e.g., atropine).

Monitoring:

1. Status of pregnancy; uterine contractions.
2. Fetal and maternal heart rate.
3. Blood pressure.
4. Glucose, potassium.
5. Signs of pulmonary edema, fluid status (monitor fluid intake to prevent fluid overload).

BIBLIOGRAPHY

Ritodrine hydrochloride. In *Drug Facts and Comparisons*, Philadelphia, 1989, JB Lippincott, p 349.

Benedetti TJ, Gonik B, Hayashi RH, Adams HJ: A multicenter evaluation of intramuscular ritodrine hydrochloride as initial parenteral therapy for preterm labor management, *J Perinatol* 1994, 14:403–407.

Kupferminc M, Lessing JB, Yaron Y, Peyser MR: Nifedipine versus ritodrine for suppression of preterm labour, *Br J Obstet Gynaecol* 1993, 100:1090–1094.

SCOPOLAMINE

Trade Names: *Transderm Scop, Isopto Hyoscine.*

Drug Action:

1. Inhibits acetylcholine muscarinic actions, resulting in decreased secretions and GI motility (anticholinergic).
2. Antiemetic (central), especially motion sickness.
3. Antiparkinsonian actions.
4. Cyclopegic.

Indications:

1. Nausea/vomiting.
2. Adjunct to anesthesia; antimuscarinic.
3. Iritis, uveitis.

Pharmacokinetics:

1. **Absorption:** SQ/PO/IM/percutaneous.
2. **Metabolism:** Liver.
3. **Excretion:** Urine.
4. **Onset:** 15–30 min after IM/SQ; several hours after percutaneous applications.
5. Mydriatic effects persist for 3–7 days.

Drug Preparations:

Transderm patch: 1 mg.
Injection: 300, 400, 1000 μg/mL.
Ophthalmic solution: 0.25%.

Dosage:

1. **Adjunct to surgery:**
   a. **Adult:** 300–600 μg IM/IV; 1 mg PO.
   b. **Pediatric:** 100–300 μg IM/IV.
2. **Antiemetic:**
   a. Adult:
      (1) 250–750 μg PO q 4–6 hr.
      (2) One transderm patch behind ear q 3 days.
      (3) 600 μg SQ initially, then 300 μg q 6 hr.

3. **Iritis/uveitis:** 1–2 drops 0.25% ophthalmic solution q day–tid.

Adverse Effects:

1. **Respiratory:** Bronchial plugs, respiratory depression.
2. **Cardiovascular:** Tachycardia, palpitations, paradoxical bradycardia.
3. **GI:** Nausea/vomiting, epigastric discomfort, dry mouth, dysphagia, constipation.
4. **GU:** Dysuria, urinary retention.
5. **Dermatologic:** Erythema, rash, dryness.
6. **Eyes:** Dilated pupils, blurred vision, photophobia, cyclopegia, increased ocular pressure, dry and itchy eyes, red eyes, acute glaucoma, ocular congestion.
7. **CNS:** Headache, drowsiness, coma, seizures, irritability, dizziness, confusion, disorientation, hallucinations, amnesia, spasticity, delirium.
8. Fever.

Drug Interactions:

1. Increased CNS depression when used with alcohol, sedatives, tranquilizers.
2. Antacids decrease absorption.
3. Additive effects with other anticholinergics.
4. Decreased GI absorption of drugs such as levodopa, ketoconazole.
5. Elevated serum digoxin level.
6. Increased risk of ulceration with GI irritants.

Monitoring: Symptoms.

BIBLIOGRAPHY

Denniston PL Jr (ed): *1995 Physicians GenRx,* Riverside, 1995, Denniston Publishing.
Physicians' Desk Reference, ed 49, Montvale, 1995, Medical Economics Data Production.
Gilman AG, Rall TW, Nies AS, Taylor P (eds): *Goodman and Gilman's The Pharmacological Basis of Therapeutics,* ed 8, New York, 1990, Macmillan.

SILVER SULFADIAZINE

Trade Names: *Silvadene, SSD Cream, Thermazene.*

Drug Action:

1. Topical antibacterial and antifungal (gram-positive and gram-negative bacteria, yeast).
2. Affects cell membranes and cell walls.

Indication:

1. Wound infection.
2. Second- and third-degree burns.

Pharmacokinetics:

1. **Absorption:** Use topically.
2. **Metabolism:** Hepatic.
3. **Excretion:** Urine.

Drug Preparations:

   Cream: 1%.

Dosage: Apply 1/16 inch cream to skin q day/bid.

Adverse Effects:

1. **Dermatologic:** Rash, pruritus, local pain.
2. **Leukopenia.**
3. **Hemolysis** (esp. in patients with G6PD deficiency).
4. **Hypersensitivity reactions.**

Drug Interactions: May inactivate topical proteolytic enzymes.

Monitoring:

1. Evaluate wound for status of infection and healing.
2. Blood cell counts.
3. Serum sulfa levels (with extensive topical use).
4. Liver function tests, BUN, creatinine.

BIBLIOGRAPHY

Silver sulfadiazine. In *Drug Facts and Comparisons,* Philadelphia, 1989, JB Lippincott, p 1911.

Silver Sulfadiazene. In *AMA Drug Evaluations,* ed 6, Philadelphia, 1986, WB Saunders, p 1506.

SODIUM BICARBONATE

Trade Names:

Parenteral: *Sodium Bicarbonate Injection.*
PO: *Citrocarbonate, Arm and Hammer Baking Soda, Soda Mint.*

Drug Action:

1. **Systemic alkalinization:** Raises blood pH by increasing plasma bicarbonate levels and buffering excess hydrogen ions.
2. **Urinary alkalinization:** Raises urinary pH by increasing excretion of free bicarbonate ions.
3. **Gastric antacid:** Reacts chemically with gastric acid.

Indications:

1. **Metabolic acidosis:** Treatment of renal disease, circulatory insufficiency, bicarbonate loss from diarrhea, severe diabetic ketoacidosis.
2. **Nephrolithiasis:** Reduces uric acid crystals and prevents crystallization during sulfonamide therapy.
3. **Gastric hyperacidity:** PO to increase gastric pH.
4. **Toxic ingestions:** May be useful in certain toxic ingestions (e.g., salicylates) to prevent GI uptake and/or to promote urinary excretion by urine alkalization.

Pharmacokinetics:

1. **Metabolism:** None.
2. **Excretion:** Renal; CO_2 formed as HCO_3^- reacts with H^+ to form H_2CO_3 is excreted by lungs.
3. **Volume of distribution:** Extracellular fluid (0.2 L/1 g).
4. **Basal circulating levels:** 24 mEq/L.
5. **Plasma half-life:** Indeterminate.

Drug Preparations:

1. **PO:**
   Effervescent sodium bicarbonate.
   Sodium bicarbonate: PO solution; tablets, 300, 325, 600, 650 mg.
2. **Parenteral:**
   Sodium bicarbonate injection: 4%–8.4% (4.8–10 mEq/10 mL)
   (undiluted), 1.5% (isotonic).

Dosage:

1. **Adult:**
   a. **PO:**
      (1) Effervescent sodium bicarbonate: 4–10 g q 6–8 hr.
      (2) Sodium bicarbonate tablets: Up to 1.0–2.0 g
          (12–24 mEq) q 2–4 hr for urinary alkalization.
          Not to exceed 16 g daily.
   b. **Parenteral:**
      (1) **Systemic alkalinization:** For severe acidosis, initial
          dose 1.0 mEq/kg, followed by 0.5 mEq/kg; adjust
          dosage as indicated by clinical condition or blood pH
          measurements. For less urgent situations, may be given
          by continuous IV infusion (2–5 mEq/kg over 4–8 hr).
      (2) **Urinary alkalinization:** 2–5 mEq/kg over 4–8 hr.
2. **Pediatric:**
   a. **PO:**
      (1) Effervescent sodium bicarbonate: Dose individualized
          by physician.
      (2) Sodium bicarbonate for PO solution: Not established.
      (3) Sodium bicarbonate tablets: Up to 10 mEq/kg body
          weight/day in divided doses q 4–6 hr.
   b. **Parenteral:** *See* Adult dosage.

Adverse Effects:

1. With excessive administration, severe metabolic alkalosis, hyperosmolality, hypokalemia, hypernatremia.
2. Irregular heartbeat, muscle cramps/pain, peripheral edema,
   mood/mental changes, obtundation (hypernatremia), heart failure, renal calculi, ionized hypocalcemia, tetany, nervousness,
   nausea/vomiting.

Drug Interactions:

1. Decreased pharmacologic effects: Benzodiazepines, ketoconazole, lithium, salicylates, sulfonylureas, tetracyclines, phenobarbital.
2. Increased pharmacologic effects: Quinidine, amphetamines, flecainide, sympathomimetics.
3. Hypokalemia enhanced: Glucocorticoids, diuretics, mineralocorticoids.

Monitoring:

1. Arterial blood pH determinations.
2. Serum bicarbonate determinations, potassium levels.
3. Urinary pH determinations.

BIBLIOGRAPHY

Gastrointestinal drugs. In *Drug Facts and Comparisons,* Philadelphia, 1996, JB Lippincott, pp 154–157.
Sodium bicarbonate. In *Drug Information for the Health Care Provider,* vol 1, ed 15, Rockville, 1995, US Pharmacopeial Convention, pp 2468–2472.

SODIUM POLYSTYRENE SULFONATE

Trade Name: *Kayexalate.*

Drug Action:

1. Cation-exchange resin.
2. Binds potassium (in exchange for sodium) in gut and prevents its absorption. Also binds small amounts of lithium, magnesium, calcium.

Indication: Hyperkalemia. Has also been anecdotally reported for use in lithium overdoses.

Pharmacokinetics:

1. **Absorption:** None.
2. **Distribution:** None.

3. **Metabolism:** None.
4. **Excretion:** Unchanged in stool.
5. **Binds** approximately 1 mEq potassium per gm Kayexalate.
6. **Onset of action:** 2–12 hr after PO administration.

Drug Preparations:

Powder: 1 pound jar (453.6 g Kayexalate).

Dosage:

1. 15–60 g PO q 6 hr prn (in 3–4 mL water, syrup, fruit juice, or soft drink per g Kayexylate; 10–20 mL 70% sorbitol helps prevent constipation).
2. 30–50 g by retention enema q 6 hr prn; mix in 100 mL aqueous vehicle, e.g., 70% sorbitol at body temperature, followed by a cleansing enema (less effective).

Adverse Effects:

Contraindications: Hypokalemia, hypersensitivity, digoxin toxicity, congestive heart failure, cirrhosis.

1. **GI:** Anorexia, nausea/vomiting, constipation, fecal impaction, gastric irritation, diarrhea (sorbitol), intestinal obstruction.
2. Electrolyte imbalance; e.g., hypokalemia, hypomagnesemia, hypocalcemia.
3. Sodium overload.
4. Metabolic alkalosis (when combined with ionic cathartics).

Drug Interactions:

1. Digitalis toxicity (hypokalemia).
2. Binds magnesium and calcium. Should not be administered with magnesium hydroxide laxatives.

Monitoring: Serum potassium, calcium, magnesium; ECG.

BIBLIOGRAPHY

Kayexalate. In *Physicians' Desk Reference,* ed 49, Montvale, 1995, Medical Economics Co., p 2212.
St. Peter WL, Halstenson CE: Pharmacologic approach in patients with renal failure. In Chernow B (ed): *The Pharmacologic Approach to the Critically Ill Patient,* ed 3, Baltimore, 1994, Williams & Wilkins, p 41.

Henry GC, Osborn H, Weisman RS: Lithium. In Goldfrank LR, Flomenbaum NE, Lewin NA, et al (eds): *Toxicologic Emergencies,* ed 5, Norwalk, 1994, Appleton & Lange, p 761.

SPIRONOLACTONE

Trade Names: *Aldactone, Alatone S.*

Drug Action:

1. Inhibits aldosterone actions on cortical collecting tubule and late distal renal tubule by direct antagonism of cytosolic mineralocorticoid receptor.
2. Increases sodium and water excretion; decreases potassium excretion (potassium-sparing diuretic).
3. Antiandrogenic.

Indications:

1. Hyperaldosterone states (e.g., primary aldosteronism, cirrhosis).
2. Hypertension (usually in combination with other agents).
3. Edema.

Pharmacokinetics:

1. **Absorption:** 90% from GI tract.
2. **Metabolism:** Liver; major active metabolite is canrenone.
3. **Excretion:** Primarily urine, some biliary.
4. **Plasma half-life:** 13–24 hr.
5. **Maximal effect:** 3 days.

Drug Preparations:

Tablets: 25, 50, 100 mg.

Dosage:

1. **Adult:** 25–200 mg/day PO in one to two doses.
2. **Pediatric:** 3.3 mg/kg/day PO in one to two doses.

Adverse Effects:

1. **GI:** Nausea, anorexia, cramping, ulceration, diarrhea.
2. **Dermatologic:** Urticaria, rash.

3. **Metabolic:** Hyperkalemia, acidosis, hyponatremia, increased BUN, menstrual irregularities, hirsutism.
4. **CNS:** Headache, drowsiness, mental confusion.
5. **Other:** Gynecomastia, dehydration, hypotension, fever, agranulocytosis.

Drug Interactions:

1. Hypotensive effects potentiated by other antihypertensives.
2. Hyperkalemia may occur when used with potassium supplements, other potassium-sparing diuretics, angiotensin converting enzyme inhibitors, salt substitutes.
3. Elevation in serum digoxin level; also interferes with radioimmunoassay for digoxin (causes elevation).
4. Diuretic effect reduced by salicylates.
5. May decrease hypoprothrombinemic effect of oral anticoagulants.

Monitoring:

1. Blood pressure, heart rate, volume status.
2. Sodium, potassium, BUN, creatinine.

BIBLIOGRAPHY

Spironolactone. In *Drug Facts and Comparisons,* Philadelphia, 1995, JB Lippincott, pp 620–622.
Spironolactone. In *Drug Information for the Health Care Professional,* Taunton, 1995, Rand McNally, pp 1152–1157.

STREPTOMYCIN

Trade Name: generics.

Drug Action:

1. Inhibition of protein biosynthesis through binding to 30S ribosomal subunits (aminoglycoside).
2. Spectrum of activity includes mycobacteria, *Yersinia pestis, Francisella tularensis, Brucella* spp., others.

Indications:

1. As single agent:
   a. Plague.
   b. Tularemia.
2. In combination:
   a. With INH, rifampin, etc., in tuberculosis.
   b. With penicillins against streptococcal and enterococcal infections.
   c. With tetracycline in brucellosis.

Pharmacokinetics:

1. **Absorption:** Well absorbed after IM administration.
2. **Serum half-life:** 2–3 hr.
3. **Excretion:** Renal.

Drug Preparations:

Vials: 1, 5 g for IM use.

Dosage:

1. **Normal renal function:**
   a. **Adult:** 0.5–1 g q 12 hr IM.
   b. **Pediatric:** 10–15 mg/kg q 12 hr IM.
2. **Impaired renal function:**

Dose (g)	Creatinine Clearance	Interval (hr)
0.5–1	>80	12
	80–50	24
	50–10	24–72
	<10 (anuria)	72–96

3. **Hemodialysis:** Supplemental dose of 5 mg/kg after each dialysis.

Adverse Effects:

1. Nephrotoxicity.
2. Circumoral or peripheral paresthesias with flushing.
3. Curare-like effect when given intraperitoneally, intrapleurally, IV.

4. Ototoxicity primarily vestibular (vertigo).
5. Headache, lethargy, diarrhea, neuromuscular blockade, hypersensivity reactions, agranulocytosis.

Monitoring:

1. Serial audiograms.
2. Clinical monitoring for vestibulotoxicity.
3. Serum levels: Peak, 15–40 mg/L; trough, <5 mg/L.

SUCCINYLCHOLINE

WARNING: Before using any neuromuscular relaxant, one should be totally familiar with its actions and be able to perform tracheal intubation and totally control ventilation in the patient.

Trade Names: *Anectine, Quelicin, Sucostrin, Sux-Cert, Suxamethonium.*

Drug Action:

1. Succinylcholine combines with the postsynaptic cholinergic receptor of the neuromuscular junction of skeletal muscle and depolarizes the motor end plate. As the muscle fibers randomly depolarize, fasciculations occur, followed rapidly by flaccid paralysis. Succinylcholine is rapidly hydrolyzed by serum pseudocholinesterase, and the duration of paralysis is brief, usually 4–6 min. Normal motor function returns as the myocyte repolarizes.
2. Succinylcholine does not cross the intact blood-brain barrier and has no known direct effect on cerebral function. However, succinylcholine is known to indirectly cause EEG activation and increase cerebral blood flow and intracranial pressure in lightly anesthetized humans and dogs. These effects are attributed to activation of muscle spindle afferents with subsequent CNS activation.

Indications:

1. Facilitation of tracheal intubation.
2. Surgical relaxation.

3. Postextubation vocal cord adduction (laryngospasm) that does not respond to gentle positive-pressure ventilation.
4. Short therapeutic procedures requiring muscle relaxation (e.g., electroconvulsive therapy, orthopedic manipulation).

Pharmacokinetics:

1. **Onset of action:** 45–60 sec if administered IV; 2–4 min if IM.
2. **Distribution:** Plasma and extracellular fluid.
3. **Metabolism:** >90% is hydrolyzed by plasma pseudo-cholinesterase to succinic acid and choline.
4. **Excretion:** <5% is renally excreted unchanged.
5. **Half-life:** 90 sec with normal pseudocholinesterase levels.

Drug Preparations:

Vials: 5 or 10 mL, with 20 mg/mL or 100 mg/mL, for injection.
Sterile Powder Flo-Pack: 1 g; mix with 500–1000 mL D_5W/ saline solution, for continuous IV drip.

Dosage:

1. **IV:** 1–1.5 mg/kg.
2. **IM:** 2–4 mg/kg (pediatric use only).

Adverse Effects: A myriad of adverse effects may occur with administration of succinylcholine; however, the frequency of significant problems is low.

1. Most serious problem is massive cellular potassium release, with resultant serum potassium rapidly reaching levels in excess of 6.5 mEq/L. This can occur following third-degree burn, trauma, intraabdominal sepsis, and denervation injuries, and in patients with paraplegia, quadriplegia, and upper motor neuron lesions. Normally, serum potassium does not rise more than 0.5–1.0 mEq/L after IV administration.
2. **Duration of action** of succinylcholine is significantly prolonged to 20–30 min in patients heterozygous for atypical pseudocholinesterase, and for several hours in patients homozygous for the atypical enzyme. Approximately 1 : 800 and 1 : 3200 people are heterozygous and homozygous, respectively, for the atypical enzyme. Although seldom a clinical problem, pregnancy, malnutrition, prolonged illness, liver disease, cancer, and other conditions may decrease serum levels

of pseudocholinesterase and mildly prolong the duration of action of succinylcholine.

3. **Other significant adverse effects:**
   a. Dysrhythmias (e.g., sinus bradycardia, junctional rhythms, even PVCs).
   b. Myalgias and myoglobinuria as a result of fasciculations.
   c. Increased intraocular pressure, especially of concern with penetrating eye injury.
   d. Prolonged muscular contraction in patients with various myotonias, which may interfere with ventilation.
   e. Possible increases in intracranial pressure (*see* Drug Action), which may be of concern in patients with elevated intracranial pressure secondary to trauma or other causes.
   f. Since intragastric pressures may increase, concern for aspiration exists, and appropriate preventive measures such as cricoid pressure must be taken when succinylcholine is used in a patient with a full stomach.
   g. Diffuse erythematous rash and histamine release are occasionally noted.
   h. Rare in the ICU setting, malignant hyperthermia has been associated with use of succinylcholine in genetically susceptible individuals.

Drug Interactions:

1. Echothiopate and some organophosphate insecticides may irreversibly bind to pseudocholinesterase and greatly retard the metabolism of succinylcholine.
2. Magnesium sulfate and aminoglycosides may prolong muscle relaxation.
3. PO contraceptives may be associated with decreased levels of pseudocholinesterase.
4. Reversible inhibition of pseudocholinesterase by various drugs (e.g., neostigmine, edrophonium, pyridostigmine, trimethaphan, local anesthetics, MAO inhibitors, chlorpromazine) may prolong paralysis.

Monitoring:

1. Flaccidness, tetany, and train-of-four are easily evaluated with standard muscle twitch monitors.

2. If abnormal pseudocholinesterase is suspected, a dibucaine number, an expression of the activity of the typical and atypical enzyme, may be determined or electrophoresis may be used to assess the quantity of normal and abnormal enzyme.
3. Respiratory status, cardiovascular status.

BIBLIOGRAPHY

Denniston PL Jr. (ed): *1995 Physicians GenRx,* Riverside, 1995, Denniston Publishing.
Physicians' Desk Reference, ed 49, Montvale, 1995, Medical Economics Data Production.
Gilman AG, Rall TW, Nies AS, Taylor P (eds): *Goodman and Gilman's The Pharmacological Basis of Therapeutics,* ed 8, New York, 1990, Macmillan.
Miller RD (ed): *Anesthesia,* ed 4, New York, 1994, Churchill Livingstone.
Stoelting RK: *Pharmacology and Physiology in Anesthetic Practice,* ed 2, Philadelphia, 1987, JB Lippincott.

SUCRALFATE

Trade Name: *Carafate.*

Drug Action: Exact mechanism remains elusive.

1. Forms ulcer-adherent complex with mucosal proteins and proteinaceous exudate at ulcer site (when gastric acid present).
2. Adsorbs pepsin.
3. Adsorbs bile salts.
4. Increases synthesis of mucosal prostaglandins.
5. Has no effect on gastric acid secretion.

Indications:

1. Peptic ulcer disease.
2. Stress ulcer prophylaxis.
3. Topical treatment of stomatitis.
4. Esophagitis.

Pharmacokinetics:

1. **Absorption:** Only 5% systemically.
2. **Duration of action:** 5 hr; onset 1–2 hr.
3. **Excretion:** Feces (small amounts unchanged in urine).
4. **Metabolism:** Not metabolized.

Drug Preparations:

Tablets: 1 g.
Liquid suspension: 1 g/10 mL.

Dosage:

1. **Acute peptic ulcer disease:**
   a. 1 g PO qid 30 min before meals and q hs.
   b. Alternatively, 2 g PO bid 30 min before breakfast and q hs.
   c. **Maintenance:** 1 g PO bid 30 min before breakfast and q hs.
2. **Stress ulcer prophylaxis:**
   a. 1–2 g PO q 4–6 hr.
   b. Can be given via NG tube as slurry dissolved in 10–15 mL water, or suspension.
3. Stomatitis: 1 g/10 mL suspension; swish and spit or swish and swallow. qid.

Adverse Effects:

1. Dizziness, vertigo.
2. Renal impairment: Aluminum toxicity (e.g., dementia, osteodystrophy).
3. Hypophosphatemia.
4. May decrease gastric emptying, constipation, diarrhea, nausea, gastric discomfort.

Drug Interactions:

1. Sucralfate decreases bioavailability of cimetidine, ranitidine, phenytoin, tetracyclines, fat-soluble vitamins (A, D, E, K), digoxin, theophylline, ciprofloxacin, itraconazole, ketoconazole, norfloxacin.
2. Concomitant antacids decrease sucralfate effectiveness (ulcer adherence). Requires gastric acid for action.

BIBLIOGRAPHY

Clearfield H, et al: International perspectives on acid-peptic disorders, *Pract Gastroenterol* 1988, May–June (suppl):1–40.

Cytoprotective agents. In *AMA Drug Evaluations,* ed 6, Philadelphia, 1986, WB Saunders, p 954.

Brogden RN, Heel RC, Speight TM, Avery GS: Sucralfate—a review of its pharmacodynamic properties and therapeutic use in peptic ulcer disease, *Drugs* 1984, 27:194–209.

Tryba M, Zevounou F, Torok M, et al: Prevention of acute stress bleeding with sucralfate, antacids, or cimetidine, *Am J Med* 1985, 79(suppl 2C):55–61.

SUFENTANIL

Trade Name: *Sufenta.*

Drug Action: Sufentanil has five to 10 times the potency of fentanyl and 500–1000 times the potency of morphine.

Indications:

1. Adjunct to local, regional, or inhalation anesthesia.
2. Primary component in nitrous oxide–narcotic-relaxant anesthesia.
3. Can be the predominant anesthetic when used in "high-dose" techniques such as with cardiac anesthesia.
4. Seldom used in treating postoperative pain.

Pharmacokinetics:

1. **Absorption:** IV onset of action 30–90 sec.
2. **Metabolism:** Approximately 98% undergoes *N*-dealkylation or *O*-demethylation in liver. Hepatic disease warrants decreasing dosage of sufentanil.
3. **Excretion:** Urine and feces.
4. **Half-life:** Approximately 2.5 hr.

Drug Preparations:

50 µg/mL in 1, 2, 5 mL ampules.

Dosage:

1. **Adjunct to inhalation anesthesia:** 1–2 μg/kg IV.
2. **Primary anesthetic in surgical procedures:** 2–10 μg/kg IV, with N$_2$O and muscle relaxant.
3. **Major cardiovascular/neurosurgical cases, debilitated patients:** 10–25 μg/kg IV, with 100% oxygen and muscle relaxant.
4. **Postoperative pain:** Like fentanyl, sufentanil is highly lipid soluble and has a brief duration of action; thus, its use in pain control is limited.

Adverse Effects:

1. Respiratory depression and potential for elevation in intracranial pressure.
2. Bradycardia frequently occurs, but hemodynamic compromise is seldom a problem, except occasionally with large doses used for cardiac anesthesia.
3. Concurrent use of sufentanil and vecuronium (muscle relaxant) may result in profound bradycardia.
4. Like fentanyl, there is no histamine release, even with large doses.
5. Muscle rigidity.

Drug Interactions: As with other narcotics, sufentanil may potentiate or be potentiated by other drugs that produce sedation, somnolence, or respiratory depression.

Monitoring: Respiratory rate, heart rate, blood pressure, mental status.

BIBLIOGRAPHY

Gilman AG, Goodman LS, Rall TW, et al (eds): *Goodman and Gilman's The Pharmacological Basis of Therapeutics,* ed 7, New York, 1985, Macmillan.

McEvoy GK (ed): *AHFS Drug Information 89,* Bethesda, 1989, American Society of Hospital Pharmacists.

Stoelting RK: *Pharmacology and Physiology in Anesthetic Practice,* Philadelphia, JB Lippincott, 1987.

SULFONAMIDES

Trade Names: *Thiosulfil, Urobiotic, Gantanol, Gantrisin.*

Drug Action:

1. Inhibition of growth by competitive antagonism of *p*-aminobenzoic acid (PABA), preventing incorporation of PABA into the folic acid molecule, resulting in inhibition of folic acid synthesis.
2. Spectrum of activity includes both gram-positive and gram-negative aerobes.

Indications:

1. **As single agent:**
   a. Uncomplicated urinary tract infections.
   b. Nocardiosis.
   c. Rheumatic fever prophylaxis.
   d. Alternative agent in chlamydial pneumonia.
   e. Ulcerative colitis (salicylazosulfapyridine).
2. **In combination** with other antimicrobials:
   a. With pyrimethamine against toxoplasmosis.

Pharmacokinetics:

1. **Absorption:** Generally used only in PO form; well absorbed.
2. **Excretion:** Renal.
3. **Serum half-life:** Variable depending on preparation.

Drug Preparations: Sulfisoxazole/sulfamethoxazole:

Tablets: 500 mg.
Suspension: 500 mg/5 mL.

Dosage:

1. **Sulfisoxazole:**
   a. **Adult:** 0.5–1 g PO q 6 hr.
   b. **Pediatric:** 37.5 mg/kg PO q 6 hr.
2. **Sulfamethoxazole:**
   a. **Adult:** 1 g PO q 8–12 hr.
   b. **Pediatric:** 25–35 mg/kg PO q 12 hr.

Adverse Effects:

1. **Allergic/hypersensitivity reactions:** Rash, fever, photosensitization, Stevens-Johnson syndrome.
2. **Hematotoxicity:** Hemolytic anemia in G6PD deficiency, agranulocytosis, thrombocytopenia, eosinophilia, methemoglobinemia.
3. **Nephrotoxicity:** Hypersensitivity, glomerular damage or obstructive nephropathy secondary to crystalluria.
4. **Kernicterus:** Displacement of bilirubin from albumen; **avoid in last trimester of pregnancy, in neonates, and while nursing.**
5. **Other:** Hepatotoxicity, neurotoxicity, vasculitis, systemic lupus erythematosus–like picture, anorexia, diarrhea, nausea/vomiting.

Drug Interactions:

1. PO anticoagulants: Increased anticoagulant effect.
2. Digoxin: Possible decreased digoxin effect with sulfasalazine.
3. Hypoglycemics, sulfonylurea: Increased hypoglycemic effect.
4. Methotrexate: Possible increased methotrexate effect.
5. Phenytoin: Increased phenytoin effect.
6. Thiopental sodium: Increased pental effect.
7. Methenamine: Increased risk of insoluble urinary precipitate formation.

SULFONYLUREAS

Trade Names:

Acetohexamide: *Dymelor*.
Chlorpropamide: *Chloronase, Diabinese, Glucamide*.
Glyburide: *DiaBeta, Euglucon, Micronase, Glynase*.
Glipizide: *Glucotrol*.
Tolazamide: *Diabewas, Tolinase, Tolamide*.
Tolbutamide: *Orinase*.

Drug Action:

1. **PO hypoglycemic:** Lowers glucose by increasing insulin secretion and action; reduces glucose output from the liver; antidiabetic.
2. **Antidiuretic:** Chlorpropamide (potentiates antidiuretic hormone [ADH] effect).
3. **Uricosuric:** Acetohexamide.
4. **Mild diuretic effect:** Glipizide, glyburide, tolazamide, acetohexamide.

Indications:

1. Hyperglycemia (type II diabetes mellitus).
2. Partial diabetes insipidus (chlorpropamide).

Pharmacokinetics:

1. **Absorption:** PO.
2. **Metabolism:** Hepatic; acetohexamide has active metabolite.
3. **Excretion:** Primarily renal, some biliary.
4. **Hepatic/renal disease:** Reduce dosage.
5. **Crosses placenta:** Acetohexamide.

	Time to Peak Effect (hr)	Half-life (hr)	Duration of Action (hr)
Tolbutamide (PO)	1–3	4–9	6–24
IV	30 min	4–9	3
Glipizide	1–3	2–4	12–24
Tolazamide	4–8	7	12–24
Glyburide	3–4	10	24
Chlorpropamide	3–6	5–16	24–48

Drug Preparations:

Tablets:
Acetohexamide: 250, 500 mg.
Chlorpropamide: 100, 250 mg.
Glipizide: 5, 10 mg.
Glyburide: 1.25, 1.5, 2.5, 3, 5 mg.
Tolazamide: 100, 250, 500 mg.
Tolbutamide: 250, 500 mg tablets; injection 1 g/20 mL

Dosage:

1. **Equivalent dosage:** 1000 mg tolbutamide = 500 mg acetohexamide = 250 mg tolazamide = 250 mg chlorpropamide =
   5 mg glyburide = 5 mg glipizide.
2. **Hyperglycemia (dose of agent should be adjusted on basis
   of dietary intake):**
   a. Acetohexamide: 250–500 mg q day–bid (max. 2 g/day).
   b. Chlorpropamide: 100–250 mg q day–bid.
   c. Glyburide: 1.25–10 mg q day–bid (max. 20 mg/day).
   d. Tolazamide: 100–500 mg q day–bid.
   e. Tolbutamide: 0.5–1.5 g q day–bid PO; IV bolus 1 g over
      2–3 min.
   f. Glipizide: 5–20 mg q day–bid (max. 40 g/day).
3. **Neurogenic diabetes insipidus:**
   a. Chlorpropamide: 125–250 mg/day

Adverse Effects:

1. Hypoglycemia. Symptoms include confusion, agitation,
   headache, nausea, tachycardia, diaphoresis, seizures, coma,
   lethargy.
2. **CNS:** Headache, dizziness, weakness, paresthesias.
3. **GI:** Nausea/vomiting, diarrhea, constipation, heartburn,
   cholestatic jaundice, hepatitis.
4. **Allergic reactions:** skin rash, hives, photosensitivity.
5. **Hematologic:** Leukopenia, agranulocytosis, thrombocytopenia, hemolytic anemia, aplastic anemia.
6. **Chlorpropamide:** Water intoxication, hyponatremia, syndrome of inappropriate secretion of ADH, edema.
7. Failure to control hyperglycemia or prevent ketosis under
   stress.

Drug Interactions:

1. **Decreased hypoglycemic effect:** β-adrenergic blockers, calcium channel blockers, estrogens, ethanol, glucocorticoids,
   isoniazid, nicotinic acid, phenobarbital, phenytoin, rifampin,
   sympathomimetics, thiazides, thyroxine, urinary alkalinizers,
   cholestyramine, diazoxide, charcoal.
2. **Increased hypoglycemic effect:** Anabolic steroids, allopurinol, β-adrenergic blockers, chloramphenicol, H_2 antagonists,

clofibrate, gemfibrozil, coumarin, ethanol, fenfluramine, guanethidine, halofenate, insulin, MAO inhibitors, methyldopa, fluconazole, miconazole, nonsteroidal anti-inflammatory drugs (e.g., phenylbutazone, salicylates), probenecid, ranitidine, sulfinpyrazone, sulfonamides, urinary acidifiers, tricyclic antidepressants.
3. Increased concentrations of PO anticoagulants.
4. Disulfiram-like reaction when combined with ethanol.
5. Increased metabolism of digoxin.

Monitoring:

1. Serum/blood glucose level.
2. Glycosylated hemoglobin.
3. Serum sodium, potassium level.
4. Urine glucose/ketones.

BIBLIOGRAPHY

Kahn CR, Shechter Y: Insulin, oral hypoglycemic agents, and the pharmacology of the endocrine pancreas. In Gilman AG, et al (eds): *Goodman and Gilman's The Pharmacological Basis of Therapeutics,* ed 8, New York, 1993, McGraw-Hill, pp 1463–1495.

Groop LC: Sulfonylureas in NIDDM, *Diabetes Care* 1992, 15: 737–754.

Zaloga GP, Chernow B: Insulin and oral hypoglycemics. In Chernow B (ed): *The Pharmacologic Approach to the Critically Ill Patient,* ed 3, Baltimore, 1994, Williams & Wilkins, pp 758–776.

SUMATRIPTAN SUCCINATE

Trade Name: *Imitrex.*

Drug Actions: Selective agonist for 5-hydroxytryptamine-1 receptors

Indications: Acute migraine attacks (not for basilar or hemiplegic migraine).

Pharmacokinetics:

1. **Absorption:** Give SQ.
2. **Onset of action:** 10 min.
3. **Metabolism:** Converted to inactive indole acetic acid metabolite.
4. **Excretion:** 22% unchanged in urine; remainder as metabolites.
5. **Half-life:** Terminal half-life 115 min.

Drug Preparations:

Injection: 6 mg (12 mg/dL).

Dosage: Subcutaneous 6 mg (may give second injection 1 hr later); max. dose 12 mg in 24 hr; do not give to patients with ischemic heart disease.

Adverse Effects: Transient increase in blood pressure, pain at injection site, hypersensitivity reactions;
common: Chest, jaw, neck tightness, sensations of warmth, cold, tingling, pressure, burning, numbness, tightness, flushing, fatigue, dizziness, drowsiness, weakness, muscle cramps, headache, anxiety;
rare: Coronary vasospasm, angina, myocardial infarction, stroke, seizures, intracranial bleed, arrhythmias, TIAs.

Drug Interactions: Augmented effect: MAO inhibitors, α-adrenergic agonists, ergot drugs (i.e., ergotamine)

Monitoring: Blood pressure, signs of coronary ischemia, signs of cerebrovascular insufficiency.

BIBLIOGRAPHY

Larey LF, Hussey EK, Fowler PA: Single dose pharmacokinetics of sumatriptan in healthy volunteers, *Eur J Clin Pharmacol* 1995, 47:543–548.

Akpunonu BE, Mutgi AB, Federman DJ, et al: Subcutaneous sumatriptan for treatment of acute migraine in patients admitted to the emergency department: a multicenter study, *Ann Emerg Med* 1995, 25:464–469.

Plosker GL, McTavish D: Sumatriptan: a reappraisal of its pharmacology and therapeutic efficacy in the acute treatment of migraine and cluster headache, *Drugs* 1994, 47:622–651.

TEICOPLANIN

Trade Name: *Targocid.*

Drug Actions:

1. Impairs bacterial cell wall synthesis by inhibiting glycopeptide polymerization.
2. Spectrum of activity similar to vancomycin with activity against only gram-positive organisms.

Indications:

1. Effective alternative to vancomycin for treatment of infections caused by gram-positive organisms, including methicillin-resistant *Staphylococcus aureus* (MRSA) and methicillin-resistant coagulase-negative staphylococci in patients who have had allergic reactions or neutropenia with vancomycin.
2. May be used in some vancomycin-resistant enterococci (VRE) infections (more often when the enterococcal strain is VanB phenotype).

Pharmacokinetics:

1. **Absorption:** IM/IV.
2. **Metabolism:** Greater lipophilicity than vancomycin, resulting in better tissue and intracellular penetration.
3. **Excretion:** Renal.
4. **Half-life:** 40–70 hr (protein binding may be as high as 90%).
5. **Therapeutic level:** For treatment of *S. aureus* endocarditis, trough levels of >20 μg/mL are required.

Drug Preparations:

Vials: 200 mg.

Dosage: 400 mg q day (teicoplanin may need to be given in larger dosages, e.g., 10–12 mg/kg/day, to maximize efficacy).

Adverse Effects: Generally well tolerated, but ototoxicity has been reported. Teicoplanin does not appear to cause the dose- or infusion rate–related histamine release associated with vancomycin.

Drug Interactions: Concomitant use of an aminoglycoside may increase the incidence of nephrotoxicity.

BIBLIOGRAPHY

Fekety R: Vancomycin and teicoplanin. In Mandell GL, Bennett JE, Dolin R (eds): *Mandell, Douglas and Bennett's Principles and Practice of Infectious Diseases,* ed 4, New York, 1995, Churchill Livingstone, pp 346–354.

Glew RH: Vancomycin. In Gorbach SL, Bartlett JG, Blacklow NR (eds): *Infectious Diseases,* Philadelphia, 1992, WB Saunders, pp 231–239.

Teicoplanin. In *Drug Facts and Comparisons,* ed 49, New York, 1995, JB Lippincott, p 3220.

TETRACYCLINES

Trade Names: *Achromycin, Sumycin*, generics.

Drug Action:

1. Inhibition of protein synthesis by binding to 30S ribosomal subunits.
2. Spectrum of activity includes wide range of bacteria, rickettsiae, mycoplasmas.

Indications:

1. Ricksettial infections.
2. Chlamydial infections.
3. *Mycoplasma pneumoniae* infections.
4. Acne.
5. Lyme borreliosis.
6. Actinomycosis (alternative to penicillin).
7. Syphilis (alternative to penicillin).
8. Brucellosis (with aminoglycoside).
9. Other: Gonorrhea, nonspecific urethritis, bronchitis, prostatitis.

Pharmacokinetics:

1. **Absorption:** Impaired by polyvalent cations (Ca, Al, Mg, Fe) found in common antacids, milk products, etc.
   a. Best to take in fasting state.

2. **Penetration:** Good into most tissues, including CNS.
3. **Metabolism:** Enterohepatic circulation.
4. **Excretion:** Renal.
5. **Serum half-life:** 8.5 hr.

Drug Preparations:

Capsules: 250, 500 mg.
Suspension: 125 mg/5 mL.
Vials: 100, 250, 500 mg.

Dosage:

1. **Normal renal function:**
   a. **Adult:** 250–500 mg PO q 6 hr, or 125–500 mg IM/IV q 6–12 hr.
   b. **Pediatric:** 6.25–12.5 mg/kg PO q 6 hr, or 2.5–5 mg/kg IM/IV q 6 hr.
2. **Impaired renal function:** Not recommended.

Adverse Effects:

1. Hypersensitivity reactions.
2. **GI:** Nausea/vomiting, diarrhea.
3. Esophageal ulcerations: Take with water 2–3 hr before lying down.
4. Dental damage: Avoid in pregnancy, infants, and children <8 yr.
5. Bone damage: Avoid in pregnancy, children <12 yr.
6. Phototoxicity.
7. Hematotoxicity: Rare but reported, involving all elements.
8. Pseudotumor cerebri–like syndrome: Increased intracranial pressure, headache, meningeal irritation (benign).
9. Nephrotoxicity.
10. Anti-anabolic effects: Accentuated prerenal azotemia by inhibition of protein synthesis.
11. Fanconi's syndrome with outdated drug.
12. Hepatotoxicity with IV drug.

Drug Interactions:

1. PO antacids: Decreased absorption of tetracycline.
2. PO anticoagulants: Increased anticoagulant effect.
3. Bismuth subsalicylate: Decreased tetracycline effect.

4. PO contraceptives: Decreased contraceptive effect.
5. Digoxin: Increased digoxin effect.
6. PO iron: Decreased tetracycline absorption.
7. Lithium: Increased lithium toxicity.
8. Phenformin: Increased lactic acidosis.
9. Zinc sulfate: Decreased tetracycline absorption.

Monitor: Renal function.

THEOPHYLLINE COMPOUNDS

Trade Names:

Theophylline: *Aerolate, Bronkodyl, Constant-T, Elixophyllin, Quibron-T, Slo-bid, Slo-phyllin, Somophyllin-T, Sustaire, Theobid, Theoclear, Theo-Dur, Theolair, Theophyl, Theospan-SR, Theo-24, Theovent, Uniphyl.*

Aminophylline (ethylenediamine salt of theophylline): *Amoline, Phyllocontin, Somophyllin, Truphylline.*

Drug Action:

1. Inhibits phosphodiesterase, elevating cAMP levels.
2. Antagonizes adenosine receptors.
3. Improves intracellular calcium availability.
4. Increases sensitivity of medullary centers to CO_2.
5. Improves diaphragmatic function.
6. Relaxes bronchial smooth muscle.
7. Increases myocardial contractility and rate.
8. Increases gastric secretion, decreases lower esophageal sphincter pressure.
9. Increases renal salt and water excretion.
10. Reduces seizure threshold and brain blood flow.
11. Anti-inflammatory action (impairs white cell function).

Indication: Bronchospasm.

Pharmacokinetics:

1. **Absorption:** Well absorbed from GI tract; rate of absorption depends on specific form. Peak levels occur 1–2 hr after ad-

ministration; sustained-release preparations produce peak levels 5–12 hr after administration
2. **Distribution:** Extracellular fluid.
3. **Therapeutic serum level:** 10–20 μg/mL.
4. **Metabolism:** Liver.
5. **Serum half-life:** 7–9 hr in adults, 4–5 hr in smokers, 3–5 hr in children, 20–30 hr in premature infants. Decreased clearance in heart failure, liver dysfunction, alcoholism, pulmonary edema, chronic obstructive pulmonary disease.
6. **Excretion:** Renal, 10% unchanged in urine.

Drug Preparations:

1. **Theophylline:**

   Capsules: 50, 100, 200, 250 mg.
   Extended release capsules: 50–300 mg.
     Ultra-slow-release preparations
     Theo-24
     Uniphyl
   Elixir: 27, 50 mg/5 mL.
   PO solution: 27, 53 mg/5 mL.
   PO suspension: 100 mg/5 mL.
   Syrup: 27, 50 mg/5 mL.
   Tablets: 100–300 mg.
   Extended-release tablets: 100–500 mg.
2. **Aminophylline** (79% theophylline):

   Injection: 250, 500 mg vials.
   PR suppositories: 250, 500 mg.
   Liquid: 105 mg/5 mL.
   Tablets: 100, 200 mg.
   Controlled-release tablets: 225 mg.

Dosage:

1. **Aminophylline:** IV (mix in D_5W or saline solution):
   a. Loading dose:
      (1) Patients not previously receiving theophylline: 5–6 mg/kg (ideal body weight) IV over 20 min, followed by continuous infusion.

(2) Patients taking theophylline: Theophylline blood level is indicated, and dosage should be based on this level. Give 1 mg/kg IV to increase blood level by 2 μg/mL.

b. Maintenance infusion:
   (1) Young adult smokers: 0.8 mg/kg/hr.
   (2) Healthy nonsmokers: 0.5 mg/kg/hr.
   (3) Patients >60 yr: 0.3 mg/kg/hr.
   (4) Patients with heart failure or liver disease: 0.2 mg/kg/hr.

2. **Theophylline:**
   a. Loading dose:
      (1) Patients not previously receiving theophylline: 5–6 mg/kg (ideal body weight) anhydrous theophylline PO.
      (2) Patients taking theophylline: *See* Aminophylline. Give 1 mg/kg ideal body weight theophylline to increase serum level by 2 μg/mL.
   b. Maintenance dose:
      (1) Young adult smokers: 4 mg/kg q 6 hr PO.
      (2) Healthy nonsmoking adults: 3 mg/kg q 6 hr PO.
      (3) Patients >60 yr: 2 mg/kg q 8 hr PO.
      (4) Patients with heart failure or liver disease: 2 mg/kg q 12 hr PO.

Adverse Effects:

1. **CNS:** Irritability, restlessness, headache, insomnia, dizziness, seizures, depression.
2. **Cardiovascular:** Palpitations, tachycardia, hypotension, arrhythmias.
3. **GI:** Nausea/vomiting, epigastric pain, diarrhea, anorexia, reflux, bleeding.
4. **Other:** Tachypnea, fever, rash, urinary retention, hyperglycemia.

Drug Interactions:

1. Theophylline increases excretion of lithium.
2. Theophylline serum levels increased by cimetidine, allopurinol, propranolol, erythromycin, PO contraceptives, troleandomycin (due to decreased hepatic clearance).
3. Barbiturates, phenytoin, aminoglutethimide, cigarette/marijuana smoking enhances hepatic metabolism.
4. Antagonized by β-adrenergic blockers.

5. Theophylline potentiates effects of sympathomimetics, digitalis, halothane, ketamine.

Monitoring:

1. Serum level (normal 10–20 μg/mL); Theophylline kinetics are variable, both within and between patients. It is essential that theophylline levels be monitored to determine optimal dosage.
2. Vital signs (e.g., heart rate, blood pressure).

Overdose: Empty stomach, activated charcoal.

BIBLIOGRAPHY

Drugs used in bronchial disorders. In *AMA Drug Evaluations,* ed 6, Philadelphia, 1986, WB Saunders, pp 393–418.
Respiratory drugs. In *Drug Facts and Comparisons,* Philadelphia, 1989, JB Lippincott, pp 730–744.

THIAMINE (VITAMIN B₁)

Trade Names: *Betalin, Biamine.*

Drug Actions: Essential coenzyme in carbohydrate metabolism; component of thiamine pyrophosphate.

Indications:

1. Treatment of thiamine deficiency including beriberi, Wernicke's encephalopathy.
2. Alcoholic patients with altered sensorium.

Pharmacokinetics:

1. **Absorption:** Adequate GI absorption; rapid & complete IM.
2. **Onset of action:** 1–2 hr.
3. **Metabolism:** Cellular.
4. **Excretion:** Renal.
5. **Half-life:** Uncertain.
6. **Therapeutic level:** 1.6–4 mg/dL.
7. **Recommended daily allowance:** Adults 1–1.5 mg; children 7–14 yr 1–1.3 mg, 1–7 yr 0.7–1 mg, birth–1 yr 0.3–0.4 mg.

Drug Preparations:

> *Injection:* 100 mg/mL.
> *Tablets:* 20, 50, 100, 250, 500 mg.

Dosage:

1. Thiamine deficiency (beriberi): Adults 5–30 mg IM or IV tid, then PO 5–30 mg/day (single or divided dose) × 1 mo; children 10–25 mg IM or IV daily or 10–50 mg PO daily for 2 wk, then 5–10 mg daily × 1 mo.
2. Wernicke's encephalopathy: Adults 100 mg IV, then 50–100 mg/day IM or IV until consuming complete diet.

Adverse Effects:

1. Cardiovascular collapse, death.
2. Warmth, tingling, rash, angioedema, hypersensitivity reactions.
3. Nausea, vomiting, diarrhea.
4. Restlessness.

Monitoring: Deficiency is best diagnosed by assessing erythrocyte transketolase activity, urine thiamine excretion, or blood pyruvate levels.

BIBLIOGRAPHY

Bortenschlager L, Zaloga GP: Vitamins. In Chernow B (ed): *The Pharmacologic Approach to the Critically Ill Patient,* ed 3, Baltimore, 1994, Williams & Wilkins, pp 805–819.

Marcus R, Couston AM: Water soluble vitamins. In Gilman AG, et al (eds): *The Pharmacological Basis of Therapeutics,* ed 8, New York, 1993, McGraw-Hill, pp 1530–1552.

THIOPENTAL

Trade Name: *Pentothal.*

Drug Action:

1. Barbiturate, hypnotic, anesthetic, direct depressant of reticular activating system, decreases pre- and postsynaptic excitation.
2. Many effects mediated via GABA, receptors.

Indications:

1. General anesthesia.
2. Seizures.
3. Increased intracranial pressure.

Pharmacokinetics:

1. **Absorption:** Do not give enterally; give IV (onset <1 min) or PR (onset 8–10 min).
2. **Distribution:** Total body fluid; lipid soluble, crosses blood-brain barrier; 80% protein bound.
3. **Metabolism:** Liver.
4. **Plasma half-life:** 3–8 hr.
5. **Duration of action:** Depends on tissue redistribution. Usually consciousness returns within 20–30 min after single IV dose. Repeated doses/infusion cause accumulation. Slow release from lipid storage sites results in prolonged anesthesia, somnolence, respiratory depression.

Drug Preparations: Thiopental is supplied as a sterile lyophilized powder in a variety of containers, including multiuse bottles and single-use syringes. It can be reconstituted with sterile water, 0.9% NaCl, or 5% dextrose injections. Clinical concentrations can range from 2% to 5% solutions. Typically, 2.5% (25 mg/mL) solutions are used when inducing general anesthesia. Solutions should be prepared aseptically and unused portions discarded after 24 hr.

1. **General anesthetic:** 2–3 mL 2.5% solution (50–75 mg) IV q 20–40 sec until desired effect reached; give additional 50–100 mg prn.
2. **Anesthesia:**
   a. **Adult:** 2–4 g PR.
   b. **Pediatric:** 1–1.5 g PR.
3. **Induction:**
   a. **Adult:** 3–4 mg/kg IV.
   b. **Pediatric/elderly:** 2–3 mg IV.
4. **Seizures:** 75–125 mg IV.

Adverse Effects:

1. **CNS:** Anxiety, restlessness, retrograde amnesia, somnolence.
2. **Cardiovascular:** Hypotension, tachycardia, myocardial depression, dysrhythmias.

3. **GI:** Nausea/vomiting.
4. **Respiratory:** Respiratory depression, apnea, laryngospasm, bronchospasm.
5. **Local effects:** Pain, swelling, ulceration, vasospasm, gangrene, necrosis.
6. Allergic reactions, shivering.
7. **Contraindications:** Porphyria, status asthmaticus.

Monitoring:

1. Blood pressure, heart rate, respiratory rate.
2. ECG.
3. CNS status.
4. Intracranial pressure.

BIBLIOGRAPHY

Denniston PL Jr (ed): *1995 Physicians GenRx,* Riverside, 1995, Denniston Publishing.
Miller RD (ed): *Anesthesia,* ed 4, New York, 1994, Churchill Livingstone.
Stoelting RK: *Pharmacology and Physiology in Anesthetic Practice,* ed 2, Philadelphia, JB Lippincott.
Gilman AG, Rall TW, Nies AS, Taylor P (eds): *Goodman and Gilman's The Pharmacological Basis of Therapeutics,* ed 8, New York, 1990, Macmillan.

THIORIDAZINE

Trade Name: *Mellaril.*

Drug Action: Antipsychotic effect thought to be caused by blockade of dopamine receptors in the forebrain and basal ganglia.

Indications: Treatment of psychotic symptoms/agitation resulting from a variety of psychiatric or medical illnesses.

Drug Preparations:

Tablets: 10, 15, 25, 50, 100, 200 mg.
Syrup: 10 mg/5 mL.

PO concentrate: 30, 100 mg/mL.
Suspension: 25, 100 mg/5 mL.

Dosage:

1. **Adult:** Initially, 50–100 mg PO q 8 hr; may gradually increase to 800 mg/day.
2. **Elderly/debilitated patients:** One third–one half adult dose.

Pharmacokinetics:

1. **Metabolism:** Hepatic with active metabolites.
2. **Half-life:** Unknown, probably >60 hr.
3. **Excretion:** (?)Renal/hepatic.
4. **Dialyzable:** (?)Limited.
5. **Renal failure:** Reduce dosage.
6. **Hepatic failure:** Use with extreme caution at greatly reduced dosage.

Adverse Effects:

1. Sedation, extrapyramidal reactions (e.g., dystonias, akathisia, parkinsonism), anticholinergic effects (e.g., dry mouth, blurred vision, urinary retention, constipation), orthostatic hypotension.
2. Rarer: allergic, hematologic, neuroendocrine, respiratory, cardiac effects.
3. Neuroleptic malignant syndrome.
4. Tardive dyskinesia.

Drug Interactions:

1. Enhances effects of other CNS depressants.
2. Additive effect with other anticholinergic drugs.
3. Antagonizes antihypertensive effect of guanethidine and other centrally active hypertensives.

Monitoring: Blood levels for routine therapeutic monitoring are currently unavailable.

BIBLIOGRAPHY

Antipsychotic drugs. In *AMA Drug Evaluations,* ed 6, Philadelphia, 1986, WB Saunders, pp 111–130.
Antipsychotic drugs. In Schatzberg A, Cole J: *Manual of Clinical Psychopharmacology,* Washington, 1986, American Psychiatric Press, pp 67–106.

THIOTHIXENE

Trade Name: *Navane.*

Drug Action: Antipsychotic effect thought to be caused by blockade of dopamine receptors in the forebrain and basal ganglia.

Indications: Treatment of psychotic symptoms/agitation resulting from a variety of psychiatric or medical illnesses.

Drug Preparations:

Capsules: 1, 2, 5, 10, 20 mg.
Solution: 2.5 mg/mL.
Injection: 2, 5, mg/mL.

Dosage:

1. **Acute active psychosis: Adult:** 4 mg IM bid–qid until symptoms are controlled.
2. **Adult:** Initially 2–5 mg PO bid–tid in divided doses; optimal dose 20–30 mg/day.
3. **Elderly/debilitated patients:** One third–one half adult dose.

Pharmacokinetics:

1. **Metabolism:** (?)Hepatic.
2. **Half-life:** ?
3. **Excretion:** (?)Renal/hepatic.
4. **Dialyzable?:** Limited.
5. **Renal failure:** Reduce dosage.
6. **Hepatic failure:** Use with extreme caution at reduced dosage.

Adverse Effects:

1. Sedation, extrapyramidal reactions (e.g., dystonias, akathisia, parkinsonism), anticholinergic effects (e.g., dry mouth, blurred vision, urinary retention, constipation), orthostatic hypotension.
2. Rarer: allergic, hematologic, neuroendocrine, respiratory, cardiac effects.
3. Neuroleptic malignant syndrome.
4. Tardive dyskinesia.

Drug Interactions:

1. Enhances effects of other CNS depressants.
2. Additive effect with other anticholinergic drugs.
3. Antagonizes antihypertensive effect of guanethidine.

Monitoring: Blood levels for routine therapeutic monitoring are currently unavailable.

BIBLIOGRAPHY

Antipsychotic drugs. In *AMA Drug Evaluations,* ed 6, Philadelphia, 1986, WB Saunders, pp 111–130.

Antipsychotic drugs. In Schatzberg A, Cole J: *Manual of Clinical Psychopharmacology,* Washington, 1986, American Psychiatric Press, pp 67–106.

THROMBOLYTICS

Trade Names:

Recombinant tissue plasminogen activator (rtPA): Altephase: *Activase.*

Streptokinase (SK): *Kabikinase, Streptase.*

Urokinase (UK): *Abbokinase, Abbokinase Open-Cath.*

Drug Action: Thrombolytic agents dissolve existing thrombi. They act directly/indirectly as endogenous plasminogen activators, converting plasminogen to proteolytic enzyme plasmin (Fig. 2). Plasmin dissolves clot by degrading fibrinogen and fibrin clot.

NOTE: rtPA has greater affinity for fibrin-bound plasminogen than for plasma plasminogen and is less likely to induce a generalized "lytic" state.

Indications: Dissolution of existing thrombi in several clinical settings.

1. Treatment of pulmonary emboli.
2. Acute myocardial infarction.
3. Deep venous thrombosis.
4. Peripheral artery thrombosis.
5. Occlusion of arteriovenous catheters.

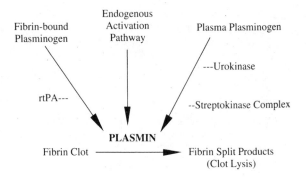

FIG 2.
Action of thrombolytic agents.

Pharmacokinetics: *See* Table 21.

Dosage:

1. **Streptokinase:**
   a. **Preparation:** 250,000, 600,000, 750,000 IU vials. Reconstitute powder with isotonic sodium chloride or D_5 W. **Avoid shaking,** which causes foaming and flocculation.
   b. **Lysis of coronary artery thrombi.**
      (1) **Selective coronary arterial infusion:** Bolus with 20,000 IU, followed by maintenance infusion of 2000 IU/min ×60 min.
      (2) **IV infusion:** 750,000 IU given as 10-min load; remainder of 1–1.5 million IV infused over following 60 min.
   c. **Deep vein thrombosis/pulmonary emboli:**
      (1) **Loading dose:** 250,000 IU IV over 30 min.
      (2) **Maintenance infusion:** 100,000 IU/hr for up to 24–72 hr as dictated by clinical response.
   d. **Arteriovenous catheter occlusion:**
      (1) 250,000 IU in 2 mL solution; fill catheter for 2 hr, remove, flush with saline solution.
2. **Urokinase:**
   a. **Preparation:** 5000 IU/mL and 250,000 IU vials. May be reconstituted only with sterile water for injection, USP, with-

TABLE 21.

Pharmacokinetics

	Streptokinase	Urokinase	rtPA
Molecular weight (daltons)	47,000	34,500–54,000	63,000–65,000
Half-life (min)			
Initial	13–23	16	5–8
Terminal	83	Prolonged in liver failure	39–53 Prolonged in liver failure
Metabolism	Unknown	Liver	Liver
Generalized proteolytic state	+4	+3	+1/+2
Activity acceleration*	6×	10×	1,400×
Bleeding complications	+4	+4	+4
Allergic potential	+3	0/+1	0
Source	Group C β-hemolytic streptococci	Embryonic human kidney cells	Recombinant DNA technology
Relative cost	+1	+3	+4
Stability after reconstitution	24 hr at 2°–4°C	<24 hr at 2°–4°C	8 hr

*Increase in activity over baseline.

out preservatives. **Avoid shaking,** which will cause filament formation.
   b. **Lysis of coronary artery thrombi:**
      (1) **Selective coronary arterial infusion:** 6000 IU/min for up to 2 hr. Average dose to achieve lysis 500,000 IU.
   c. **Pulmonary emboli:**
      (1) **Loading dose:** 4400 IU/kg IV over 10 min.
      (2) **Maintenance infusion:** 4400 IU/kg/hr for 12 hr.
   d. **Catheter clearance:**
      (1) Urokinase in final concentration of 5000 IU/mL is prepared and injected via tuberculin syringe in a volume equal to catheter "dead space."
3. **rtPA:**
   a. **Preparation:** 20, 50 mg vials. May be reconstituted only with sterile water for injection, USP, without preservatives. May be administered as reconstituted at 1.0 mg/mL. Slight foaming is not unusual. Use within 8 hr of reconstitution.

b. **Lysis of coronary artery thrombi:**
  (1) IV rtPA appears to have equal efficacy as intracoronary streptokinase. Total dose 100 mg is administered: 60 mg in first hour (of which 10 mg is given as bolus over 2 min), 20 mg in second hour, 20 mg in third hour.
c. **Pulmonary emboli:**
  (1) IV infusion of up to 90 mg is as effective as infusion directly into pulmonary artery; 50 mg rtPA is given over 2 hr, followed by additional 40 mg over next 4 hr.

NOTE: Dosage and protocols for administration of all thrombolytics are under intense investigation and review to minimize hemorrhagic complications. Consult individual institutional protocols or most recent literature information to administer these drugs in compliance with accepted, current standards.

Adverse Effects:

1. **Hemorrhage:** Serious bleeding is the most common complication of thrombolytic therapy and occurs with a frequency of approximately 5%. Oozing and hematoma formation at sites of minor recent trauma (e.g., venipuncture) are increased.
2. Contraindications to initiation of therapy may be absolute or relative:
   a. **Absolute contraindications:**
     (1) Active ongoing bleeding.
     (2) Stroke or intracranial/intraspinal surgery within 2 mo.
     (3) Intracranial neoplasm.
   b. **Relative contraindications:**
     (1) Major surgery/biopsy within 10 days.
     (2) GI bleeding/biopsy within 10 days.
     (3) Recent trauma/CPR.
     (4) Pregnancy/postpartum state.
     (5) Diabetic retinopathy.
     (6) Uncontrolled arterial hypertension.
     (7) Severe hepatic/renal disease.
     (8) Active malignancy.

Overall status and condition of the patient must be assessed carefully before initiating therapy.

2. **Allergic reactions:** Most common with streptokinase; include anaphylaxis, rash, fever.

3. **Arrhythmias:** Rapid lysis of coronary thrombi frequently causes reperfusion-induced ventricular dysrhythmias.

Drug Interactions:

1. Increased risk of severe bleeding with concomitant administration of heparin, warfarin, antiplatelet drugs (aspirin).
2. Inhibited by aminocaproic acid (incomplete).

Monitoring:

1. Full battery of coagulation tests (fibrinogen, fibrin, degradation products, PT, PTT, thrombin time [TT]) plus hematocrit should be performed before initiation of therapy. During thrombolytic drug infusion, decreases in plasminogen and fibrinogen levels and increase in concentration of fibrin degradation products are expected. TT performed 3–4 hr after initiation of infusion should confirm existence of a lytic state. Degree of prolongation of TT does not predict fibrinolytic efficacy or risk of bleeding.
2. ECG for arrhythmias; blood pressure, heart rate, bleeding tendency.

Drug Reversal: Serious bleeding mandates immediate cessation of therapy and direct pressure where applicable. Use of fresh-frozen plasma or cryoprecipitate may be required to restore circulating fibrinogen levels. In extreme circumstances, epsilon-aminocaproic acid (Amicar) may be considered, although no proved protocol exists for such administration. Amicar is an antifibrinolytic agent and should inhibit any further effect on the hemostatic plug.

BIBLIOGRAPHY

Eisenberg PR, Jaffe AS: Thrombolytic therapy. In Chernow B (ed): *The Pharmacologic Approach to the Critically Ill Patient,* ed 2, Baltimore, 1988, Williams & Wilkins, pp 287–301.

Hirsh J, Cairns JA: Antithrombotic therapy in acute myocardial infarction and unstable angina, *J Intensive Care Med* 1987, 2:299–312.

Loscalzo J, Braunwald E: Tissue plasminogen activator, *N Engl J Med* 1988, 319:925–931.

Marder VJ, Sherry S: Thrombolytic therapy: current status. Part I, *N Engl J Med* 1988, 318:1512–1520.

Marder VJ, Sherry S: Thrombolytic therapy: current status. Part II, *N Engl J Med* 1988, 318:1585–1595.

O'Reilly R: Anticoagulant, antithrombotic, and thrombolytic drugs. In Gilman AG, Goodman LS, Rall TW, et al (eds): *The Pharmacologic Basis of Therapeutics,* ed 7, New York, 1985, Macmillan, pp 1338–1359.

THYROID HORMONE

Trade Names:

Levothyroxine (T_4): *Synthroid, Levoxine, Levothroid.*

Liothyronine (T_3): *Cytomel, Triostat.*

Desiccated thyroid (contains both T_4 and T_3; amounts vary between preparations): *Armour Thyroid, Dathroid, Delcoid, S-P-T, Thyrar.*

Drug Action: Thyroid hormone synthesis and release are regulated by thyroid-stimulating hormone (TSH) secreted from the anterior pituitary. TSH secretion is controlled by hypothalamic release of thyrotropin-releasing hormone (TRH). Thyroid hormone (principally T_3) acts by binding to intracellular (nuclear) receptors, where it alters genetic expression. Thyroid hormone affects RNA and protein synthesis, enzyme activity, cell differentiation, growth, metabolic rate, cardiac contraction, and numerous other functions in all cells of the body.

Indications: Hypothyroidism, suppression of nontoxic goiter nodules.

Pharmacokinetics:

1. **Absorption:** Small bowel; T_4 is 50%–80% absorbed, T_3 95% absorbed.
2. **Metabolism:** Monodeiodination in peripheral tissues, liver, kidneys, Gi tract.
3. **Excretion:** Feces, 20% T_4.

4. **Volume of distribution:** T_4 10 L (primarily extracellular); T_3 38 L.
5. **Metabolic clearance rate:** T_4 1.1 L/day; T_3, 21 L/day.
6. **Serum half-life:** T_4 6–7 days; T_3 1–2 days.
7. **Serum concentration:** T_4 5–11.5 µg/dL; T_3 80–190 ng/dL.

Drug Preparations:

1. **T_4:**

   Tablets: 25, 50, 75, 88, 100, 112, 125, 137, 150, 175, 200, 300 µg.

   Vials: 200, 500 µg for IV use.

2. **T_3:**

   Tablets: 5, 25, 50 µg. Injection: 10 µg/mL (1 mL).

3. **Desiccated thyroid:** (Beef/pork)

   Tablets: 15, 30, 60, 90, 120, 180, 240, 300 mg.

   NOTE: 25 µg T_3 = 100 µg T_4 = 65 mg desiccated thyroid.

Dosage:

1. **Mild hypothyroidism**
   a. **T_4:**
      (1) **Adult:** Initially 50 µg/day PO; increase by 25–50 µg/day q 2–4 wk until desired response achieved. Average maintenance dose 100–150 µg/day.
      (2) **Elderly/patients with cardiac disease:** Begin with 25 µg/day PO; increase by 25 µg/day q 3–4 wk.
      (3) **Pediatric:**
         (a) **0–6 mo:** Initially 25–50 µg/day PO (8–10 µg/kg).
         (b) **6–12 mo:** 50–75 µg/day PO.
         (c) **>1 yr:** 75–100 µg/day PO.

   Reduce dose by 20%–50% when administering IV.
   b. **T_3:**
      (1) **Adult:** Initially 25 µg/day PO; increase by 12.5–25 µg/day q 1–2 wk until desired response reached. Maximum 100 µg/day.
      (2) **Elderly/patients with cardiac disease:** Begin with 2.5–5 µg/day PO; increase by 2.5–5 µg/day q 2–3 wk. Usual maintenance dose 50–100 µg/day; may be given in divided doses bid–tid.

    (3) Congenital hypothyroidism: 5 μg/day PO, increase by 5 μg/day every 3 days. Usual dose 20 μg/day for infants, 50 μg/day for children 1–3 yr.

  c. **Thyroid extract:**

    (1) **Adult:** Initially 30–60 mg/day PO; increase by 30–60 mg/day q 3–4 wk until desired response reached. Usual maintenance dose 60–180 mg/day.

    (2) **Elderly/patients with underlying cardiac disease:** Begin with 15 mg/day PO; increase by 15–30 mg/day q 3–4 wk.

2. **Severe hypothyroidism** (myxedema):

  a. T_4 **Adult:** Initially 12.5–25 μg/day PO; increase by 25–50 μg/day q 2–4 wk, IV or IM: Reduce dose by 20%–50%.

  b. T_3: Initially 5 μg/day PO; increase by 5–10 μg/day q 1–2 wk.

3. Myxedema coma:

  a. T_4: 200–500 μg IV bolus once. Maintenance 50–200 μg/day.

  b. T_3: May add to T_4 if inadequate peripheral conversion of T_4 to T_3 is suspected, in doses of 10–100 μg/day IV.

Adverse Reactions:

1. **CNS:** Nervousness, tremor, insomnia, headache, psychosis, seizures.

2. **Cardiovascular:** Palpitations, tachycardia, hypertension, chest pain, myocardial infarction, arrhythmias.

3. **GI:** Nausea, vomiting, anorexia, weight loss, diarrhea, abdominal cramps.

4. **General:** Diaphoresis, heat intolerance, fever, increased appetite, bone loss, muscle aches, hair loss, shortness of breath, hypoglycemia.

5. **Allergy** to beef/pork in thyroid extract/base (ie.., tartrazine) in T_4/T_3.

6. **Adrenal insufficiency:** Use with caution. Thyroid hormone increases need for glucocorticoids and may precipitate adrenal insufficiency.

7. **Elderly/patients with cardiac disease:** Use with caution; may precipitate ischemia.

Drug Interactions:

1. Potentiates effect of anticoagulants, tricyclic antidepressants, sympathomimetics.
2. Increased need for insulin, PO hypoglycemics, digitalis (metabolism increased).
3. Estrogens raise binding proteins and increase need for thyroid hormone.
4. Phenytoin (and other hepatic enzyme inducers) stimulates metabolism of thyroid hormones.
5. Cholestyramine and colestipol bind thyroid hormones in the gut and decrease absorption.
6. Salicylates displace T_4 and T_3 from protein binding sites.

Monitoring:

1. Heart rate, blood pressure.
2. Serum levels of TSH, T_4, T_3 (use minimum amount required to suppress TSH).
3. Estrogens (and some diseases) increase binding proteins and total T_4 and T_4 levels; may need to measure free (unbound) hormones.

Treatment of Overdosage:

1. **Chronic, non–life-threatening:** Reduce dosage.
2. **Acute massive overdose:** Reduce GI absorption (e.g., gastric lavage, activated charcoal). β-Adrenergic blockers can blunt sympathetic effects. Prophylthiouracil and glucocorticoids can decrease T_4 to T_3 conversion. Control fever, hypoglycemia, fluid loss.

BIBLIOGRAPHY

Burman KD: Thyroid hormones. In Chernow B (ed): *The Pharmacologic Approach to the Critically Ill Patient,* ed 3, Baltimore, 1994, Williams & Wilkins, pp 741–757.

Haynes RC: Thyroid and antithyroid drugs. In Gilman AG, et al (eds): *The Pharmacological Basis of Therapeutics,* ed 8, New York, 1993, McGraw-Hill, pp 1361–1383.

Roti E, Minelli R, Gardini E, Braverman LE: The use and misuse of thyroid hormone, *Endocr Rev* 1993, 14:401–423.

TICARCILLIN

Trade Name: *Ticar.*

Drug Action:

1. Inhibition of cell wall synthesis (penicillin).
2. Spectrum of activity includes non–β-lactamase-producing gram-positive aerobes (streptococci but not staphylococci), most gram-negative aerobes (including *Pseudomonas aeruginosa* but not *Klebsiella*), and anaerobes (including *Bacteroides fragilis*).

Indications: Infections caused by susceptible organisms, particularly those involving *P. aeruginosa* (synergistic with aminoglycosides) and mixed aerobes/anaerobes.

Pharmacokinetics:

1. **Absorption:** IM/IV.
2. **Excretion:** Renal.
3. **Disodium salt:** 5.2 mEq sodium/g.
4. **Serum half-life:** 70 min.

Drug Preparations:

   Vials: 1, 3, 6 g for parenteral use.

Dosage:

1. **Normal renal function: Adults,** 200–300 mg/kg/day IV/IM in divided doses q 4–6 hr (3 g q 4–6 hr); **children,** 37.5–50 mg/kg q 4–6 hr IV/IM.
2. **Impaired renal function:**

Dose (g)	Creatinine Clearance	Interval (hr)
3	>80	4–6
3	80–50	4–6
2–3	50–10	6–8
2	<10 (anuria)	12

3. **Dialysis:**
   a. **Hemodialysis:** Supplemental dose of 3 g after each dialysis.
   b. **Peritoneal:** 3 g q 12 hr IV/IM.

Adverse Effects:

1. Similar to penicillin, including hypersensitivity reactions, GI problems (e.g., nausea/vomiting, diarrhea), cytopenias, neurotoxicity, interstitial nephritis.
2. Sodium overload, hypokalemia.
3. Qualitative platelet defect, bleeding.

Drug Interactions: Aminoglycoside inactivation by ticarcillin if administered in same bottle.

Monitoring: Serial bleeding times in patients at risk; potassium, sodium levels; neurologic status; blood cell counts.

TICARCILLIN AND CLAVULANIC ACID

Trade Name: *Timentin.*

Drug Action:

1. Ticarcillin inhibits cell wall synthesis; clavulanic acid acts as β-lactamase inhibitor.
2. Spectrum of activity includes gram-positive aerobes (including staphylococci because of clavulanic acid), most gram-negative aerobes (including *Pseudomonas aeruginosa*), and anaerobes (including *Bacteroides fragilis*).

Indications: Infections caused by susceptible organisms, especially involving *P. aeruginosa.*

Pharmacokinetics: Similar to ticarcillin.

Drug Preparations:

Vials: 3.1 g vial for parenteral use, containing 3 g ticarcillin disodium and 0.1 g clavulanate potassium. 3.2 g, containing twice the clavulanate component.

Dosage:

1. **Normal renal function:** 3.1 g q 4–6 hr IV.

2. **Impaired renal function:**

Dose (g)	Creatinine Clearance	Interval (hr)
3.1	>60	4
2	60–30	4
2	30–10	8
2	<10	12

3. **Hepatic dysfunction:** 2 g q 24 hr.
4. **Dialysis:**
   a. **Peritoneal:** 3.1 g q 12 hr.
   b. **Hemodialysis:** 2 g q 12 hr, supplemented with 3.1 g after each dialysis.

Adverse Effects:

1. Same as with ticarcillin.
2. False-positive Coombs test secondary to clavulanate component.

TICLOPIDINE

Trade Name: *Ticlid.*

Drug Actions: Inhibitor of platelet function, prolongs bleeding time.

Indications: Prevent thrombosis (stroke, aortocoronary bypass grafts, deep venous thrombosis).

Pharmacokinetics:

1. **Absorption:** PO.
2. **Onset of action:** Within 6 hr, peak effect 3–5 days.
3. **Metabolism:** Liver.
4. **Half-life:** 24 hr.

Drug Preparations:

   Tablets: 250 mg.

Dosage:

Adult: 250 mg PO bid.

Adverse Effects:

1. Hypersensitivity reactions, rash.
2. Bleeding, epistaxis.
3. Diarrhea, nausea/vomiting, GI upset, hepatic injury.
4. Neutropenia, thrombocytopenia.
5. Tinnitus.

Drug Interactions:

1. Synergistic effect on platelet function and prolongation of bleeding time when used with other antiplatelet agents or anti-coagulants.
2. Decreased effect with antacids, corticosteroids.
3. Decreased effect of digoxin, cyclosporine.
4. Increased effect of NSAIDs, cimetidine, theophylline, antipyrine, anticoagulants, aspirin.

Monitoring: Clinical response, bleeding.

BIBLIOGRAPHY

Schror K: Antiplatelet drugs. A comparative review, *Drugs* 1995, 50:7–28.
Desager JP: Clinical pharmacokinetics of ticlopidine, *Clin Pharmacokinet* 1994, 26:347–355.

TOBRAMYCIN

Trade Name: *Nebcin.*

Drug Action:

1. Inhibition of protein synthesis through binding to 30S ribosomal subunits (aminoglycosides).
2. Spectrum of activity includes staphylococci (but not streptococci, including pneumococci), enterococci (with penicillin or vancomycin), most gram-negative aerobes (especially *Pseudomonas aeruginosa*), and **no** anaerobes.

Indications:

1. Infections caused by susceptible organisms, especially involving *P. aeruginosa,* usually in combination with an antipseudomonal penicillin such as ticarcillin.
2. Effective against *Escherichia coli, Proteus, Klebsiella, Enterobacter, Serratia, Staphylococcus aureus, Citrobacter.*

Pharmacokinetics:

1. **Absorption:** IV/IM.
2. **Excretion:** Renal.
3. **Penetration:** Poor into CSF.
4. **Serum half-life:** 2–2.75 hr.

Drug Preparations:

Vials: 80 mg/2 mL, 20 mg/2 mL.
Syringes: 60 mg/1.5 mL.

Dosage:

1. **Normal renal function:**
   a. **Adults:** 1–1.7 mg/kg q 8 hr IV/IM.
   b. **Pediatric:** 2–2.5 mg/kg q 8 hr.
2. **Impaired renal function:**

Dose (mg/kg)	Creatinine Clearance	Interval (hr)
1.5	>80	8
	80–50	8–12
	50–10	12–24
	<10 (anuria)	24–48

3. **Dialysis:**
   a. **Hemodialysis:** Supplemental dose of 1 mg/kg after each dialysis.
   b. **Peritoneal:** 1 mg/2 L of dialysate removed.

Adverse Effects: Similar to other aminoglycosides.

1. Nephrotoxicity: Proximal tubular necrosis.
2. Ototoxicity.
3. Neuromuscular blocking effect.

Drug Interactions:

1. Amphotericin B: Increased nephrotoxicity.
2. Loop diuretics: Increased ototoxicity.
3. Antipseudomonal penicillins: Aminoglycoside inactivation.
4. Cephalosporins (cephalothin): Increased nephrotoxicity.
5. Potentiates neuromuscular blocking effect of neuromuscular blocking agents.

Monitoring:

1. Serial serum levels: Peak 5–12 μg/mL, trough <1–2 μg/mL.
2. Serial renal function studies.
3. Serial clinical monitoring (signs and symptoms: e.g., tinnitus, dizziness, vertigo) and audiometry (early loss of high frequency), for ototoxicity.

TOCAINIDE

Trade Name: *Tonocard.*

Drug Actions: Amine analog of lidocaine, class IB antiarrhythmic, decreases Na and K conductance across membranes, decreasing excitability of myocardial cells

Indications: Ventricular arrhythmias.

Pharmacokinetics:

1. **Absorption:** PO, 100% bioavailable.
2. **Onset of action:** Peak levels 0.5–2 hr.
3. **Metabolism:** Hepatic.
4. **Excretion:** 40% unchanged in urine.
5. **Half-life:** 15 hr.
6. **Therapeutic level:** 4–10 μg/mL.

Drug Preparations:

  Tablets: 400, 600 mg.

Dosage: Individualize dose, initial dose: 400 mg q 8 hr PO (decrease for hepatic and renal impairment).

Adverse Effects:

1. *Blood dyscrasias:* Agranulocytous, bone marrow depression, leukopenia, neutropenia, aplastic/hypoplastic anemia, thrombocytopenia.
2. *Pulmonary:* fibrosis: Interstitial pneumonitis, pulmonary edema. *cardiac:* decrease in cardiac contraction (may aggravate heart failure), may increase mortality when used long term; may increase arrhythmias in some patients, may accelerate ventricular rate in patients with A fib/flutter Hypotension, bradycardia, palpitations, conduction disorders; rash; contraindications: Hypersensitivity, second-, third-degree AV block (without pacemaker); *GI:* hepatic toxicity, nausea/vomiting (8%), anorexia, diarrhea; *CNS:* Seizures, obtundation/coma, dizziness, vertigo (15%—most common), agitation, tremor, paresthesia, fatigue, blurred vision, tinnitus, confusion, disorientation, hallucinations, anxiety, ataxia.

Drug Interactions: Additive effects on heart with β-blockers.

Monitoring: Blood counts (including WBC, plt), pulmonary status, clinical and ECG response

BIBLIOGRAPHY

Lucas WJ, Maccioli GA, Mueller RA: Advances in oral anti-arrhythmic therapy—implications for the anesthetist, *Can J Anaesth* 1990, 37:94–101.
Snyder DW: Class IB antiarrhythmic drugs: tocainide, mexiletine, and moricizine, *J La State Med Soc* 1989, 141:21–25.

TORSEMIDE

Trade Name: *Demadex.*

Drug Actions: Inhibits sodium and chloride reabsorption in thick ascending limb of loop of Henle by blocking the chloride site of the Na-K-2Cl cotransporter.

Indications:

1. Edema: Congestive heart failure, cirrhosis, nephrotic syndrome.
2. Pulmonary edema.
3. Hypertension, usually in combination with other agents; not considered a first-line agent in essential hypertension.

Pharmacokinetics:

1. **Absorption:** Rapid with peak serum level reached in 1 hr.
2. **Onset of action:** IV, 10 min; PO, 60 min.
3. **Metabolism:** Hepatic via P-450 system.
4. **Excretion:** 70%–80% excreted in urine.
5. **Half-life:** 210 min (longer than other loop diuretics).

Drug Preparations:

Tablets: 5, 10, 20, 100 mg.
Injection: 10 mg/mL in 2 and 5 mL ampules.

Dosage: Diuretic IV 10–20 mg once daily. Dose may be titrated upward, but single doses >200 mg have not been adequately studied. Diuretic PO: same dose as IV because of high bioavailability. Hypertension: 5 mg once daily. May be increased to 10 mg daily if blood pressure not controlled within 4 wk.

Adverse Effects: Hypotension, dizziness, headache (7.3%), hypokalemia (2%–4%), hyponatremia, hyperuricemia, nausea, diarrhea, constipation. No known reports of ototoxicity or effects on serum glucose or lipid levels.

Drug Interactions: Concurrent NSAID administration may reduce the diuretic and natriuretic effects of torsemide.

Monitoring: Blood pressure, serum electrolytes, BUN, creatinine, hearing examinations.

BIBLIOGRAPHY

Diuretics and cardiovasculars. In *Drug Facts and Comparisons,* New York, 1995, JB Lippincott, pp 607–615.
Torsemide. In *Micromedex Drug Evaluation Monographs,* 1996, Micromedex.

Fowler SF, Murray KM: Torsemide—a new loop diuretic. Am J
Health-System Pharmacy 1995, 52:1771–1780.

TRIFLUOPERAZINE

Trade Name: *Stelazine.*

Drug Action: Antipsychotic effect is thought to be caused by
blockade of dopamine receptors in forebrain and basal ganglia.

Indications: Treatment of psychotic symptoms/agitation resulting from a variety of psychiatric or medical illnesses.

Drug Preparations:

> *Tablets:* 1, 2, 5, 10 mg.
> *PO concentrate:* 10 mg/mL.
> *Injection:* 2 mg/mL.

Dosage:

1. **Acute psychosis:**
   a. **Adult:** 1–2 mg IM q 4–6 hr prn (total daily dose about 6
      mg) or 2–4 mg PO bid; may gradually increase to 10
      mg/day.
   b. **Elderly/debilitated patients:** One third–one half adult
      dose.

Pharmacokinetics:

1. **Metabolism:** Hepatic, with active metabolites.
2. **Half-life:** Probably >60 hr.
3. **Excretion:** (?)Hepatic, renal.
4. **Dialyzable?:** Limited.
5. **Renal failure:** Reduce dosage.
6. **Hepatic failure:** Use with extreme caution at greatly reduced
   dosage.

Adverse Effects:

1. Sedation, extrapyramidal reactions (e.g., dystonias, akathisia,
   parkinsonism), anticholinergic effects (e.g., dry mouth, blurred

vision, urinary retention, constipation), orthostatic hypotension.
2. Rarer: Allergic, hematologic, neuroendocrine, respiratory, cardiac effects.
3. Neuroleptic malignant syndrome.
4. Tardive dyskinesia.

Drug Interactions:

1. Enhances effects of other CNS depressants.
2. Additive effect with other anticholinergic drugs.
3. Antagonizes antihypertensive effect of guanethidine and other centrally active antihypertensives.

Monitoring: Blood levels for routine therapeutic monitoring are currently unavailable.

BIBLIOGRAPHY

Antipsychotic drugs. In *AMA Drug Evaluations,* ed 6, Philadelphia, 1986, WB Saunders, pp 111–130.
Antipsychotic drugs. In Schatzberg A, Cole J: *Manual of Clinical Psychopharmacology,* Washington, 1986, American Psychiatric Press, pp 67–106.

TRIMETHAPHAN

Trade Name: *Arfonad.*

Drug Action:

1. Autonomic ganglionic blockade. Decreased blood pressure and increased heart rate with no change in serum catecholamine levels or renin levels.
2. Direct peripheral vasodilation.
3. Histamine release.

Indications:

1. Treatment of hypertensive crisis.
2. Management of autonomic hyperreflexia.
3. Use in induced hypotension.

4. Use in dissecting aortic aneurysm. Trimethaphan leads to decreased blood pressure and decreased left ventricle wall tension, which produces less stress on the aortic wall during ejection.
5. Treatment of hypertension in patients with increased intracranial pressure (ICP). Trimethaphan has quaternary ammonia group, which does not allow the compound to penetrate the CNS. This would allow lowering of systemic blood pressure, decreasing cerebral blood flow without increasing ICP.

Pharmacokinetics:

1. **Metabolism:** Probably metabolized by plasma cholinesterases.
2. **Excretion:** Kidneys.
3. **Plasma half-life:** Minutes; clinical effect lasts longer.
4. **Onset time:** Almost immediate.

Drug Preparations:

Ampules: 500 mg/10 mL.

Dosage: 500 mg/500 mL =1 mg/mL solution. Dose range 0.3–6 mg/min. Start at 0.3 mg/min and titrate infusion rate to effect.

Adverse Effects:

1. Marked hypotension, tachycardia.
2. Constipation, nausea/vomiting.
3. Paralytic ileus.
4. Urinary retention.
5. Cycloplegia.
6. Reduction in cerebral blood flow while cerebral metabolic rate remains unchanged.
7. Weakness, respiratory distress.

Drug Interactions:

1. Enhanced hypotensive effects with antihypertensive agents.
2. By binding to plasma cholinesterases, may prolong neuromuscular blocking agents, e.g., succinylcholine.

Monitoring:

1. Hypotension.
2. Beware of tachyphylaxis.

BIBLIOGRAPHY

Stoelting RK: Peripheral vasodilators. In *Pharmacology and Physiology in Anesthetic Practice,* Philadelphia, 1987, JB Lippincott, pp 311–317.

Taylor P: Ganglionic stimulating and blocking agents. In Gilman AG, Goodman LS, Gilman A (eds): *The Pharmacological Basis of Therapeutics,* ed 6, New York, 1980, Macmillan, pp 215–217.

TRIMETHOPRIM

Trade Names: *Proloprim, Trimpex,* generics.

Drug Actions:

1. Trimethoprim binds to and reversibly inhibits dihydrofolate reductase, preventing reduction of dihydrofolate to tetrahydrofolate (which interferes with microbial folic acid synthesis and, ultimately, bacterial nucleotide production—humans do not synthesize folic acid but require it in their diet).
2. Spectrum of activity: Some gram-positive cocci (namely coagulase-negative staphylococci, including *Staphylococcus saprophyticus*) and most gram-negative rods (but not *Pseudomonas aeruginosa* and *Bacteroides* spp.). Trimethoprim (with dapsone) can be used to treat *Pneumocystis carinii* pneumonia.

Indications:

1. Uncomplicated urinary tract infections.
2. Prophylaxis of uncomplicated urinary tract infections.
3. *P. carinii* pneumonia: Trimethoprim plus dapsone can be used as an alternative to trimethoprim/sulfamethoxazole in AIDS patients allergic/intolerant to sulfa drugs. (There is, however, an approximately 50% cross-reactivity between sulfa drugs and dapsone, which is a sulfone.)

Pharmacokinetics:

1. **Absorption:** PO.
2. **Metabolism:** 10%–20% is metabolized (primarily in the liver); the remainder is excreted unchanged in the urine.

3. **Half-life:** 8–10 hr (half-life is increased with severely impaired renal function).

Drug Preparations:

Tablets: 100, 200 mg.

Dosage:

100 mg PO bid.

For *P. carinii* treatment: 20 mg/kg/day divided q 6 hr (and used with dapsone).

Adverse Effects:

1. Rash (usually pruritic) occurs in 2.9%–6.7%.
2. Trimethoprim competes with creatinine for renal tubular secretion, with a resultant decrease in clearance and increase in serum creatinine (reversible).

Drug Interactions: Inhibits hepatic metabolism of phenytoin (increasing phenytoin half-life by 51% and decreasing phenytoin clearance rate by 30%).

BIBLIOGRAPHY

Physicians' Desk Reference, ed 50, Montvale, 1996, Medical Economics Co.
Sanford JP, Gilbert DN, Sande MA (eds): *The Sanford Guide to Antimicrobial Therapy,* ed 26, Dallas, 1996, Antimicrobial Therapy.

TRIMETHOPRIM AND SULFAMETHOXAZOLE

Trade Names: *Bactrim, Septra, Cotrimoxazole,* generics.

Drug Action:

1. Blockage of two consecutive steps in biosynthesis of nucleic acids and proteins essential to many organisms:
   a. Sulfamethoxazole (SMX), by competitive inhibition, blocks conversion of *p*-aminobenzoic acid to dihydrofolate (folic acid).

  b. Trimethoprim (TMP) binds to and reversibly inhibits dihydrofolate reductase, blocking conversion of folic acid to folinic acid.
2. Broad spectrum of activity, including most gram-positive and gram-negative aerobes (some methicillin-resistant *Staphylococcus aureus* but not *Pseudomonas aeruginosa*); effective against *Escherichia coli, Klebsiella, Enterobacter, Proteus, Haemophilus influenzae, Streptococcus pneumoniae, S. aureus, Acinetobacter, Salmonella, Shigella, Pneumocystis carinii;* no clinically useful antianaerobic activity.

Indications:

1. Urinary tract infections: treatment/prophylaxis.
   a. Cystitis, pyelonephritis, prostatitis.
2. Respiratory tract infections:
   a. Bronchitis.
   b. *P. carinii* pneumonitis.
   c. Otitis media.
3. Enteric infections: Shigellosis, salmonellosis.
4. Other:
   a. Infections caused by *Pseudomonas* spp. other than *P. aeruginosa: P. multophilia, P. cepacia, P. pseudomallei.*
   b. Brucellosis.
   c. Nocardiosis.
   d. Gram-negative bacillary meningitis (especially *Acinetobacter*).

Pharmacokinetics:

1. **Absorption:** Well absorbed PO.
2. **Penetration:** Excellent, including CSF.
3. **Metabolism:** Liver.
4. **Excretion:** Renal.
5. **Serum half-life:** 10 hr.

Drug Preparations:

Regular strength tablets: 80 mg TMP/400 mg SMX.
Double-strength tablets: 160 mg TMP/800 mg SMX.
Suspension: 40 mg TMP/200 mg SMX/5 mL.
Ampules: 5 mL: 80 mg TMP/400 mg SMX. 10 mL: 160 mg TMP/800 mg SMX.

Dosage:

1. **Normal renal function:**
   a. **Adult: PO:** 2 tabs (160 mg TMP/800 mg SMX) q 12 hr or 1 tab q 6 hr. **Parenteral:** 4–5 mg/kg (based on TMP) q 6–12 hr.
   b. **Pediatric: PO/parenteral:** 4–5 mg/kg (based on TMP) q 6–12 hr.
2. **Impaired renal function:**

Dose (mg/kg)	Creatinine Clearance	Interval (hr)
4–5	>80	6–12
	80–50	12
	50–10	18
	<10 (anuria)	24–48

3. **Dialysis:**
   a. **Hemodialysis:** Supplemental dose of 4–5 mg/kg (as TMP) after each dialysis.
   b. **Peritoneal:** Daily dose 0.16/0.8 g q 48 hr.

Adverse Effects:

1. Same as sulfonamides. Seizures, hepatotoxicity, mental depression.
2. Most frequent: Nausea/vomiting, diarrhea, anorexia, hypersensitivity reactions (especially rashes).
3. Cytopenias (along with increased rash in HIV-infected patients).
4. Renal dysfunction (infrequent, reversible).
5. Increase in measured serum creatinine.
6. Potential for teratogenesis and kernicterus; contraindicated in pregnant/nursing women.

Drug Interactions:

1. Same as sulfonamides.
2. Cyclosporin: Increased nephrotoxicity (synergistic with TMP).
3. Enhances anticoagulant effects. Potentiates hypoglycemic effects of sulfonylureas.

Monitor: Blood cell counts, renal/hepatic function.

TRIMETREXATE

Trade Name: *NeuTrexin.*

Drug Actions:

1. A derivative of methotrexate, trimetrexate acts as a folic acid antagonist through inhibition of microbial dihydrofolate reductase.
2. Trimetrexate must be used with leucovorin (folinic acid), which protects the patient's bone marrow from the cytotoxic effects of trimetrexate. (Leucovorin is selectively taken up by mammalian host cells and not *Pneumocystis carinii* organisms.)

Indications: Alternative therapy for treatment of moderate to severe *P. carinii* pneumonia in immunocompromised patients, including AIDS patients, who are intolerant of or refractory to trimethoprim/sulfamethoxazole (TMP/SMX) therapy or for whom TMP/SMX is contraindicated.

Pharmacokinetics:

1. **Absorption:** IV.
2. **Metabolism:** Metabolized by liver and excreted by kidney. 10%–30% of administered dose is excreted unchanged in urine.
3. **Half-life:** 11 hr.

Drug Preparations:

   Vials: 5 mL (contains trimetrexate glucuronate equivalent to 25 mg trimetrexate).

Dosage: *See* Table 22.

   45 mg/m^2 IV q day (recommended duration of therapy is 21 days).

   Leucovorin must be administered daily (20 mg/m^2 IV or PO qid—oral dosage should be rounded up to next higher 25 mg increment) during treatment and for 72 hr after last dose of trimetrexate.

Adverse Effects: Neutropenia: Absolute neutrophil count ≤1000/mm^3 (30.3%); increased AST (13.8%), increased ALT

TABLE 22.

Dose Modifications for Hematologic Toxicity

Toxicity Grade	Neutrophils (Polys and Bands)	Platelets	Recommended Dosages of	
			NeuTrexin	Leucovorin
1	>1000/mm^3	>75,000/mm^3	45 mg/m^2 once daily	20 mg/m^2 q6h
2	750–1000/mm^3	50,000–75,000/mm^3	45 mg/m^2 once daily	40 mg/m^2 q6h
3	500–749/mm^3	25,000–49,999/mm^3	22 mg/m^2 once daily	40 mg/m^2 q6h
4	<500/mm^3	<25,000/mm^3	Day 1–9 Discontinue Day 10–21 Interrupt up to 96 hr*	40 mg/m^2 q6h

*If grade 4 hematologic toxicity occurs prior to day 10, NeuTrexin should be discontinued. Leucovorin (40 mg/m^2, q6h) should be administered for an additional 72 hr. If grade 4 hematologic toxicity occurs at day 10 or later, NeuTrexin may be held up to 96 hr to allow counts to recover. If counts recover to grade 3 within 96 hr, NeuTrexin should be administered at a dose of 22 mg/m^2 and leucovorin maintained at 40 mg/m^2, q6h. When counts recover to grade 2 toxicity, NeuTrexin dose may be increased to 45 mg/m^2, but the leucovorin dose should be maintained at 40 mg/m^2 for the duration of treatment. If counts do not improve to ≤grade 3 toxicity within 96 hr, NeuTrexin should be discontinued. Leucovorin at a dose of 40 mg/m^2, q6h should be administered for 72 hours following the last dose of NeuTrexin.

(11.0%), thrombocytopenia (10.1%), fever (8.3%), anemia (7.3%), rash/pruritus (5.5%), and others.

Drug Interactions:

1. Agents that induce the cytochrome P-450 system (e.g., rifampin, rifabutin, and others) may decrease plasma concentrations of trimetrexate.
2. Erythromycin, clotrimazole, ketoconazole, miconazole, and other drugs that inhibit the cytochrome P-450 system may increase levels of trimetrexate.

Monitoring: Patients receiving trimetrexate with leucovorin protection should be seen frequently by a physician and have CBC with differential, BUN and creatinine, and liver function tests at least twice weekly.

BIBLIOGRAPHY

Physicians' Desk Reference, ed 50, Montvale, 1996, Medical Economics Co.

TROMETHAMINE

Trade Names: *Tham Solution, Talatrol.*

Drug Action:

1. **Proton binding:** Corrects acidosis by actively binding hydrogen ions. Binds cations of fixed or metabolic acids as well as hydrogen ions of carbonic acid.
2. **Osmotic diuresis:** Acts as an osmotic diuretic. Increases urinary pH, urine flow, excretion of fixed acids and electrolytes and carbon dioxide.

Indications:

1. Metabolic acidosis associated with cardiac bypass surgery. Can be used to correct acidosis occurring during/after cardiopulmonary bypass.
2. Metabolic acidosis from banked blood.
3. Metabolic acidosis during cardiac arrest and hypoperfusion states.

Pharmacokinetics:

1. **Metabolism:** Minimal.
2. **Excretion:** Rapidly excreted in urine, probably greater than 90% excreted unchanged.
3. **Volume of distribution:** Distributes to volume greater than extracellular fluid. After equilibration, appears to distribute to total body water.
4. **Plasma half life:** Approximately 3–5 hr.

Drug Preparations: Tham is supplied in a single-dose 500 mL glass container as a 0.3 mol/L solution. pH is adjusted to 8.6 with glacial acetic acid. Each 100 mL contains 3.6 g (30 mEq) in water for injection.

Dosage: Tham should be administered by slow venous infusion to avoid overtreatment and resultant metabolic alkalosis. Dose should be limited to amount sufficient to correct pH to 7.35–7.45. IV dosage can be estimated from base deficit by means of Siggaard-Andersen nomogram, with the following formula as a guideline:

Tham (mL of 0.3 mol/L) = Body weight (kg) × Base deficit (mEq/L) × 1.1. Average dose in cardiac bypass surgery is 0.32 gm/kg.

The 1.1 correction factor accounts for the approximate 10% reduction in buffering capacity due to the presence of the acetic acid used to lower the pH of 0.3 mol/L solution to approximately 8.6.

Adverse Effects:

1. **Respiratory:** Ventilatory depression can result from binding of carbonic acid and lowering of PCO_2 in blood. This effect may be more pronounced in patients with chronic hypoventilation.
2. **Vascular:** May cause local tissue damage and sloughing if perivascular infiltration occurs. Chemical phlebitis and venospasm have been reported.
3. **Hypoglycemia:** Can result in transient depression of blood glucose level.
4. **Coagulation abnormalities:** Has been noted to cause increases in coagulation time in animal experiments.
5. Hypokalemia, alkalosis, cardiac arrhythmias.

Drug Interactions:

1. **Decreased pharmacologic effects:** Benzodiazepines, keto-conazole, lithium, salicylates, sulfonylureas, tetracyclines, phenobarbital.
2. **Increased pharmacologic effects:** Quinidine, amphetamines, flecainide, sympathomimetics.
3. **Hypokalemia enhanced:** Glucocorticoids, diuretics, miner-alocorticoids.

Monitoring:

1. Arterial blood gas (pH).
2. Serum electrolytes and bicarbonate.
3. Blood glucose level.
4. Coagulation studies.

BIBLIOGRAPHY

Tromethamine. In *Drug Facts and Comparisons,* Philadelphia, 1996, JB Lippincott, pp 160–161.

Nahas GG: The clinical pharmacology of Tham, *Clin Pharmacol Ther* 1963, 4:784.

Wolf AL, Levi L, Marmarou A, et al: Effect of THAM upon outcome in severe head injury. *J Neurosurg* 78(1):54–59, 1993.

VALACYCLOVIR (VALACICLOVIR)

Trade Name: *Valtrex.*

Drug Actions:

1. Valacyclovir is the hydrochloride salt of L-valyl ester of acy-clovir. It is rapidly converted to acyclovir and L-valine by first-pass intestinal and/or hepatic metabolism. Acyclovir ultimately inhibits viral replication after a series of biochemical steps: it is first converted by virus-encoded thymidine kinase to a monophosphate and then cellular enzymes further convert the drug to its triphosphate form, which interferes with the functions of viral DNA polymerase. (Neither valacyclovir nor acy-clovir metabolism is associated with liver microsomal enzymes.)

2. Spectrum of activity: Herpes simplex viruses (HSV) types 1 and 2 and varicella-zoster virus (VZV).

Indications:

1. Herpes zoster (shingles) in immunocompetent adults.
2. Episodic treatment of recurrent genital herpes in immunocompetent adults.

Pharmacokinetics:

1. **Absorption:** PO; rapidly absorbed from GI tract and may be taken without regard to meals.
2. **Excretion:** Renal.
3. **Half-life:** 2.5–3.3 hr.

Drug Preparations:

Caplets: 500 mg.

Dosage:

1. Herpes zoster: 1 q PO tid for 7 days (most effective when given within 48 hr of onset of zoster rash).
2. Recurrent genital herpes: 500 mg PO bid for 5 days (should be initiated within 24 hr of symptom/sign onset).
3. Reduction in dosage is recommended for patients with renal insufficiency.

Adverse Effects:

1. Thrombotic thrombocytopenic purpura (TTP)/hemolytic uremic syndrome (HUS) has occurred in patients with HIV disease and also in bone marrow transplant and renal transplant recipients receiving high-dose valacyclovir. Valacyclovir should *not* be given to immunocompromised patients.
2. Headache (17%), nausea (6%), diarrhea (4%), dizziness (3%), and others.

Drug Interactions: Cimetidine and probenecid increase concentrations of acyclovir.

BIBLIOGRAPHY

Physicians' Desk Reference, ed 50, Montvale, 1996, Medical Economics Co.

VALPROIC ACID

Trade Names: *Depakene, Depakote.*

Drug Action: Valproic acid has antiepileptic activity against a wide variety of seizure types. It is more useful in absence and generalized tonic-clonic seizures. It has been suggested that valproic acid increases the level of GABA by inhibiting GABA transaminase, thereby increasing neuronal inhibition.

Indications: Valproic acid is particularly effective in treatment of absence seizures and helps in a variety of other seizures, including myoclonic and tonic-clonic seizures. It is less effective in controlling partial seizures, but may be used as adjunctive therapy.

Pharmacokinetics:

1. **Metabolism:** Rapidly absorbed after PO administration. Peak levels occur in 1–4 hr. Most of the drug is converted to the conjugate ester of glucuronic acid. Some metabolites have anticonvulsant activity.
2. **Excretion:** Urinary excretion of unchanged compound is 1.8% ±2.4%.
3. **Volume of distribution:** 0.13 ± 0.04 L/kg.
4. **Basal clearance:** 0.11 ± 0.02 mL/min/kg.
5. **Therapeutic level:** 55–100 µg/mL.
6. **Plasma half-life:** 14 ± 3 hr.
7. **Compatibilities:**
   a. In combination with phenobarbital, concentration of the barbiturate may rise as much as 40%.
   b. Phenytoin concentrations may fall when patient is concurrently receiving valproic acid.
   c. Concurrent administration of valproic acid and clonazapam has been associated with development of absence status epileptic state.
   d. Valproic acid potentiates effects of alcohol.

Drug Preparations:

1. Depakene (valproic acid):
   Capsules: 250 mg.
2. Depakote (divalproex sodium):

Tablets: 125, 250, 500 mg.
PO syrup: 250 mg sodium valproate/5 mL.

Dosage:

1. **Adult:** Usual daily dose 15–45 mg/kg in two to four doses, depending on serum level.
2. **Pediatric:** Usual daily dose 15–16 mg/kg. It is suggested that the initial dosage be 15 mg/kg/day in divided doses bid–tid, with weekly increases of 5–10 mg/kg/day until therapeutic levels are obtained. Max. recommended dose 60 mg/kg/day.

Adverse Reactions:

1. GI symptoms occur in as much as 16% of patients; more common with acid form of the compound.
2. Hair loss and skin rashes have been reported.
3. Sedation, ataxia, tremor, appetite stimulation, and elevation of hepatic enzymes may occur in 15%–30% of patients.
4. Fulminant, often fatal, hepatitis may occur at an incidence of 1/20,000–1/40,000 patients. 85% of those with this severe complication are using multiple drugs. Fatal hepatitis is more likely in the very young patient who is being treated with multiple agents.
5. Thrombocytopenia, bone marrow suppression, prolongation of PT and PTT, decreased serum fibrinogen have been reported.

Drug Interactions: Potentiates MAO inhibitors, antidepressants, PO anticoagulants.

Monitoring:

1. Blood levels are available via high-pressure liquid chromatography analysis in most large hospital laboratories and reference laboratory facilities.
2. Therapeutic level 55–100 µg/mL.
3. Monitor liver function, platelet counts, blood cell counts, PT.

BIBLIOGRAPHY

Cohen S, Armstrong M: *Drug Interactions: A Handbook for Clinical Use,* Baltimore, 1974, Williams & Wilkins.
Drug Information for the Health Care Professional, ed 8, Rockville, 1988, US Pharmacopeial Convention.

Evans WE, Oellerich M: *Therapeutic Drug Monitoring Clinical Guide,* ed 2, Irving, 1984, Abbott Laboratories Publications.

Gilman A, Goodman L, Rall T, et al (eds): *The Pharmacological Basis of Therapeutics,* ed 7, New York, 1985, Macmillan.

Johnson G: *Blue Book of Pharmacologic Therapeutics,* Philadelphia, 1985, WB Saunders.

McEvoy GK: *Drug Information 88,* Bethesda, 1988, American Society of Hospital Pharmacists.

VANCOMYCIN

Trade Names: *Vancocin, Vancoled, Vancor.*

Drug Action:

1. Interferes with glycopeptide polyerization as a result of interference with transfer of disaccharide-pentapeptide from a membrane lipid carrier to a cell wall acceptor in second stage of cell wall synthesis.
   a. May alter permeability or plasma membrane and inhibit RNA synthesis.
2. Spectrum of activity only against **gram-positive** bacteria, particularly aerobes.

Indications:

1. Staphylococcal infections, including methicillin-resistant *Staphylococcus aureus.*
   a. Patients allergic to β-lactams.
2. Streptococcal infections.
3. Enterococcal infections (with aminoglycoside in penicillin-allergic patients).
4. Diphtheroid infections.
5. Multiple sites, including heart, CNS, foreign bodies.
6. Pseudomembranous colitis associated with *Clostridium difficile* toxin: Use PO.

Pharmacokinetics:

1. **Absorption:** Not absorbed PO.
2. Not tolerated IM (muscule necrosis).
3. **Excretion:** Renal.
4. **Serum half-life:** 4–8 hr.
5. Minimal amounts removed by dialysis.

Drug Preparations:

Vials: 500 mg for IV use.
Capsules: 125, 250 mg.

Dosage:

1. **Normal renal function:**
   a. **Adult:**
      (1) PO: 0.125–0.5 g q 6 hr.
      (2) Parenteral: 15 mg/kg q 12 hr or 6.5–8 mg/kg q 6 hr.
   b. **Pediatric:**
      (1) PO: 12.5 mg/kg q 6 hr.
      (2) Parenteral: 10 mg/kg q 6 hr.
2. **Impaired renal function:** Dose should be adjusted by following serum levels, with troughs 5–15 μg/mL. Approximate dose adjustment: Creatinine <1.5 mg/dL, 1 g q 12 hr; Cr 1.5–5 mg/dL, 1 g q 3–6 days; >5 mg/dL, 1 g q 10–14 days.

Adverse Effects:

1. Hypersensitivity reactions, nausea/vomiting.
2. Phlebitis: 17% (lessened by rotating sites, increasing interval, etc.)
3. Fever.
4. Ototoxicity: Major side effect with levels >80 μg/mL.
5. Nephrotoxicity: Uncommon.
6. Neutropenia.
7. **Red neck syndrome:** Tingling at infusion site, dizziness, erythematous pruritic rash involving face, neck, upper trunk, upper extremities.
   a. Histamine mediated.
   b. Dose and infusion rate related.
8. Hypotension (after rapid IV infusion).

Drug Interactions: Increased ototoxicity and nephrotoxicity when used with aminoglycosides and other nephrotoxic drugs.

Monitoring:

1. Serial drug levels: Peak no higher than 30–40 µg/mL, trough 5–10 µg/mL.
2. Observe renal function, blood cell counts.

VASOPRESSIN

Trade Names:

Vasopressin: *Pitressin*.
Vasopressin tannate in oil: *Pitressin tannate*.
Lypressin: *Diapid*.

Drug Action:

1. **Antidiuretic:** Decreases free water excretion. Increases cyclic adenosine monophosphate levels in kidney.
2. **Antihemorrhagic:** Decreases hepatic blood flow and portal venous pressure; increases clotting and hemostasis.
3. **Vasopressor.**
4. **Peristaltic stimulant:** Stimulates GI smooth muscle.

Indications:

1. Neurogenic diabetes insipidus.
2. Upper GI bleeding (esophageal varices).
3. Postoperative abdominal distention.
4. Abdominal roentgenography to dispel gas shadows.

Pharmacokinetics:

1. **Absorption:** Destroyed in GI tract; give intranasally or parenterally. Vasopressin in oil is absorbed more slowly than aqueous solution.
2. **Distribution:** Extracellular fluid.
3. **Metabolism:** Liver, kidneys.
4. **Excretion:** Renal; 5% of SQ dose excreted unchanged in urine.
5. **Serum half-life:** 10–20 min.

6. **Duration of action:**
   a. Vasopressin tannate in oil IM: 24–72 hr.
   b. Aqueous vasopressin IM/SQ: 2–8 hr.
   c. Lypressin (nasal): 3–4 hr (onset 1 hr).

Drug Preparations:

1. Aqueous vasopressin: *Ampules:* 0.5, 1.0 mL, 20 pressor U/mL.
2. Vasopressin tannate in oil: **Do not give IV or intra-arterially.** *Suspension in peanut oil:* 1 mL ampules, 5 pressor U/mL.
3. Lypressin: *Solution* (spray): 5 mL containers, 50 pressor U/mL; 1 spray equals approximately 2 pressor units.

Dosage:

1. **Diabetes insipidus (titrate to effect on basis of serum/urine sodium and osmolality):**
   a. **Adult:**
      (1) Aqueous vasopressin 5–10 U IM/SQ bid–qid.
      (2) Vasopressin tannate in oil: 2.5–5 U IM/SQ q 1–3 days.
      (3) Lypressin: 1–4 sprays/nostril bid–qid.
   b. **Pediatric:**
      (1) Aqueous vasopressin: 2.5–10 IM/SQ bid–qid.
      (2) Vasopressin tannate in oil: 1.25–2.5 U IM q 1–3 days.
2. **Postoperative abdominal distention:** Aqueous vasopressin: 5–10 U IM initially, then q 3–4 hr.
3. **Upper GI bleeding:** Aqueous vasopressin: 0.2–0.4 U/min IV, or 0.1–0.5 U/min intra-arterially. Titrate dose to effect. If bleeding stops, continue at same dose for 12 hr, then taper off over 24–48 hr.

Adverse Effects:

1. **CNS:** Tremor, dizziness, headache, weakness, coma, confusion, seizures, stroke.
2. **Cardiovascular:** Angina, vasospasm (leading to tissue necrosis), hypertension, infarction, bradycardia, arrhythmias, heart failure.
3. **Dermatologic:** Skin necrosis and gangrene (at injection site), hypersensitivity, pallor, urticaria.
4. **GI:** Abdominal cramps, nausea/vomiting, diarrhea, hyperactivity, rare bowel infarction.
5. Water intoxication, oliguria, hyponatremia.

6. Bronchial constriction, shortness of breath.
7. CAUTION: Cardiac disease, vascular disease, hypertension, epilepsy, renal disease.

Drug Interactions:

1. Potentiates antidiuretic effect: Carbamazepine, chlorpropamide, clofibrate, phenformin, fludrocortisone.
2. Decreases antidiuretic effect: Demeclocycline, lithium, norepinephrine, epinephrine, alcohol, heparin.
3. Increases plasma cortisol levels.
4. Antagonizes action of antihypertensive/antianginal drugs.

Monitoring:

1. Serum sodium and osmolality, fluid balance, urine output, urine osmolality or specific gravity, daily weight.
2. Blood pressure, heart rate, ECG.

BIBLIOGRAPHY

Hayes RM: Agents affecting the renal conservation of water. In Gilman AG, et al (eds): *The Pharmacological Basis of Therapeutics,* ed 8, New York, 1993, McGraw-Hill, pp 732–742.

Robertson GL: Diabetes insipidus, *Endocrinol Metab Clin North Am* 1995, 24:549–572.

Zaloga GP: Hormones—vasopressin, growth hormone, glucagon, somatostatin, prolactin, G-CSF, CM-CSF. In Chernow B (ed): *The Pharmacologic Approach to the Critically Ill Patient,* ed 3, Baltimore, 1994, Williams & Wilkins, pp 700–714.

VERAPAMIL

Trade Names: *Calan, Isoptin.*

Drug Action: Intracellular calcium is important in excitation-contraction coupling process in cardiac muscle, in the generation of action potentials in SA and AV nodal tissue, and in smooth muscle contraction. Intracellular calcium levels are increased when extracellular calcium passes through specific membrane calcium channels. These drugs block slow (voltage-sensitive) calcium channels.

1. SA/AV node: Decreased rate of spontaneous diastolic depolarization, increased membrane threshold; negative chronotropy (slow conduction velocity).
2. Negative inotropic action.
3. Smooth muscle relaxation: Coronary and peripheral vasodilation.
4. Improved diastolic relaxation, which improves myocardial compliance and aids in relieving myocardial ischemia.
5. May suppress early and late afterdepolarizations.

Indications:

1. Myocardial ischemia.
2. Supraventricular arrhythmias, especially AV nodal reentry.
3. Rapid ventricular response in atrial flutter/fibrillation.
4. Hypertrophic cardiomyopathy: Relieves obstruction by improving relaxation.
5. Hypertension.

Pharmacokinetics:

1. **Absorption:** PO/IV. Peak effect 1–2 hr after PO intake, 4–8 hr with extended-release tablets.
2. **Metabolism:** Hepatic.
3. **Excretion:** Renal 70%.
4. **Protein binding:** 90%.
5. **Onset of action:** 2–3 min IV.
6. **Plasma half-life:** 110 min IV, 4.5–10 hr PO.

Drug Preparations:

Tablets: 80, 120, 240 mg (extended release).
Ampules: 5 mg/2 mL, 10 mg/4 mL.
Vials: 10 mg/4 mL.

Dosage:

1. **Supraventricular arrhythmias:**
   a. **Adult:** 0.075–0.15 mg/kg bolus over 2 min. Repeat in 10 min if no response.
   b. **Pediatric:** 0.1–0.3 mg/kg IV over 2 min.
   c. **PO:** 80–120 mg tid–qid.
   d. **Maintenance of heart rate in atrial fibrillation/flutter:** Infusion at 0.005 mg/kg/min, taper to effect.

2. **Angina pectoris:**
   a. **Adult:** 80–120 mg PO q 6–8 hr.
3. **Hypertension:**
   a. **Adult:** 80–120 mg PO tid or 240 mg extended-release PO q d–bid.

Adverse Effects:

1. Hypotension, bradycardia, dizziness, headache, fatigue.
2. Heart block.
3. Congestive heart failure (CHF).
4. May increase ventricular rate in Wolff-Parkinson-White syndrome.
5. Ventricular tachycardia may degenerate into ventricular fibrillation. Use with caution in wide QRS tachycardias.
6. Constipation, nausea, hepatotoxicity.

Drug Interactions:

1. Increases digoxin levels by approximately 60%; also increases carbamazepine levels.
2. Combination with β-blockers can produce congestive heart failure or heart block.
3. Potentiates neuromuscular blocking drugs and antihypertensive drugs.
4. Accentuate cardiac depression in association with halothane anesthesia.

Monitoring: Blood pressure, heart rate, ECG, liver function.

BIBLIOGRAPHY

Antman EM, Stone P, Muller JE, et al: Calcium channel blocking agents in the treatment of cardiovascular disorders. I: Basic and clinical electrophysiologic effects, *Ann Intern Med* 1980, 93:875–885.

Braunwald E: Mechanism of action of calcium channel blocking agents, *N Engl J Med* 1982, 307:1618–1627.

Stone PH, Antman EM, Muller JE, et al: Calcium channel blocking drugs in the treatment of cardiovascular disorders. II: Hemodynamic and clinical applications, *Ann Intern Med* 1980, 93:886–904.

VITAMIN B₁₂ (CYANOCOBALAMIN)

Trade Names: *Cobex,* others.

Drug Actions: Coenzyme for various metabolic functions, including fat-carbohydrate-protein metabolism, required for cell replication (i.e., hematopoiesis) and CNS integrity.

Indications:

1. Treatment of pernicious anemia (megaloblastic anemia).
2. Vitamin B₁₂ deficiency.

Pharmacokinetics:

1. **Absorption:** Terminal ileum, requires intrinsic factor.
2. Water soluble.
3. **Metabolism:** Tissues.
4. **Excretion:** Bile, urine, enterohepatic cycle (stool).
5. Tissue stores adequate for 1–2 yr.
6. **Normal serum level:** 150–750 pg/mL.

Drug Preparations:

Injection: 30, 100, 1000 μg/mL (1, 10, 30 mL).
Tablets: 25, 50, 100, 250, 500, 1000 μg.

Dosage:

1. RDA: Adults 3 μg, children 0.3–2 μg.
2. Pernicious anemia: Adults 100 μg/day for 1–2 wk (IM, SQ), then 100 μg every other day for 2 wk (IM or SQ), then 100 μg q 3 days for 2–3 wk (IM, SQ); maintenance 100 μg/mo (for life) (IM, SQ).
3. Vitamin B₁₂ deficiency: Adults 30 μg/day for 5–10 days, maintenance 100–200 μg/mo (give IM or SQ).

Adverse Effects:

1. Metabolic: hypokalemia.
2. Dermatologic: Itching, urticaria.
3. Gastrointestinal: Diarrhea.
4. Cardiovascular: Peripheral vascular thrombosis, anaphylaxis.
5. Polycythemia.

Monitoring:

1. Serum potassium (treatment may result in severe hypokalemia).
2. RBC (especially mean corpuscular volume), reticulocyte count, Hb, Hct.
3. Vitamin B$_{12}$ level: 150–750 pg/mL (normal range).

BIBLIOGRAPHY

Bortenschlager L, Zaloga GP: Vitamins. In Chernow B (ed): *The Pharmacologic Approach to the Critically Ill Patient,* ed 3, Baltimore, 1994, Williams & Wilkins, pp 805–819.

Hillman RS: Hematopoietic agents—growth factors, minerals, and vitamins. In Gilman AG, et al (eds): *The Pharmacological Basis of Therapeutics,* ed 8, New York, 1993, McGraw-Hill, pp 1294–1302.

VITAMIN D

Trade Names:

Ergocalciferol: *Calciferol, Drisdol.*
Calcifediol (25-hydroxyvitamin D): *Calderol.*
Calcitriol (1,25-dihydroxyvitamin D): *Rocaltrol.*

Drug Action: Antihypocalcemic agent. Vitamin D is absorbed in the diet or made in the skin. It is 25-hydroxylated to calcifediol in the liver, and 1-hydroxylated to calcitriol in the kidney. Calcitriol is the active form of the vitamin. Calcitriol increases gut absorption, bone resorption, and renal reabsorption of calcium. In conjunction with parathyroid hormone, vitamin D regulates calcium homeostasis.

Indications:

1. Chronic hypocalcemia.
2. Hypoparathyroidism.
3. Rickets, osteomalacia.

Pharmacokinetics: *See* Table 23.

Drug Preparations:

1. Ergocalciferol (1.25 mg = 50,000 units of activity):

    Capsules or Tablets: 0.625 mg (25,000 U), 1.25 mg (50,000 U).
    Liquid: 8000 U/mL.
    Injection: 12.5 mg (500,000 U)/mL.
2. Calcifediol:

    Capsules: 20, 50 μg.
3. Calcitriol:

    Capsules: 0.25, 0.50 μg.
    Injection: 1, 2 μg/mL.

Dosage: NOTE: Dosage must be individualized and adequate intake of calcium assured.

1. Ergocalciferol (each μg = 40 USP units):
    a. **Adults/children with rickets or osteomalacia:** 25–125 μg/day PO.
    b. **Malabsorption:** 0.25–7.5 mg/day PO, or 250 μg IM q day.
       Hypoparathyroidism/hypocalcemia: 0.625–2.5 mg/day; increase dosage until desired effect obtained. RDA adults = 200 U.
2. Calcifediol: Initially 50 μg/day PO; increase by 50 μg/day q 4 wk until desired effect obtained. Useful in severe liver disease.
3. Calcitriol: Initially 0.25 μg/day PO; increase by 0.25 μg/day q 2–4 wk until desired effect obtained. Usual maintenance dose 0.25–1.25 μg/day. Useful in patients with renal disease.

Adverse Effects: Effects result from hypercalcemia.

1. **CNS:** Headache, irritability, somnolence, coma, seizures, psychosis.
2. **ENT:** Conjunctivitis, photophobia, rhinorrhea, tinnitus.
3. **GI:** Nausea/vomiting, constipation, anorexia, metallic taste, pancreatitis, hepatotoxicity.
4. **GU:** Polyuria, nephrocalcinosis, renal stones, renal failure.
5. **Cardiovascular:** Hypertension, AV nodal block, arrhythmias, bradycardia, flushing.
6. **Musculoskeletal:** Bone pain, weakness, myopathy, bone demineralization.

TABLE 23.
Pharmacokinetics

	Ergocalciferol*	Calcifediol	Calcitriol
1. **Absorption:**	Small bowel	Small bowel	Small bowel
Vitamin D is fat soluble and requires bile for absorption. Absorption is reduced in liver or biliary disease.			
2. **Distribution:**			
Vitamin D is stored in liver; also found in fat, muscle, skin, brain, spleen, bones.			
3. **Metabolism:**	Liver, kidney	Liver, kidney	Liver, kidney
4. **Excretion:**	Bile, urine	Bile, urine	Bile, urine
5. **Serum level:**	10 ng/mL	30 ng/mL	0.03 ng/mL
6. **Serum half-life:**	30 days	15 days	3–8 hr
Serum half-life of calcifediol is prolonged with renal disease.			
7. **Duration:**	60 days	30 days	3–5 days

*40,000 U vitamin D activity =1 mg ergocalciferol.

7. Ectopic calcification, pruritus, polydipsia, hypersensitivity re-actions.

Drug Interactions:

1. Absorption decreased by antacids, cholestyramine, colestipol, mineral oil.
2. Metabolism increased by barbiturate,s phenytoin, primidone.
3. Hypercalcemia potentiates digitalis effect, may cause toxicity.
4. Thiazides decrease calcium excretion in urine.
5. Corticosteroids inhibit drug action.
6. May antagonize effect of calcium channel blockers.

Monitoring:

1. Serum calcium (ionized calcium is best), phosphate.
2. 24-hr urine calcium.
3. Calcifediol and calcitriol levels.
4. Maintain constant dietary calcium intake.
5. BUN, creatinine.

BIBLIOGRAPHY

Zaloga GP, Chernow B: Divalent ions: calcium, magnesium, and phosphorus. In Chernow B (ed): *The Pharmacologic Approach to the Critically Ill Patient,* ed 3, Baltimore, 1994, Williams & Wilkins, pp 777–804.

Bortenschlager L, Zaloga GP: Vitamins. In Chernow B (ed): *The Pharmacologic Approach to the Critically Ill Patient,* ed 3, Baltimore, 1994, Williams & Wilkins, pp 805–819.

Marcus R, Couston AM: Fat soluble vitamins. In Gilman AG, et al (eds): *The Pharmacological Basis of Therapeutics,* ed 8, New York, 1993, McGraw-Hill, pp 1553–1571.

VITAMIN K

Trade Names:

1. Menadiol sodium diphosphate (K_4) (water soluble): generics.
2. Phytonadione (K_1): *Aquamephyton, Konakion, Mephyton.*

Drug Action: Promotes hepatic formation of coagulation factors II, VII, IX, X.

Indications:

1. Vitamin K deficiency states (e.g., malabsorption, drug therapy).
2. Reversal of PO anticoagulant action.
3. Hemorrhagic disease of newborn.

Pharmacokinetics:

1. **Absorption:** Phytonadione requires bile for absorption (enters lymphatics); menadiol does not require bile (enters bloodstream directly).
2. **Metabolism:** Liver, menadiol is metabolized to menadione.
3. **Excretion:** Feces (bile), urine.
4. Concentrated in liver.
5. **Onset:**
   a. **IV administration:** 1–2 hr for phytonadione; 8–24 hr for menadiol.
   b. **PO administration:** 6–10 hr for phytonadione.
6. **Minimal daily requirements:** 70–140 µg for adults; 15–100 µg for children.
7. Crosses placenta.

Drug Preparations:

1. Phytonadione (lipid-soluble synthetic):
   Tablets: 5 mg.
   Injection: 2, 10 mg/mL.
2. Menadiol (water-soluble derivative):
   Tablets: 5 mg.
   Injection: 5, 10, 37.5 mg/mL.

Dosage:

1. **Vitamin K deficiency** (adults/children):
   a. Menadiol/phytonadione: 5–25 mg/day PO, or 5–10 mg IV/IM/SQ q day–bid.
   b. If no other route is feasible, may give IV; administer slowly (<1 mg/min). Use menadiol for IV administration.
2. **Reversal of anticoagulant-induced hypoprothrombinemia:**
   a. Phytonadione: 2.5–10 mg SQ/IM/IV/PO; taper to effect.
   b. Menadiol is ineffective.

3. **Long-term total parenteral nutrition:** Phytonadione: 5–10 mg/wk SQ/IM.
4. **Hemorrhagic disease of newborn:** Phytonadione: Prophylaxis, 0.5–2 mg IM in single dose, treatment, 1–2 mg/day SQ/IM.
5. **IV Administration:** Dilute in normal saline, D_5W, D_5NS and infuse slowly (<1 mg/min). Use this route only if another route is not feasible.

Adverse Effects:

1. **Respiratory:** Bronchospasm, dyspnea.
2. **Cardiovascular:** Hypotension after IV administration, tachycardia, arrhythmias.
3. **GI:** Nausea/vomiting, GI upset, hyperbilirubinemia in neonates.
4. **Dermatologic:** Rash, pruritus, urticaria, erythema, pain/swelling (local).
5. **CNS:** Headache, dizziness, seizures.
6. **Other:** Sweating, flushing, cramps, hypersensitivity reactions, anaphylaxis, hemolysis in G6PD deficiency and rarely in neonates.
7. **Severe reactions,** including death, have occurred rarely after phytonadione has been given IV.

Drug Interactions:

1. Broad-spectrum antibiotics decrease gut bacterial production of vitamin K, increase requirements for exogenous vitamin K.
2. Decreased absorption with mineral oils, cholestyramine.
3. Vitamin K antagonizes effects of PO anticoagulants.

Monitoring: PTT.

BIBLIOGRAPHY

Bortenschlager L, Zaloga GP: Vitamins. In Chernow B (ed): *The Pharmacologic Approach to the Critically Ill Patient,* ed 3, Baltimore, 1994, Williams & Wilkins, pp 805–819.

Marcus R, Couston AM: Fat soluble vitamins. In Gilman AG, et al (eds): *The Pharmacological Basis of Therapeutics,* ed 8, New York, 1993, McGraw-Hill, pp 1553–1571.

Marks J: *A guide to the vitamins,* Baltimore, 1975, University Park Press, pp 67–72.

WARFARIN SODIUM

Trade Names:

Warfarin: *Coumadin, Sofarin.*

1. Warfarin is the coined generic name for 3-(α-acetonylbenzyl)-4-hydroxycoumarin, based on this drug's development at the Wisconsin Alumni Research Foundation (WARF).
2. *Dicumarol:* PO coumarin anticoagulant with a different chemical structure than warfarin group.

Drug Action: Blocks vitamin K–dependent posttranslational modification of factors II, VII, IX, X (acting at glutamatic acid residues in amino acid sequence of these protein clotting factors) in liver.

Indications: PO anticoagulation in venous thrombosis, atrial fibrillation with embolization, pulmonary embolism, prosthetic cardiac valves.

Pharmacokinetics:

1. **Absorption:** Warfarin is rapidly and completely absorbed from GI tract, peaking within 1 hr after ingestion.
   a. Dicumarol is incompletely absorbed and has a dose-dependent half-life of 1–4 days.
2. **Metabolism:** Hepatic, with enterohepatic circulation of inactive metabolites.
3. **Excretion:** Hepatic (bile), renal.
4. **Distribution:** Bound 99% to albumin, limiting distribution to "albumin space." However, only free drug is biologically active.
5. **Plasma half-life:** Approximately 36 hr. Duration of action 2–5 days.

Drug Preparations:

a. Warfarin:
   Tablets: 2, 2.5, 5, 7.5, 10 mg.
   Vials: 50 mg for injection.
b. Dicumarol:
   Tablets: 25, 50 mg.

Dosage:

1. **Warfarin:** Large loading doses are no longer recommended. Initiate therapy with 10–15 mg PO q day, then reduce subsequent daily doses to 2.5–10 mg/day. Initially, **daily** prothrombin times (PTs) are required to titrate doses. Since time to peak anticoagulant effect is 36–72 hr, prolongation of PT will reflect effect of the **preceding** day's warfarin dose. Appropriate dosing for each patient must be individualized and titrated. Warfarin may also be given IM/IV.
2. **Dicumarol:** Initiate therapy with 200–300 mg PO q day, then titrate maintenance daily doses to 25–200 mg.

Adverse Effects:

1. **Hemorrhage:** Bleeding may occur even when PT is maintained within therapeutic range. Patients who are poorly compliant, hypertensive, or alcoholic; have had recent surgery or trauma; or have a history of gastric ulcers are at increased risk for hemorrhagic complications.
2. **Teratogenicity:** Warfarin crosses the placenta and has been associated with birth defects, especially involving CNS. One third of infants exposed during the first trimester of pregnancy will be affected.
3. **Skin necrosis:** Necrotic lesions (unrelated to skin hemorrhage) may occur in fat-rich tissues of the buttocks, breasts, thighs as a result of depression of protein C levels. It is reported that heparinization prior to initiation of warfarin therapy greatly reduces the risk of dermal necrosis. Rash, urticaria may also develop.
4. **Early thrombosis due to protein C deficiency:** This hereditary or acquired condition, which should be suspected if there is a history of recurrent episodes of thromboembolic disorders, has been associated with increased risk for necrosis following warfarin administration. It has been reported that concurrent anticoagulation therapy with heparin for 5–7 days during initiation of therapy may minimize the incidence of this reaction. Warfarin therapy should be discontinued when warfarin is suspected to be the cause of developing necrosis, and heparin therapy may be considered for anticoagulation.
5. Leukopenia, agranulocytosis, fever.

Treatment of Overdosage/Hemorrhage:

1. **Mild/non–life-threatening** (incidence 15%–18%): Vitamin K_1 PO (10–20 mg) or IV (5–10 mg at rate not to exceed 1 mg/min) will reverse warfarin effects within 4–24 hr. Repeat doses may be required.
2. **Serious/life-threatening** (incidence <5%): Fresh-frozen plasma will immediately replenish factors II, VII, IX, X. Three units fresh-frozen plasma is usually adequate to return PT to levels of 14–15 sec.

Drug Interactions: Drug interactions are **frequent** and significantly alter pharmacokinetics/pharmacodynamics of warfarin. Certain disease states may alter anticoagulant potency. Table 24 summarizes the qualitative effect of some of these numerous interactions.

Drug Monitoring: Quick one-stage PT is used to monitor effects of warfarin therapy. Factor VII levels are depressed most quickly and profoundly at initiation of warfarin therapy, and act as the primary PT determinant during the first few days of treatment. PT peaks at 1–3 days. Therapeutic range is generally one and one half to two times baseline control values.

BIBLIOGRAPHY

Agents used for anticoagulant therapy. In *AMA Drug Evaluations,* ed 6, Philadelphia, 1986, WB Saunders, pp 603–616.

Anticoagulants. In Stoelting RK: *Pharmacology and Physiology in Anesthetic Practice,* Philadelphia, 1987, JB Lippincott, pp 444–453.

Nanfro J: Anticoagulants in critical care medicine. In Chernow B (ed): *The Pharmacologic Approach to the Critically Ill Patient,* ed 2, Baltimore, 1988, Williams & Wilkins, pp 511–535.

O'Reilley R: Anticoagulant, antithrombotic, and thrombolytic drugs. In Gilman AG, Goodman LS, Rall TW, et al (eds): *The Pharmacologic Basis of Therapeutics,* ed 7, New York, 1985, Macmillan, pp 1338–1359.

TABLE 24.

Drug/Disease Interactions with Warfarin

Drug	Disease
Augmented anticoagulant effect	
Allopurinol	Cancer
Anesthetics	Collagen disorders
Aspirin	Congestive heart failure
Chloramphenicol	Hepatitis
Cimetidine	Hyperthyroidism
Clofibrate	Steatorrhea
Heparin	Vitamin K deficiency
Ibuprofen	
Methyldopa	
MAO inhibitors	
Phenytoin	
Propylthiouracil	
Quinidine	
Tolbutamide	
Inhibited anticoagulant effect	
Adrenocorticosteroids	Edema
Antacids	Hereditary resistance
Barbiturates	Hypothyroidism
Cholestyramine	
Colchicine	
Haloperidol	
PO contraceptives	
Rifampin	
Tetracycline	
Vitamin C	

ZOLPIDEM

Trade Name: *Ambien.*

Drug Actions: Imidazopyridine (nonbenzodiazepine) hypnotic for oral administration. Schedule IV controlled substance.

Indications: Hypnotic indicated for short-term treatment of insomnia.

Pharmacokinetics:

1. **Absorption:** Rapid absorption from GI tract.
2. **Onset of action:** Peak serum concentrations in 1.5 hr.
3. **Metabolism:** Hepatic metabolism to inactive metabolites.
4. **Excretion:** Primarily renal excretion of metabolites.
5. **Half-life:** 2.5 hr.
6. **Therapeutic level:** Not established.

Drug Preparations:

Tablets: 5, 10 mg.

Dosage: 10 mg PO before bedtime. Decrease dose in patients with hepatic insufficiency. Peak concentration, T1/2, AUC increase 50% in patients >70 yr old.

Adverse Effects: Infrequent. Most common are drowsiness (0.5%), dizziness (0.4%), headache (0.5%), nausea (0.5%).

Drug Interactions: Enhanced effect with other CNS-depressant drugs. However, no apparent interaction with haloperidol.

Monitoring: Daytime drowsiness, amnesia.

BIBLIOGRAPHY

Salva P, Costa J: Clinical pharmacokinetics and pharmacodynamics of zolpidem. Therapeutic implications, *Clin Pharmacokinet* 1995, 29:142–153.

Durand A, Thenot JP, Bianchetti G, Morselli PL: Comparative pharmacokinetic profile of two imidazopyridine drugs: zolpidem and alpidem, *Drug Metab Rev* 1992, 24:239–266.

APPENDIXES

3

Appendix A

TREATMENT OF SPECIFIC INFECTIONS

I. **Skin and soft tissues:**
   A. **Acne**
      1. Moderate or inflammatory:
         a. Topical clindamycin (expensive) or erythromycin.
         b. PO doxycycline or erythromycin.
      2. Severe and/or cystic:
         a. Isotretinoin (contraindicated in pregnancy).
   B. **Recurrent boils:**
      1. Generally secondary to *Staphylococcus aureus* carriage.
         a. Eliminate nasal carriage with either rifampin plus cloxacillin/dicloxacillin or ciprofloxacin. Mupirocin applied topically can eradicate nasal carriage of *S. aureus,* including methicillin-resistant *S. aureus* (MRSA).
   C. **Breast abscess or mastitis:**
      1. Postpartum *S. aureus.*
         a. Penicillinase-resistant penicillin or first-generation cephalosporin.
         b. In penicillin-allergic patients: Vancomycin.
      2. Nonpuerperal (*S. aureus* and anaerobes, if subareolar).
         a. Cefoxitin, cefotetan, ampicillin/sulbactam, or equivalent parenterally, plus surgical drainage.
         b. PO alternatives: Amoxicillin/clavulanic acid and clindamycin.
   D. **Impetigo:**
      1. Bullous (*S. aureus*):
         a. PO penicillinase-resistant penicillin or erythromycin.
         b. Alternatives: First-generation cephalosporin or clindamycin.
      2. Nonbullous (group A streptococci and *S. aureus*):
         a. PO penicillinase-resistant penicillin, erythromycin, or first-generation cephalosporin.
         b. Alternatives: Clindamycin and amoxicillin/clavulanic acid.

E. **Bites:**
   1. Human (mouth anaerobes, group A streptococci, *S. aureus, Eikenella corrodens*).
      a. X-ray clenched fist injuries.
      b. PO amoxicillin/clavulanic acid.
      c. Parenteral ampicillin/sulbactam, cefoxitin, cefotetan.
   2. Cat (*Pasteurella multocida, S. aureus,* DF-2 gram negative):
      a. May also transmit tularemia.
      b. PO amoxicillin-clavulanic acid or tetracycline.
      c. Parenteral ampicillin/sulbactam, ceftriaxone.
   3. Dog (*P. multocida,* streptococci, staphylococci, anaerobes, DF-2 and EF-4):
      a. Consider antirabies treatment.
      b. PO amoxicillin/clavulanic acid.
      c. Tetracycline or ceftriaxone.
   4. Rat (*Streptobacillus moniliformis* or *Spirillum minus*):
      a. Ampicillin (or tetracycline).
F. **Decubitus ulcer** (*S. aureus,* group A streptococci, anaerobes, gram-negative enterics plus *Pseudomonas aeruginosa*).
   1. Clindamycin plus an aminoglycoside or ticarcillin/clavulanic acid.
   2. Alternatives: β-Lactam and aminoglycoside combinations covering pathogens.
G. **Facial cellulitis:**
   1. Adult (group A streptococci, *S. aureus*):
      a. Penicillinase-resistant penicillin or first-generation cephalosporin.
      b. Vancomycin or clindamycin in penicillin-allergic patients.
   2. Children (*Haemophilus influenzae*):
      a. PO amoxicillin/clavulanic acid or cefuroxime axetil in less severe cases.
      b. Parenteral cefuroxime or ampicillin/sulbactam.
H. **Burns** (*S. aureus* and resistant gram-negative organisms, including *P. aeruginosa*).
   1. Anti-*Pseudomonas* penicillin plus aminoglycoside.
   2. Alternatives: Advanced-generation cephalosporin plus aminoglycoside or imipenem alone.

I. **Traumatic wounds** (*S. aureus,* group A streptococci, clostridiae, and Enterobacteriaceae).
1. Antitetanus prophylaxis.
2. Amoxicillin/clavulanic acid if less severe.
3. Ampicillin/sulbactam, cefoxitin, cefotetan, or equivalent parenterally.
4. Clindamycin with or without penicillin for invasive group A streptococci.

J. **Postoperative wounds:**
1. Nonsystemic (*S. aureus,* group A streptococci, and gram-negative organisms):
    a. First-generation cephalosporin or amoxicillin/clavulanic acid.
2. Septic:
    a. Penicillinase-resistant penicillin plus aminoglycoside or imipenem.
3. Involving GI or female genital tract (anaerobes and others):
    a. Clindamycin plus an aminoglycoside, ticarcillin/clavulanic acid, or imipenem.

K. **Orbital cellulitis:**
1. Children (*S. aureus, H. influenzae*):
    a. Cefuroxime with/without penicillinase-resistant penicillin.
    b. Advanced-generation cephalosporin or trimethoprim/sulfamethoxazole (TMP/SMX).
2. Adults (*S. aureus,* Enterobacteriaceae):
    a. Penicillinase-resistant penicillin plus aminoglycoside.
    b. Alternatives: Ampicillin/sulbactam, ticarcillin/clavulanic acid, or advanced-generation cephalosporin with/without vancomycin or penicillinase-resistant penicillin.

II. **Respiratory tract:**
A. **Ears:**
1. Malignant otitis externa (*P. aeruginosa*):
    a. Antipseudomonal penicillin plus an aminoglycoside, followed by ciprofloxacin for extended period, depending on need for surgical drainage, presence of osteomyelitis, etc.

2. Otitis media:
   a. Neonatal (pneumococci, *H. influenzae, S. aureus,* group A streptococci, Enterobacteriaceae):
      (1) Ampicillin plus gentamicin (or another regimen based on results of tympanocentesis).
   b. Infants, children, adults (pneumococci, *H. influenzae, Moraxella catarrhalis, S. aureus,* and group A streptococci):
      (1) Ampicillin, amoxicillin, erythromycin (plus sulfonamide in children <4 yr), or newer macrolides (e.g., clarithromycin).
         (a) Failure rates related to β-lactamase production of *H. influenzae* and *M. catarrhalis.*
      (2) Amoxicillin/clavulanic acid, cefaclor, cefprozil, cefuroxime, or TMP/SMX (not effective against group A streptococci).
3. Acute mastoiditis (pneumococci and *H. influenzae*):
   a. Cefuroxime, amoxicillin/clavulanic acid, or TMP/SMX.
   b. Chronic mastoiditis should be treated on basis of microbiology of surgical specimen.

B. **Sinusitis:**
   1. Acute (pneumococci, *H. influenzae,* group A streptococci, anaerobes, and rarely staphylococci):
      a. Ampicillin with low β-lactamase prevalence.
      b. Amoxicillin/clavulanic acid, cefaclor, cefuroxime, TMP/SMX with β-lactamase high prevalence.
      c. Newer macrolides (clarithromycin, azithromycin).
   2. Chronic (anaerobes):
      a. Clindamycin or ampicillin/sulbactam.
      b. PO amoxicillin/clavulanic acid.

C. **Pharyngitis:**
   1. Exudative (group A streptococci; *Arcanobacterium haemolyticum,* with scarlatiniform rash in teenagers).
      a. Other causes are infectious mononucleosis and
      · viruses.
      b. Penicillin (benzathine G IM or penicillin V PO for 10 days).
      c. Alternative: Erythromycin for 10 days.

  2. Membraneous (*Corynebacterium diphtheriae*):
     a. Diphtheria antitoxin plus tracheostomy gear at ready.
     b. Erythromycin.
     c. Alternatives include penicillin and rifampin.
 D. **Epiglottiditis** (*H. influenzae*):
  1. Cefuroxime or advanced-generation cephalosporin.
  2. Chloramphenicol as alternative.
 E. **Laryngitis** (most cases caused by viruses and need no therapy, except *M. catarrhalis,* which produces β-lactamase, common in adults): *Chlamydia pneumoniae.*
  1. Amoxicillin/clavulanic acid, TMP/SMX, cefaclor, cefuroxime, doxycycline, erythromycin (or a newer macrolide).
 F. **Bronchitis:**
  1. Infants/children (bronchiolitis secondary to respiratory syncytial virus):
     a. Consider aerosolized ribavirin if ICU required (contraindicated if patient is intubated and on respirator).
  2. Acute in adolescents and adults (*Mycoplasma pneumoniae,* viruses, or *Bordetella pertussis*):
     a. Erythromycin or newer macrolide.
     b. Alternative: Tetracycline.
  3. Chronic in adult smokers (pneumococci, *H. influenzae, M. catarrhalis*):
     a. Amoxicillin/clavulanic acid, TMP/SMX.
     b. Alternatives: PO cephalosporins (cefaclor, cefuroxime), tetracyclines, or newer macrolides.
 G. **Aspiration pneumonia:**
  1. No treatment initially mandated, and may select resistant suprainfection:
  2. Putrid abscess (anaerobes including *Bacteroides* spp.):
     a. Clindamycin.
     b. Alternatives: High-dose penicillin, cefoxitin, cefotetan, ampicillin/sulbactam.
 H. **Bronchopneumonia:**
  1. Neonatal:
     a. <5 days of age at onset (*Escherichia coli,* group A or B streptococci):
        (1) Ampicillin plus gentamicin.

   b. >5 days of age at onset (group A or B streptococci, *S. aureus, Chlamydia trachomatis, E. coli,* others):
      (1) Penicillinase-resistant penicillin plus gentamicin.
      (2) Erythromycin (or sulfisoxazole) with *C. trachomatis.*
         (a) Afebrile with staccato cough.
2. Infants and children to 2 yr of age (group A or B streptococci, *S. aureus,* gram-negative organisms):
   a. Penicillinase-resistant penicillin plus cefuroxime or advanced-generation cephalosporin.
3. Community-acquired:
   a. No underlying problems (pneumococci, *M. pneumoniae, Legionella* spp., and *C. pneumoniae*).
      (1) Erythromycin or newer macrolide.
      (2) Alternative: Tetracycline (perhaps better with *C. pneumoniae*).
   b. Chronic bronchitis (pneumococci, *H. influenzae, M. catarrhalis,* others):
      (1) Amoxicillin/clavulanic acid or TMP/SMX.
      (2) Alternatives: Tetracycline, cefaclor, cefuroxime.
   c. Chronic obstructive pulmonary disease (COPD), diabetes mellitus, alcoholism, nursing home (pneumococci, *H. influenzae,* group A streptococci, *Klebsiella* spp., staphylococci, *Legionella* spp., *C. pneumoniae,* others):
      (1) First- or second-generation cephalosporin plus aminoglycoside; penicillinase-resistant penicillin or vancomycin plus advanced-generation cephalosporin; imipenem; or ticarcillin/clavulanic acid.
         (a) Any regimen also includes erythromycin.
4. Hospital-acquired:
   a. Nonneutropenic:
      (1) Tracheostomy, previous antibiotics, etc. (resistant gram-negative bacilli, including *P. aeruginosa* plus *S. aureus*):
         (a) Penicillinase-resistant penicillin or vancomycin plus advanced-generation cephalosporin; advanced-generation

cephalosporin plus aminoglycoside; or
imipenem.
   (b) May be able to switch to PO ciprofloxacin.
a. Defective cell-mediated immunity (e.g., lymphoma
but not AIDS):
   (a) In addition to above pathogens, *Legionella, Nocardia,* and *Pneumocystis.*
   (b) Penicillinase-resistant penicillin plus
aminoglycoside plus erythromycin
with/without TMP/SMX.
b. Neutropenic (same pathogens as nonneutropenic,
fungi):
   (1) Penicillinase-resistant penicillin plus aminoglycoside or advanced-generation cephalosporin
plus erythromycin with/without TMP/SMX.
      (a) Amphotericin B added with no response or
if fungi found.
5. HIV infection (*Pneumocystis carinii,* cytomegalovirus
(CMV), herpes simplex virus (HSV), *Legionella* spp.,
Mycobacterium tuberculosis, and fungi):
a. TMP/SMX plus erythromycin.
b. If treating *P. carinii* pneumonia, add prednisone (if
Po_2 <70 on room air arterial blood gases).

I. **Lobar pneumonia:**
1. Community-acquired:
   a. No underlying disease (pneumococci, group A
streptococci):
      (1) Penicillin or ampicillin.
      (2) Alternatives: Erythromycin or newer macrolide,
or first-generation cephalosporin.
   b. Underlying disease such as COPD, diabetes mellitus, alcoholism (pneumococci, *H. influenzae,* group
A streptococci, *Klebsiella* spp., *S. aureus,* other
gram-negative organisms):
      (1) First- or second-generation cephalosporin plus
aminoglycoside; advanced-generation
cephalosporin; imipenem; ticarcillin/clavulanic
acid; or ampicillin/sulbactam (where
Pseudomonas not present).

III. **Bone and joint infections:**
  A. Osteomyelitis:
    1. Newborn (*S. aureus,* group A or B streptococci, or Enterobacteriaceae):
       a. Penicillinase-resistant penicillin plus advanced-generation cephalosporin.
    2. Children <3 yr (*H. influenzae,* streptococci):
       a. Cefuroxime or advanced-generation cephalosporin.
    3. Children >3 yr to adult (*S. aureus*):
       a. Penicillinase-resistant penicillin.
       b. Alternatives: Clindamycin, first-generation cephalosporin, vancomycin, or ciprofloxacin (only in adults).
    4. Drug addicts or postoperatively (*S. aureus,* Enterobacteriaceae, *P. aeruginosa*):
       a. Ciprofloxacin.
       b. Alternatives: Antistaphylococcal agent (e.g., first-generation cephalosporin or penicillinase-resistant penicillin) plus antipseudomonal agent (e.g., aminoglycoside or advanced-generation cephalosporin); imipenem.
    5. Adult with hemoglobinopathy (*S. aureus, Salmonella* spp., Enterobacteriaceae):
       a. Ampicillin/sulbactam or penicillinase-resistant penicillin plus ampicillin.
       b. Alternatives: First-generation cephalosporin or ciprofloxacin.
  B. **Arthritis:**
    1. Infants <3 mo (*S. aureus,* group B streptococci, Enterobacteriaceae):
       a. Penicillinase-resistant penicillin plus advanced-generation cephalosporin.
    2. Children 3 mo–2 yr (*H. influenzae, S. aureus, pneumococci*):
       a. Cefuroxime with/without penicillinase-resistant penicillin.
       b. Alternative: Vancomycin plus cefuroxime.

3. Children >2 yr (*S. aureus, H. influenzae,* group A streptococci):
   a. Cefuroxime with/without penicillinase-resistant
      penicillin.
4. Adult (gonococci, *S. aureus, H. influenzae,* group A
   streptococci, Enterobacteriaceae):
   a. Ceftriaxone as first choice with sexually transmitted
      disease exposure.
   b. Alternatives: Imipenem or penicillinase-resistant
      penicillin plus aminoglycoside.
5. Prosthetic joint, postoperative, post–intra-articular injection (*Staphylococcus epidermidis* or *S. aureus,* Enterobacteriaceae, *P. aeruginosa*):
   a. Vancomycin plus ceftazidime, aztreonam, or amino-
      glycoside.
   b. Alternatives: Imipenem or ciprofloxacin.

IV. **Intra-abdominal Infections:**
   A. **Dysentery** (*Shigella* spp., *Campylobacter jejuni, Salmo-
      nella* spp., *E. coli,* others):
      1. Ciprofloxacin.
      2. Alternatives: TMP/SMX (*C. jejuni* resistant).
   B. **Traveler's diarrhea** (enterotoxigenic *E. coli, Salmonella*
      spp., *Shigella* spp., *Campylobacter* spp., others):
      1. Ciprofloxacin.
      2. Alternatives: TMP/SMX and doxycycline.
   C. **Pseudomembranous colitis** (*Clostridium difficile*):
      1. Metronidazole.
      2. PO vancomycin.
   D. **Perirectal abscess:**
      1. Normal host (Enterobacteriaceae, anaerobes, entero-
         cocci):
         a. Rule out Crohn's disease.
         b. Surgical drainage plus ampicillin/sulbactam, cefox-
            itin, or cefotetan.
         c. Alternative antibiotic regimen of penicillin plus
            clindamycin plus aminoglycoside.
      2. HIV-infected patients (Enterobacteriaceae, anaerobes,
         enterococci):
         a. Rule out HSV infection and non-Hodgkin's lym-
            phoma.

   b. Same as above.
3. Neutropenic patients (same as above plus *P. aeruginosa*):
   a. Antipseudomonal penicillin plus aminoglycoside.
E. **Biliary tract infections,** including cholecystitis, cholangitis, and biliary sepsis (Enterobacteriaceae, anaerobes, and enterococci):
   1. Ampicillin/sulbactam, ticarcillin/clavulanic acid, or imipenem.
   2. Alternatives: Aminoglycoside plus cefoxitin or cefotetan.
F. **Hepatic abscess** (Enterobacteriaceae, enterococci, anaerobes, *S. aureus*):
   1. Rule out amebiasis serologically.
   2. Imipenem; ampicillin/sulbactam plus aminoglycoside; ticarcillin/clavulanic acid plus metronidazole.
   3. Alternative regimens according to microbiology.
G. **Diverticulitis** (Enterobacteriaceae, anaerobes, enterococci):
   1. TMP/SMX plus metronidazole.
   2. Alternatives: Ampicillin/sulbactam, cefoxitin, or cefotetan; clindamycin plus aminoglycoside.
H. **Peritonitis:**
   1. Primarily due to cirrhotic or nephrotic condition (pneumococci, group A streptococci, Enterobacteriaceae, *S. aureus*):
      a. Ampicillin/sulbactam, cefoxitin, cefotetan, or ticarcillin/clavulanate.
   2. Secondary to bowel perforation:
      a. Community-acquired (Enterobacteriaceae, enterococci, anaerobes):
         (1) Ampicillin/sulbactam, cefoxitin, cefotetan, or ticarcillin/clavulanic acid.
      b. Hospital-acquired or after antibiotic therapy (more resistant Enterobacteriaceae plus above):
         (1) Ampicillin/sulbactam, cefoxitin, cefotetan, or clindamycin plus aminoglycoside.
         (2) Alternatives: Imipenem, ticarcillin/clavulanic acid, metronidazole plus aminoglycoside.

      c. Associated with chronic ambulatory peritoneal dialysis (*S. epidermidis* or *S. aureus,* streptococci, Enterobacteriaceae):

        (1) Rule out candidal infection, which requires amphotericin B. Vancomycin plus tobramycin in dialysate (plus IV if patient systemically ill).

        (2) Cefuroxime or ceftazidime in dialysate.

V. Urinary tract infections:

A. **Acute urethral syndrome** (*C. trachomatis,* occasionally Enterobacteriaceae or gonococci):

    1. Doxycycline or tetracycline.

B. **Acute cystitis** (Enterobacteriaceae, almost always *E. coli; Staphylococcus saphrophyticus*):

    1. TMP/SMX or ampicillin/amoxicillin.

C. **Pyelonephritis:**

    1. Nonseptic (Enterobacteriaceae):

      a. TMP/SMX.

      b. Alternatives: Ampicillin, ciprofloxacin, norfloxacin, others.

    2. Septic or after urologic procedure (Enterobacteriaceae, *P. aeruginosa*):

      a. Ampicillin plus aminoglycoside; imipenem; advanced-generation cephalosporin, e.g., ceftazidime or cefoperazone; ticarcillin/clavulanic acid; or a quinolone, e.g., norfloxacin or ciprofloxacin.

D. **Prostatitis**

    1. Acute (Enterobacteriaceae, *P. aeruginosa*):

      a. Fluoroquinolone (ciprofloxacin or ofloxacin) or TMP/SMX.

      b. Alternatives: Tetracycline/doxycycline or ampicillin without *Pseudomonas.*

    2. **Chronic (Enterobacteriaceae):**

      a. TMP/SMX or ciprofloxacin.

VI. **CNS infections:**

A. **Brain abscess:**

    1. Secondary to sinusitis or cyanotic congenital heart disease (streptococci):

      a. High-dose penicillin.

      b. Advanced-generation cephalosporin.

2. Secondary to otitis media, mastoiditis, or lung abscess (anaerobes and Enterobacteriaceae):
   a. High-dose penicillin plus metronidazole plus advanced-generation cephalosporin.
3. Postoperative or posttraumatic (*S. aureus,* Enterobacteriaceae):
   a. Nafcillin plus advanced-generation cephalosporin.

B. **Meningitis:**
1. Infants <1 mo (multiple pathogens possible, including group B or D streptococci, Enterobacteriaceae, *Listeria, H. influenzae,* meningococci, pneumococci):
   a. Ampicillin plus aminoglycoside or advanced-generation cephalosporin.
2. Infants 1–3 mo (*H. influenzae,* pneumococci, meningococci, and group B streptococci):
   a. Ampicillin plus advanced-generation cephalosporin.
   b. Some authorities recommend dexamethasone in addition to antibiotics.
3. Children >3 mo–<10 yr (*H. influenzae,* pneumococci, and meningococci):
   a. Vancomycin plus advanced-generation cephalosporin (ceftriaxone, cefotaxime, ceftazidime):
   b. Alternatives: Cefuroxime or ampicillin plus chloramphenicol.
   c. Some authorities recommend dexamethasone in addition to antibiotics.
4. Adult:
   a. Noncompromised (meningococci, pneumococci, group A streptococci):
      (1) Vancomycin plus advanced-generation cephalosporin (ceftriaxone, cefotaxime, ceftazidime).
      (2) Alternatives: Chloramphenicol, advanced-generation cephalosporin.
      (3) Some authorities recommend dexamethasone in addition to antibiotics.
   b. Compromised: Immunosuppression, alcoholism, elderly (above plus Enterobacteriaceae, *H. influenzae, P. aeruginosa, Listeria*):

(1) Ceftazidime plus aminoglycoside.

(2) Ampicillin added with *Listeria.*

5. Postoperative (*S. aureus, P. aeruginosa,* Enterobacteriaceae):

a. Vancomycin (nafcillin if not MRSA) plus ceftazidime plus aminoglycoside (and consider also intrathecal gentamicin if ventriculitis present).

6. Posttraumatic:

a. Early: onset within 3 days (pneumococci, group A streptococci):

(1) Vancomycin (and await cultures and discontinue vancomycin if alternative options).

(2) Alternative: Chloramphenicol.

b. Late: Onset after 3 days (same as postoperative):

(1) Vancomycin (nafcillin if not MRSA) plus ceftazidime plus aminoglycoside.

Appendix B
TETANUS PROPHYLAXIS

TABLE B–1.

Characteristics of Tetanus Prone Wounds

Wound age >6 hr
Devitalized tissue present
Wound contamination
Deep wound (>1 cm)
Nonlinear wound edge
Avulsion
Crush injury
Burn injury
Hypothermic injury

TABLE B–2.

Immunization Schedule

History of Tetanus Immunization	Tetanus-Prone Wound		Non–Tetanus-Prone Wound	
	TD*†	TIG	Td	TIG
Unknown or <3 doses	Yes	Yes	Yes	No
3 or more doses	No‡	No	No§	No

*Td—Tetanus and diphtheria toxoids, adsorbed (adult); TIG—tetanus immune globulin (human).
†Yes if wound >24 hr old. For children <7 yr, DPT (DT if pertussis vaccine contraindicated); for persons ≥7 yr, Td preferred to tetanus toxoid alone.
‡Yes if >5 yr since last booster.
§Yes if >10 yr since last booster.

Adapted from MMWR 1990, 39:37.

Appendix C

RABIES PREVENTION

I. **Vaccines:**
   A. **Human diploid cell rabies vaccine (HDCV):**
      1. Inactivated virus vaccine.
      2. Supplied as 1.0 mL single-dose vials of lyophilized vaccine with accompanying diluent.
   B. **Rabies vaccine, adsorbed (RVA):**
      1. Inactivated and absorbed to aluminum phosphate.
      2. Supplied as 1.0 mg single-dose vials of liquid vaccine.
II. **Rabies immune globulin, human (HRIG):**
   A. 150 international units (IU) per mL.
   B. Supplied in 2 mL (300 IU) and 10 mL (500 IU) vials for pediatric and adult use, respectively.
III. **Rabies postexposure prophylaxis guide:** The recommendations in Table C–1 are only a guide. In applying them, take into account the animal species involved, the circumstances of the bite or other exposure, the vaccination status of the animal, and the presence of rabies in the region. Local and state public health officials should be consulted if questions arise about the need for rabies prophylaxis.

BIBLIOGRAPHY

MMWR 1991, 40:RR–3.

TABLE C–1.

Rabies Postexposure Prophylaxis
All wounds should be cleaned immediately and thoroughly with
soap and water.
This has been shown to protect 90% of experimental animals!

Postexposure Prophylaxis Guide, United States, 1991

Animal Type	Evaluation and Disposition of Animal	Recommendations for Prophylaxis
Dogs, cats	Healthy and available for 10-day observation	Do not start unless animal develops sx, then immediately begin HRIG + HDCV or RVA
	Rabid or suspected rabid	Immediate vaccination
	Unknown (escaped)	Consult public health officials
Skunks, raccoons, bats, foxes, most carnivores	Regard as rabid	Immediate vaccination
Livestock, rodents, rabbits; includes hares squirrels, hamsters, guinea pigs, gerbils, chipmunks, rats, mice		Almost never require antirabies rx

Appendix D
PROPHYLAXIS OF VIRAL HEPATITIS

I. **Hepatitis A:**
   A. **Preexposure prophylaxis:**
      1. The major group for whom preexposure prophylaxis is recommended is international travelers. The risk of hepatitis A for US citizens traveling abroad varies with living conditions, length of stay, and the incidence of hepatitis A infection in areas visited. In general, travelers to developed areas of North America, western Europe, Japan, Australia, and New Zealand are at no greater risk of infection than they would be in the United States. For travelers to developing countries, risk of infection increases with duration of travel and is highest for those who live in or visit rural areas, trek in back country, or frequently eat or drink in settings of poor sanitation. Nevertheless, studies have shown that many cases of travel-related hepatitis A occur in travelers with "standard" tourist itineraries, accommodations, and food and beverage consumption behaviors. In developing countries, travelers should minimize their exposure to hepatitis A and other enteric diseases by avoiding potentially contaminated water or food. Travelers should avoid drinking water (or beverages with ice) of unknown purity and eating uncooked shellfish or uncooked fruits or vegetables that they did not prepare.
      2. Immune globulin (IG) is recommended for all susceptible travelers to developing countries. IG is especially important for persons who will be living in or visiting rural areas, eating, or drinking in settings of poor or uncertain sanitation, or who will have close contact with local persons (especially young children) in settings with poor sanitary conditions. Persons who plan

to reside in developing areas for long periods should receive IG regularly.

3. A hepatitis A vaccine is now available for use in preexposure prophylaxis.

B. **Postexposure prophylaxis:**

Hepatitis A cannot be reliably diagnosed on clinical presentation alone, and serologic confirmation of index patients is recommended before contacts are treated. Serologic screening of contacts for anti–hepatitis A virus (HAV) before they are given IG is not recommended because screening is more costly than IG and would delay its administration.

For postexposure IG prophylaxis, a single IM dose of 0.02 mL/kg is recommended. IG should be given as soon as possible after last exposure; giving IG more than 2 wk after exposure is not indicated.

Specific recommendations for IG prophylaxis for hepatitis A depend on the nature of the HAV exposure.

1. **Close personal contact.** IG is recommended for all household and sexual contacts of persons with hepatitis A.

2. **Day care centers.** Day care facilities attended by children in diapers can be important settings for HAV transmission. IG should be administered to all staff and attendees of day care centers or homes if (1) one or more children or employees are diagnosed as having hepatitis A or (2) cases are recognized in two or more households of center attendees. When an outbreak (hepatitis cases in three or more families) occurs, IG should also be considered for members of households that have children (center attendees) in diapers. In centers not enrolling children in diapers, IG need be given only to classroom contacts of an index patient.

3. **Schools.** Contact at elementary and secondary schools is usually not an important means of transmitting hepatitis A. Routine administration of IG is not indicated for pupils and teachers in contact with a patient. However, when an epidemiologic investigation clearly shows the existence of a school- or classroom-centered

outbreak, IG may be given to persons who have close contact with patients.

4. **Institutions for custodial care.** Living conditions in some institutions, such as prisons and facilities for the developmentally disabled, favor transmission of hepatitis A. When outbreaks occur, giving IG to residents and staff who have close contact with patients with hepatitis A may reduce the spread of disease. Depending on the epidemiologic circumstances, prophylaxis can be limited or can involve the entire institution.

5. **Hospitals.** Routine IG prophylaxis for hospital personnel is not indicated. Rather, sound hygienic practices should be emphasized. Staff education should point out the risk of exposure to hepatitis A and emphasize precautions regarding direct contact with potentially infective materials. Outbreaks of hepatitis A among hospital staff may occur. In outbreaks, prophylaxis of persons exposed to feces of infected patients may be indicated.

6. **Offices and factories.** Routine IG administration is not indicated under the usual office or factory conditions for persons exposed to a fellow worker with hepatitis A. Experience shows that casual contact in the work setting does not result in virus transmission.

7. **Common-source exposure.** IG use might be effective in preventing foodborne or waterborne hepatitis A if exposure is recognized in time. However, IG is not recommended for persons exposed to a common source of hepatitis infection after cases have begun to occur, since the 2-wk period during which IG is effective will have been exceeded.

If a food handler is diagnosed as having hepatitis A, common-source transmission is possible but uncommon. IG should be administered to other food handlers but is usually not recommended for patrons. However, IG administration to patrons may be considered if all the following conditions exist: (1) the infected person is directly involved in handling, without gloves, foods that will not be cooked before they are eaten; (2) the hygienic practices of the food handler are deficient or the food handler has had diarrhea; and (3) patrons can be identified and treated within 2 wk of exposure. Situations in which repeated exposures may have occurred, such as in institutional cafeterias, may warrant stronger consideration of IG use.

8. **A hepatitis A vaccine** is now available for use in post-exposure prophylaxis.

II. **Hepatitis B:**

A. **Hepatitis B prophylaxis:** Two types of products are available for prophylaxis against hepatitis B. Hepatitis B vaccines, first licensed in 1981, provide active immunization against hepatitis B virus (HBV) infection, and their use is recommended for both preexposure and postexposure prophylaxis. Hepatitis B immune globulin (HBIG) provides temporary, passive protection and is indicated only in certain postexposure settings.

1. **HBIG:** HBIG is prepared from plasma preselected to contain a high titer of anti-HBs. In the United States, HBIG has an anti-HBs titer of >100,000 by radioimmunoassay (RIA). Human plasma from which HBIG is prepared is screened for antibodies to HIV; in addition, the Cohn fractionation process used to prepare this product inactivates and eliminates HIV from the final product. There is no evidence that the causative agent of AIDS (HIV) has been transmitted by HBIG.

2. **Hepatitis B vaccine:**

a. Two types of hepatitis B vaccines are currently licensed in the United States: Genetically engineered vaccine (hepatitis B vaccine, recombinant) and plasma derived vaccine. Plasma-derived vaccine consists of a suspension of inactivated, alum-adsorbed, 22-nm, HBsAg particles that have been purified from human plasma by a combination of biophysical (ultracentrifugation) and biochemical procedures. Inactivation is a threefold process using 8M urea, pepsin at pH 2, and 1 : 4000 formalin. These treatment steps have been shown to inactivate representatives of all classes of viruses found in human blood, including HIV. Plasma-derived vaccine is no longer being produced in the United States, and use is now limited to hemodialysis patients, other immunocompromised hosts, and persons with known allergy to yeast.

b. Vaccine usage: Primary vaccination comprises three IM doses of vaccine, with the second and third doses given 1 and 6 mo, respectively, after the first. Adults and older children should be given a full 1.0 mL/dose; children <11 yr of age should usually receive one half this dose (0.5 mL). An alternative schedule of four doses of vaccine given at 0, 1, 2, and 12 mo has been approved for one vaccine for postexposure prophylaxis or for more rapid induction of immunity. However, there is no clear evidence that this regimen provides greater protection than the standard three-dose series. Hepatitis B vaccine should be given only in the deltoid muscle for adults and children or in the anterolateral thigh muscle for infants and neonates.

For patients undergoing hemodialysis and for other immunosuppressed patients, higher vaccine doses (2 mL) or increased numbers of doses are required. Persons with HIV infection have an impaired response to hepatitis B vaccine. The immunogenicity of higher doses of vaccine is unknown for this group, and firm recommendations on dosage cannot be made at this time.

Vaccine doses administered at longer intervals provide equally satisfactory protection, but optimal protection is not conferred until after the third dose. If the vaccine series is interrupted after the first dose, the second and third doses should be given separated by an interval of 3–5 mo. Persons who are late for the third dose should be given this dose when convenient. Postvaccination testing is not considered necessary in either situation.

3. **Persons for whom hepatitis B prophylaxis is recommended or should be considered:**
   a. Preexposure:
      (1) Health care and public safety workers having blood or needle-stick exposures.
      (2) Clients and staff of institutions for the developmentally disabled.
      (3) Hemodialysis patients.
      (4) Sexually active homosexual men.

(5) Users of illicit injectable drugs.

(6) Recipients of certain blood products (clotting factor concentrates).

(7) Household members and sexual contacts of HBV carriers.

(8) Members of families accepting as adoptees orphans or unaccompanied minors from countries of high or intermediate HBV endemicity. (Family members should be vaccinated if adoptee children are found to be HBsAg positive on screening laboratory examination.)

(9) Other contacts of HBV carriers (e.g., workers at child care centers where special circumstances exist such as behavior problems or medical conditions that could facilitate transmission).

(10) Members of populations with high endemicity of HBV infection (e.g., Alaskan Natives, Pacific Islanders, and immigrants and refugees from HBV-endemic areas).

(11) Inmates of long-term correctional facilities.

(12) Sexually active heterosexual persons with multiple sexual partners.

(13) International travelers (when travel to an area with high levels of endemic HBV and close contact with the local population are anticipated).

   b. Postexposure:

(1) Infants born to HBsAg-positive mothers (perinatal exposure).

(2) Persons having percutaneous or permucosal exposure to HBsAg-positive blood.

(3) Persons having sexual exposure to a HBsAg-positive person.

(4) Infants <12 mo of age exposed in the household to a primary caregiver who has acute hepatitis B.

4. **Perinatal exposure and recommendations:**

   a. Transmission of HBV from mother to infant during the perinatal period represents one of the most efficient modes of HBV infection and often leads to severe long-term sequelae. Infants born to HBsAg-positive and HBeAg-positive mothers have a 70%–90% chance of acquiring perinatal HBV infection, and 85%–90% of infected infants will become chronic HBV carriers. Estimates are that >25% of these carriers will die from primary hepatocellular carcinoma (PHC) or cirrhosis of the liver. Infants born to HBsAg-positive and HBeAg-negative mothers have a lower risk of acquiring perinatal infection; however, such infants have had acute disease, and fatal fulminant hepatitis has been reported. On the basis of 1987 U.S. data, an estimated 18,000 births occur to HBsAg-positive women each year, resulting in approximately 4000 infants who become chronic HBV carriers. Prenatal screening of all pregnant women identifies those who are HBsAg positive and allows treatment of their newborns with HBIG and hepatitis B vaccine, a regimen that is 85%–95% effective in preventing the development of the HBV chronic carrier state.

b. The following are perinatal recommendations:

(1) All pregnant women should be routinely tested for HBsAg during an early prenatal visit in each pregnancy. This testing should be done at the same time that other routine prenatal screening tests are ordered. In special situations (e.g., when acute hepatitis is suspected, when a history of exposure to hepatitis has been reported, or when the mother has a particularly high-risk behavior, such as IV drug abuse), an additional HBsAg test can be ordered later in the pregnancy. No other HBV marker tests are necessary for the purpose of maternal screening, although HBsAg-positive mothers identified during screening may have HBV-related acute or chronic liver disease and should be evaluated by their physicians.

(2) If a woman has not been screened prenatally or if test results are not available at the time of admission for delivery, HBsAg testing should be done at the time of admission, or as soon as pos-

sible thereafter. If the mother is identified as HBsAg positive >1 mo after giving birth, the infant should be tested for HBsAg. If the results are negative, the infant should be given HBIG and hepatitis B vaccine.

(3) Following all initial positive tests for HBsAg, a repeat test for HBsAg should be performed on the same specimen, followed by a confirmatory test using a neutralization assay. For women in labor who did not have HBsAg testing during pregnancy and who are found to be HBsAg positive on first testing, initiation of treatment of their infants should not be delayed by more than 24 hr for repeat or confirmatory testing.

(4) Infants born to HBsAg-positive mothers should receive HBIG (0.5 mL) IM once they are physiologically stable, preferably within 12 hr of birth. Hepatitis B vaccine should be administered IM at the appropriate infant dose. The first dose should be given concurrently with HBIG but at a different site. If vaccine is not immediately available, the first dose should be given as soon as possible. Subsequent doses should be given as recommended for the specific vaccine. Testing infants for HBsAg and anti-HBs is recommended when they are 12–15 mo of age to monitor the success or failure of therapy. If HBsAg is not detectable and anti-HBs is present, children can be considered protected. Testing for anti-HBc is not useful, since maternal anti-HBc can persist for >1 yr. HBIG and hepatitis B vaccinations do not interfere with routine childhood vaccinations. Breast-feeding poses no risk of HBV infection for infants who have begun prophylaxis.

(5) Household members and sexual partners of HBV carriers identified through prenatal screening should be tested to determine susceptibility to HBV infection, and if susceptible should receive hepatitis B vaccine.

(6) Obstetric and pediatric staff should be notified directly about HBsAg-positive mothers so that neonates can receive therapy without delay after birth and follow-up doses of vaccine can be given. Programs to coordinate the activities of persons providing prenatal care, hospital-based obstetric services, and pediatric well-baby care must be established to ensure proper follow-up and treatment both of infants born to HBsAg-positive mothers and of other susceptible household and sexual contacts.

(7) In those populations under U.S. jurisdiction in which hepatitis B infection is highly endemic (including certain Alaskan Natives, Pacific Island groups, and refugees from highly endemic areas accepted for resettlement in the United States), universal vaccination of newborns with hepatitis B vaccine is the recommended strategy for hepatitis B control. HBsAg screening of mothers and use of HBIG for infants born to HBV-carrier mothers may be added to routine hepatitis B vaccination when practical, but screening and HBIG alone will not adequately protect children from HBV infection in endemic areas. In such areas, hepatitis B vaccine doses should be integrated into the childhood vaccination schedule. More extensive programs of childhood hepatitis B vaccination should be considered if resources are available.

5. **Acute exposure to blood that contains (or might contain) HBsAg:**

For accidental percutaneous (needlestick, laceration, or bite) or permucosal (ocular or mucous membrane) exposure to blood, the decision to provide prophylaxis must include consideration of several factors: (1) whether the source of the blood is available, (2) the HBsAg status of the source, and (3) the hepatitis B vaccination and vaccine-response status of the exposed person. Such exposures usually affect persons for whom hepatitis B vaccine is recommended. For any exposure of a person not previously vaccinated, hepatitis B vaccination is recommended.

Following any such exposure, a blood sample should be obtained from the person who was the source of the exposure, and should be tested for HBsAg. The hepatitis B vaccination status and anti-HBs response status (if known) of the exposed person should be reviewed. The outline below summarizes prophylaxis for percutaneous or permucosal exposure to blood according to the HBsAg status of the source of exposure, and the vaccination status and vaccine response of the exposed person.

For greatest effectiveness, passive prophylaxis with HBIG, when indicated, should be given as soon as possible after exposure (its value beyond 7 days after exposure is unclear).

a. Source of exposure HBsAg positive:

   (1) The exposed person has not been vaccinated or has not completed vaccination. Hepatitis B vaccination should be initiated. A single dose of HBIG (0.06 mL/kg) should be given as soon as possible after exposure and within 24 hr, if possible. The first dose of hepatitis B vaccine should be given IM at a separate site (deltoid for adults) and can be given simultaneously with HBIG or within 7 days of exposure. Subsequent doses should be given as recommended for the specific vaccine. If the exposed person has begun but not completed vaccination, one dose of HBIG should be given immediately, and vaccination should be completed as scheduled.

   (2) The exposed person has already been vaccinated against hepatitis B, and anti-HBs response status is known.

      (a) If the exposed person is known to have had adequate response in the past, the anti-HBs level should be tested unless an adequate level has been demonstrated within the last 24 mo. Although current data show that vaccine-inducd protection does not decrease as antibody level wanes, most experts consider the following approach to be prudent:

(1) If anti-HBs level is adequate, no treatment is necessary.

(2) If anti-HBs level is inadequate,* a booster dose of hepatitis B vaccine should be given.

    (b) If the exposed person is known not to have responded to the primary vaccine series, he or she should be given either a single dose of HBIG and a dose of hepatitis B vaccine as soon as possible after exposure, or two doses of HBIG (0.06 mL/kg), one given as soon as possible after exposure and the second 1 mo later. The latter treatment is preferred for those who have failed to respond to at least four doses of vaccine.

(3) The exposed person has already been vaccinated against hepatitis B, and the anti-HBs response is unknown. He or she should be tested for anti-HBs.

    (a) If the exposed person has adequate antibody, no additional treatment is necessary.

    (b) If the exposed person has inadequate antibody on testing, one dose of HBIG (0.06 mL/kg) should be given immediately and a standard booster dose of vaccine given at a different site.

b. Source of exposure known and HBsAg negative:

    (1) The exposed person has not been vaccinated or has not completed vaccination. If unvaccinated, he or she should be given the first dose of hepatitis B vaccine within 7 days of exposure, and vaccination should be completed as recommended. If the exposed person has not completed vaccination, vaccination should be completed as scheduled.

*An adequate antibody level is ≥10 milli-International units (mIU)/mL, approximately equivalent to 10 sample ratio units (SRU) by RIA or positive by EIA.

      (2) The exposed person has already been vaccinated against hepatitis B. No treatment is necessary.

  c. Source of exposure unknown or not available for testing:

      (1) The exposed person has not been vaccinated or has not completed vaccination. If unvaccinated, he or she should be given the first dose of hepatitis B vaccine within 7 days of exposure, and vaccination should be completed as recommended. If the exposed person has not completed vaccination, vaccination should be completed as scheduled.

      (2) The exposed person has already been vaccinated against hepatitis B, and anti-HBs response status is known.

         (a) If the exposed person is known to have had adequate response in the past, no treatment is necessary.

         (b) If the exposed person is known not to have responded to the vaccine, prophylaxis as described earlier under "Source of exposure HBsAg positive" may be considered if the source of the exposure is known to be at high risk of HBV infection.

      (3) The exposed person has already been vaccinated against hepatitis B, and the anti-HBs response is unknown. He or she should be tested for anti-HBs.

         (a) If the exposed person has adequate anti-HBs, no treatment is necessary.

         (b) If the exposed person has inadequate anti-HBs, a standard booster dose of vaccine should be given.

6. **Sexual partners of persons with acute HBV infection:**

  a. Sexual partners of HBsAg-positive persons are at increased risk of acquiring HBV infection, and HBIG has been shown to be 75% effective in preventing such infections. Because data are limited, the period after sexual exposure during which HBIG is effective is unknown, but extrapolation from other settings makes it unlikely that this period would exceed 14 days. Before treatment, testing of sexual partners for susceptibility is recommended if it does not delay treatment beyond 14 days after last exposure. Testing for anti-HBc is the most efficient prescreening test to use in this population.

b. All susceptible persons whose sexual partners have acute hepatitis B infection or whose sexual partners are discovered to be hepatitis B carriers should receive a single dose of HBIG (0.06 mL/kg) and should begin the hepatitis B vaccine series if prophylaxis can be started within 14 days of the last sexual contact, or if ongoing sexual contact with the infected person will occur. Giving the vaccine with HBIG may improve the efficacy of postexposure treatment. The vaccine has the added advantage of conferring long-lasting protection.

c. An alternative treatment for persons who are not from a high-risk group for whom vaccine is routinely recommended and whose regular sexual partners have acute HBV infection is to give one dose of HBIG (without vaccine) and retest the sexual partner for HBsAg 3 mo later. No further treatment is necessary if the sexual partner becomes HBsAg negative. If the sexual partner remains HBsAg positive, a second dose of HBIG should be given and the hepatitis B vaccine series started.

7. **Household contacts of persons with acute HBV infection:** Since infants have close contact with primary caregivers and have a higher risk of becoming HBV carriers after acute HBV infection, prophylaxis of an infant <12 mo of age with HBIG (0.5 mL) and hepatitis B vaccine is indicated if the mother or primary caregiver has acute HBV infection. Prophylaxis for other household contacts of persons with acute HBV infection is not indicated unless they have had identifiable blood exposure to the index patient, such as by sharing toothbrushes or razors. Such exposures should be treated similarly to sexual exposures. If the index patient becomes an HBV carrier, all household contacts should be given hepatitis B vaccine.

III. **Hepatitis C:**

Hepatitis C accounts for 20%–40% of acute viral hepatitis in the United States and has epidemiologic characteristics similar to those of hepatitis B. Groups at high risk of acquiring this disease include transfusion recipients, parenteral drug users, and dialysis patients. Health care work that entails frequent contact with blood, personal contact with others who have had hepatitis in the past, and contact with infected persons within households has also been documented in some studies as risk factors for acquiring hepatitis C. However, the role of person-to-person contact in disease transmission has not been well defined, and the importance of sexual activity in the transmission of this type of hepatitis is unclear.

An average of 50% of patients who have acute hepatitis C infection later develop chronic hepatitis.

The risk of perinatal transmission of hepatitis C is not well defined but appears to be low.

The results have been equivocal in several studies attempting to assess the value of prophylaxis with IGs against hepatitis C. For persons with percutaneous exposure to blood from a patient with hepatitis C, it may be reasonable to administer IG (0.06 mL/kg) as soon as possible after exposure. In other circumstances, no specific recommendations can be made.

IV. **Hepatitis D:**

The hepatitis D virus (HDV) (also known as delta virus) is a defective virus that may cause infection only in the presence of active HBV infection. The HDV is a 35- to 37-nm viral particle, consisting of single-stranded RNA (mw 500,000) and an internal protein antigen (delta antigen [HDAg]), coated with HBsAg as the surface protein. Infection may occur as either coinfection with HBV or superinfection of an HBV carrier, each of which usually causes an episode of clinical acute hepatitis. Coinfection usually resolves, whereas superinfection frequently causes chronic HDV infection and chronic active hepatitis. Both types of infection may cause fulminant hepatitis.

HDV infection may be diagnosed by detecting various markers (HDAg, total or IgM-specific anti-HDV) in serum.

Routes of transmission of HDV are similar to those of HBV. In the United States, HDV infection most commonly affects persons at high risk of HBV infection, particularly parenteral drug abusers and persons with hemophilia.

Since HDV is dependent on HBV for replication, prevention of hepatitis B infection, either before or after exposure, will suffice to prevent HDV infection for a person susceptible to hepatitis B. Known episodes of perinatal, sexual, or percutaneous exposure to serum, or exposure to persons known to be positive for both HBV and HDV, should be treated exactly as such exposures to HBV alone.

Persons who are HBsAg carriers are at risk of HDV infection, especially if they participate in activities that put them at high risk of repeated exposure to HBV (parenteral drug abuse, male homosexual activity). However, at present no products are available that might prevent HDV infection in HBsAg carriers either before or after exposure.

V. **Hepatitis E:**

Hepatitis E is a distinct type of hepatitis acquired by the fecal-oral route. It was first identified through investigations of large waterborne epidemics in developing countries. This enterically transmitted hepatitis, which has occurred in epidemics or sporadically in parts of Asia, North and West Africa, and Mexico, is distinct from other hepatitis viruses. Young to middle-aged adults are most often affected, with an unusually high mortality rate among pregnant women.

Hepatitis E has not been recognized as an endemic disease in the United States or Western Europe. Cases have been documented among persons returning from travel to countries in which this disease occurs.

Travelers to areas having hepatitis E may be at some risk of acquiring this disease by close contact with infected persons or by consuming contaminated food or water. There is no evidence that U.S.-manufactured IG will prevent this infection. As with hepatitis A and other enteric infections, the best means of preventing hepatitis E is avoiding potentially contaminated food or water.

BIBLIOGRAPHY

Prevention of viral hepatitis, *MMWR* 1990, 39: 1-26.

Appendix E
PREVENTION OF INFECTIVE ENDOCARDITIS

TABLE E-1.
Cardiac Conditions*

Endocarditis Prophylaxis Recommended

Prosthetic cardiac valves, including bioprosthetic and homograft valves
Previous bacterial endocarditis, even in the absence of heart disease
Most congenital cardiac malformations
Rheumatic and other acquired valvular dysfunction, even after valvular surgery
Hypertrophic cardiomyopathy
Mitral valve prolapse with valvular regurgitation

Endocarditis Prophylaxis Not Recommended

Isolated secundum atrial septal defect
Surgical repair without residua beyond 6 mo of secundum atrial septal defect,
    ventricular septal defect, or patent ductus arteriosus
Previous coronary artery bypass graft surgery
Mitral valve prolapse without valvular regurgitation†
Physiologic, functional, or innocent heart murmurs
Previous Kawasaki disease without valvular dysfunction
Previous rheumatic fever without valvular dysfunction
Cardiac pacemakers and implanted defibrillators

*This table lists selected conditions but is not meant to be all-inclusive.
†Individuals who have a mitral valve prolapse associated with thickening and/or redundancy of the valve leaflets may be at increased risk for bacterial endocarditis, particularly men 45 years of age or older.

TABLE E-2.

Dental or Surgical Procedures*

Endocarditis Prophylaxis Recommended

Dental procedures known to induce gingival or mucosal bleeding, including
  professional cleaning

Tonsillectomy and/or adenoidectomy

Surgical operations that involve intestinal or respiratory mucosa

Bronchoscopy with a rigid bronchoscope

Sclerotherapy for esophageal varices

Esophageal dilatation

Gallbladder surgery

Cystoscopy

Urethral dilatation

Urethral catheterization if urinary tract infection is present†

Urinary tract surgery if urinary tract infection is present†

Prostatic surgery

Incision and drainage of infected tissue†

Vaginal hysterectomy

Vaginal delivery in the presence of infection†

Endocarditis Prophylaxis Not Recommended‡

Dental procedures not likely to induce gingival bleeding, such as simple
  adjustment of orthodontic appliances or fillings above the gum line

Injection of local intraoral anesthetic (except intraligamentary injections)

Shedding of primary teeth

Tympanostomy tube insertion

Endotracheal intubation

Bronchoscopy with a flexible bronchoscope, with or without biopsy

Cardiac catheterization

Endoscopy with or without gastrointestinal biopsy

Cesarean section

In the absence of infection for urethral catheterization, dilatation and curettage,
  uncomplicated vaginal delivery, therapeutic abortion, sterilization procedures,
  or insertion or removal of intrauterine devices

*This table lists selected procedures but is not meant to be all-inclusive.
†In addition to prophylactic regimen for genitourinary procedures, antibiotic
therapy should be directed against the most likely bacterial pathogen.
‡In patients who have prosthetic heart valves, a history of endocarditis or of
surgically constructed systemic-pulmonary shunts or conduits, physicians may
choose to administer prophylactic antibiotics even for low-risk procedures that
involve the lower respiratory, genitourinary, or GI tracts.

TABLE E-3.

Recommended Standard Prophylactic Regimen for Dental, Oral, or Upper Respiratory Tract Procedures in Patients at Risk*

Drug	Dosing Regiment†
	Standard Regimen
Amoxicillin	3.0 g PO 1 hr before procedure, then 1.5 g 6 hr after initial dose
	Amoxicillin/Penicillin-Allergic Patients
Erythromycin	Erythromycin ethylsuccinate, 800 mg, or erythromycin stearate, 1.0 g PO 2 hr before procedure, then half
or	the dose 6 hr after initial dose
Clindamycin	300 mg PO 1 hr before procedure and 150 mg 6 hr after initial dose

*Includes those with prosthetic heart valves and other high-risk patients.
†Initial pediatric doses are as follows: Amoxicillin, 50 mg/kg; erythromycin ethylsuccinate or erythromycin stearate, 20 mg/kg; clindamycin, 10 mg/kg. Follow-up doses should be one half the initial dose. Total pediatric dose should not exceed total adult dose. The following weight ranges may also be used for the initial pediatric dose of amoxicillin: <15 kg, 750 mg; 15–30 kg, 1500 mg; >30 kg, 3000 mg (full adult dose).

TABLE E-4.

Alternate Prophylactic Regimens for Dental, Oral, or Upper Respiratory Tract Procedures in Patients at Risk

Drug	Dosing Regimen†
Patients Unable to Take Oral Medications	
Ampicillin	IV or IM administration of ampicillin 2.0 g 30 min before procedure; then IV or IM administration of ampicillin, 1.0 g or PO administration of amoxicillin, 1.5 g 6 hr after initial dose
Ampicillin/Amoxicillin/Penicillin-Allergic Patients Unable to Take Oral Medications	
Clindamycin	IV administration of 300 mg 30 min before procedure and IV or PO administration of 150 mg 6 hr after initial dose
Patients Considered High Risk and Not Candidates for Standard Regimen	
Ampicillin, gentamicin, and amoxicillin	IV or IM administration of ampicillin, 2.0 g, plus gentamicin, 1.5 mg/kg (not to exceed 80 mg), 30 min before procedure; followed by amoxicillin, 1.5 g PO 6 hr after initial dose; alternatively, parenteral regimen may be repeated 8 hr after initial dose
Ampicillin/Amoxicillin/Penicillin-Allergic Patients Considered High Risk	
Vancomycin	IV administration of 1.0 g over 1 hr, starting 1 hr before procedure; no repeated dose necessary

*Initial pediatric doses are as follows: Ampicillin, 50 mg/kg; clindamycin, 10 mg/kg; gentamicin, 2.0 mg/kg; vancomycin, 20 mg/kg. Follow-up doses should be one half the initial dose. **Total pediatric dose should not exceed total adult dose.** No initial dose is recommended in this table for amoxicillin (25 mg/kg is the follow-up dose).

TABLE E-5.

Regimens for Genitourinary/Gastrointestinal Procedures

Drug	Dosing Regimen*
	Standard Regimen
Ampicillin, gentamicin, and amoxicillin	IV or IM administration of ampicillin, 2.0 g, plus gentamicin, 1.5 mg/kg (not to exceed 80 mg), 30 min before procedure; followed by amoxicillin, 1.5 g, PO 6 hr after initial dose; alternatively, the parenteral regimen may be repeated once 8 hr after initial dose
	Ampicillin/Amoxicillin/Penicillin-Allergic Patient Regimen
Vancomycin and gentamicin	IV administration of vancomycin, 1.0 g, over 1 hr plus IV or IM administration of gentamicin, 1.5 mg/kg (not to exceed 80 mg), 1 hr before procedure; may be repeated once 8 hr after initial dose
	Alternate Low-Risk Patient Regimen
Amoxicillin	3.0 g PO 1 hr before procedure, then 1.5 g 6 hr after initial dose

*Initial pediatric doses are as follows: Ampicillin, 50 mg/kg amoxicillin, 50 mg/kg; gentamicin, 2.0 mg/kg; vancomycin, 20 mg/kg. Follow-up doses should be half the initial dose. **Total pediatric dose should not exceed total adult dose.**

From Dajani AS, Birno AL, Chung KJ, et al. Prevention of bacterial endocarditis—recommendations by the American Heart Association, *JAMA* 1990, 264:2919–2922.

Appendix F

NUCLEOSIDE ANALOGUE ANTIRETROVIRALS

TABLE F-1.
Nucleoside analog antiretrovirals

	Zidovudine (AZT, ZDV)	Didanosine (ddI)	Zalcitabine (ddC)	Stavudine (d4T)	Lamivudine (3TC)
Trade name	Retrovir	Videx	Hivid	Zerit	Epivir
Usual dose (PO)	200 mg tid	(Tablet form) >60 kg: 200 mg bid <60 kg: 125 mg bid 200 mg/day (powder)	0.75 mg tid	>60 kg: 40 mg bid <60 kg: 30 mg bid	150 mg bid
Minimum effective dose	300 mg/d				
Oral bioavailability (%)	60	Tablet: 40 Powder: 30	85	86	86
Serum half-life	1.1 hr	1.6 hr	1.2 hr	1.0 hr	3–6 hr
Intracellular half-life	3 hr	12 hr	3 hr	3.5 hr	12 hr
CNS penetration (% serum levels)	60	20	20	30–40	10
Elimination	Metabolized to AZT glucuronide (GAZT) Renal excretion GAZT	Renal excretion—50%	Renal excretion—70%	Renal excretion—50% unchanged	Renal excretion—71% majority unchanged
Major toxicity	Bone marrow suppression: Anemia and/or neutropenia Subjective complaints	Pancreatitis Peripheral neuropathy	Peripheral neuropathy Stomatitis	Peripheral neuropathy	Minimal toxicity

Modified from Bartlett JG: Antiretroviral therapy in patients with HIV infection. *Infect Dis Clin Pract* 1996, 5:172–179.

Appendix G
METABOLIC ALKALOSIS/ACIDOSIS

Metabolic alkalosis results from conditions that cause base accumulation or net loss of hydrogen ions from the blood. It is usually characterized by an alkalemic pH (>7.45) and elevated serum bicarbonate (>27.0 mEq/L). Metabolic alkaloses are often classified according to whether they are responsive or unresponsive to sodium chloride administration. Responsiveness to sodium chloride administration implies that metabolic alkalosis is maintained as a consequence of intravascular volume depletion. A third, miscellaneous group is not well characterized.

I. **Sodium chloride–responsive metabolic alkalosis:**
   A. **Gastrointestinal disorders:**
      1. Vomiting.
      2. Villous adenoma.
      3. Nasogastric suctioning.
      4. Diarrhea.
   B. **Diuretic therapy.**
   C. **Post hypercapnia.**
   D. **Cystic fibrosis.**
II. **Sodium chloride–resistant metabolic alkalosis:**
   A. **Excessive mineralocorticoid activity:**
      1. Hyperaldosteronism.
      2. Licorice intoxication.
      3. Cushing's syndrome.
      4. Bartter's syndrome.
   B. **Profound potassium depletion.**
   C. **Excessive use of chewing tobacco.**
III. Miscellaneous causes of metabolic alkalosis:
   A. **Administration of alkalinizing agents.**
   B. **Milk-alkali syndrome.**
   C. **Nonparathyroid hypercalcemia.**
   D. **Massive doses of carbenicillin or penicillin.**
   E. **Hypoparathyroidism.**
   F. **Massive transfusion** (secondary to citrate metabolism).
   G. **Massive infusion of lactated IV solutions.**

Acidosis

I. **Non-anion Gap Acidosis:**
  A. **Renal bicarbonate loss:**
    1. Renal tubular acidosis/interstitial renal disease.
    2. Hypoaldosteronism.
    3. Urinary tract obstruction.
    4. Carbonic anhydrase inhibitors.
  B. **Gastrointestinal loss:**
    1. Diarrhea.
    2. Ileal loop, ureterosigmoidostomy, enteric fistula.
    3. Anion exchange resins.
  C. **Acidifying agents:**
    1. Ammonium chloride, other drugs with HCl.
  D. **Miscellaneous:**
    1. Dehydration.
    2. Hyperalimentation (with obsolete formulations).
II. **Anion Gap Acidosis:**
  A. **Toxins:**
    1. Methanol.
    2. Salicylates.
    3. Ethylene glycol.
    4. Paraldehyde.
  B. **Diabetes:**
    1. Diabetic ketoacidosis.
    2. Nonketotic hyperosmolar state.
  C. **Nondiabetic ketoacidosis:**
    1. Starvation.
    2. Ethanol intoxication.
  D. **Renal failure:**
    1. Uremic acidosis.
  E. **Lactic acidosis:**
    1. Shock (increased lactate production).
    2. Liver failure (decreased metabolism).

Appendix H
ANTIDOTES TO POISONING/OVERDOSE

I. **General treatment:**
  A. Stabilization of vital organ function and supportive care; stop offending agent if present.
  B. **Decrease absorption:**
    1. Emesis (syrup of ipecac)—selective use, primarily in home.
    2. Gastric lavage—selective use on an individual basis.
    3. Activated charcoal (routinely, except where ineffective or contraindicated).
    4. Osmotic cathartics (single dose).
  C. **Increase elimination:**
    1. Diuresis (alkaline or acid)—weak acids (ASA, barbs) or weak bases (PCP, amphetamines), respectively.
    2. Activated charcoal (routinely except where ineffective or contraindicated).
    3. Osmotic cathartics (single dose).
    4. Dialysis (with or without a charcoal-impregnated membrane).
    5. ?Whole bowel irrigation—role currently undefined.
  D. **Antidotes.**
II. **Poison (overdose)/Antidote:**
  A. **Acetaminophen:**
    1. **Acetylcysteine:**
      a. **Adult:** Load with 140 mg/kg PO diluted with water, soft drink, or juice.
        (1) **Maintenance:** 17 additional doses of 70 mg/kg q 4 hr.
        (2) IV regimens effective, but still experimental and awaiting FDA approval (*see* Acetylcysteine).
  B. **Anticholinesterases, organophosphates, carbamate pesticides:**
    1. **Atropine sulfate:**
      a. **Adult:** 2–5 mg IV; double the dose every 5–10 min until drying/clearing of secretions is clinically evident.

    b. **Pediatric:** 0.50 mg/kg IV; double the dose q 5–10 min until drying/clearing of secretions is clinically evident.

  2. **Pralidoxime chloride:**

    a. **Adult:** 1 gm IV over 30 min; may be repeated in 1 hr if clinically necessary; repeat q 6–8 hr for 48 hr or until resolution of symptoms (muscular weakness).

    b. **Pediatric:** 25–40 mg/kg IV over 30 min; repeat in 1 hr if clinically indicated, then q 6–8 hr × 48 hr or until resolution of symptoms (muscular weakness).

C. **Anticholinergics, tricyclic antidepressants, antihistamines:**

  1. **Physostigmine salicylate** (no longer used for tricyclics):

    a. **Adult:** 1–2 mg IV slowly over 3–5 min; repeat at 5–10 min intervals until anticholinergic symptoms resolve.

    b. **Pediatric:** 0.5 mg IV slowly over 3–5 min; repeat at 5–10 min intervals until anticholinergic symptoms resolve.

  2. **Sodium bicarbonate for tricyclic antidepressants:** Raise pH_a >7.50–7.55—initial adult dose 1–2 mEq/kg IV.

  3. **Multidose Activated charcoal for tricyclic antidepressants:** Increases elimination due to enterohepatic cycling. Osmotic cathartic (e.g., sorbitol) may be required more than once because of anticholinergic effects of drugs.

D. **Benzodiazepines:**

  1. Flumazenil 0.2 mg IV, then 0.1 mg IV q 30–60 sec until a clinical response or a total dose of 1.0 mg (controversial).

E. **β-Adrenergic antagonist overdose:**

  1. Catecholamine (β-agonist) infusions: Isoproterenol, epinephrine, dopamine, dobutamine.

  2. Glucagon: 50 μg/kg IV bolus.

  3. Cardiac pacing may be required to maintain heart rate.

F. **Calcium channel blockers:**

  1. **Calcium** chloride 1 g IV, repeated q 10 min × 3 additional doses as clinically indicated.

2. **Glucagon,** 50 μg/kg IV bolus for bradycardia.
3. **Atropine** 0.5–1.0 mg q 5 min to max. of 3.0 mg.
4. **Catecholamine infusions:** Dopamine, epinephrine, isoproterenol.

G. **Carbon monoxide:**
   1. **100% Oxygen** or hyperbaric oxygen.

H. **Cyanide (nitroprusside) "Cyanide Kit":**
   1. **(Step 1) Amyl nitrite pearls:** Crushed in gauze pad and inhaled for 30 sec q 1–2 min.
   2. **(Step 2) Sodium nitrite:** 10 mL of a 3% solution (300 mg) IV over 2–4 min; repeat if symptoms recur.
   3. **(Step 3) Sodium thiosulfate:** 50 mL of a 25% solution (12.5 g) IV over 10 min.
   4. **Hydroxycobalamin** 4 g IV, followed by sodium thiosulfate as above (experimental and awaiting FDA approval).

I. **Digoxin:**
   1. **Digixin immune Fab** (Digibind):
      a. **Adult:** Depends on amount to be neutralized (Digibind); if dose unknown, give 800 mg (20 vials) IV over 30 min.

J. **Ethanol:** *See* Alcohol withdrawal medications.
   1. **Thiamine.** 100 mg IV q day (technically not an antidote but administered to prevent development of Wernicke's encephalopathy).

K. **Ethylene glycol:**
   1. **Ethanol:**
      a. **Adult:** 0.6 g/kg (0.75 mL of 100% ethanol diluted to a 10% solution IV load over 20–60 min), then 70–130 mg/kg/hr infusion to achieve serum ethanol concentration of 100–150 mg/dL.
   2. **Thiamine:** 100 mg IV q day (as above).
   3. **Pyridoxine:** 50 mg q 6 hr.
   4. **Calcium** chloride 5–10 mg/kg IV for severe ionized hypocalcemia.
   5. **Bicarbonate** for severe metabolic acidosis.
   6. **Hemodialysis:** level >25 mg/dL.

L. **Heavy metals:**
   Iron:
   1. **Deferoxamine mesylate:**

a. **Adult/Pediatric:** 1000 mg IM/IV slowly, then 500 mg q 4 hr until the disappearance of pink "vin rose" urine (max. dose of 6 g/day).

Iron, lead, mercury, copper, nickle, zinc, cadmium, cobalt:
1. **Calcium disodium edetate** (EDTA):
   a. **Adult:** 1000–1500 mg/m^2/day deep IM or slow IV infusion for up to 5 days.

Mercury, arsenic, gold, lead (in combination with EDTA):
1. **Dimercaprol** (BAL):
   a. **Adult:** 3–5 mg/kg deep IM q 4 hr × 2 days; q 4–6 hr until urinary arsenic <50 µg/mL; for mercury, 4 mg/kg IM q 4 hr × 2 days, 4 mg/kg IM q 6 hr × 2 days, 2 mg/kg IM q 8 hr × 2 days, then 2 mg/kg q 12 hr × 2 days.

Arsenic, copper, mercury:
1. **D-Penicillamine:**
   a. **Adult:** 25 mg/kg (250 mg in adults) PO q 6 hr (max. 1 g/day). Administer until urinary levels decrease to insignificant values (i.e., arsenic <50 µg/L).

M. **Heparin:**
   1. **Protamine sulfate:**
      a. **Adult:** 1.0 mg protamine for each 100 U heparin administered slowly IV over 5–10 min.

N. **Hyperkalemia:**
   1. **Calcium chloride:** 5–10 mL 10% over 5 min.
   2. **Insulin and glucose:** 5–10 U regular insulin with 1 amp D$_{50}$.
   3. **Sodium bicarbonate:** 44 mEq over 5 min.
   4. **Sodium polystyrene sulfonate** (Kayexalate): 1 g binds 1 mEq K$^+$.
      a. **Oral/NG:** Give 20–50 g in 100 mL 20% sorbitol q 3–4 hr as indicated by clinical response.
      b. **Retention enema:** 50 g Kayexalate plus 50 g sorbitol in 200 mL water; retain 30–60 min; repeat hourly as indicated by clinical response.
   5. **Diuresis:** Furosemide or other loop diuretics.
   6. **Dialysis.**

O. **Hypermagnesemia:**

1. **Calcium chloride:** 5–10 mL 10% over 5–10 min.
2. **Diuresis:** Fluid loading with IV crystalloids followed by furosemide 0.5–1.0 mg/kg IV.
3. **Dialysis.**

P. **Hyperphosphatemia:**
   1. Phosphate-binding antacids.
      a. Aluminum containing (Amphogel).
   2. **Diuresis.**
   3. **Dialysis.**

Q. **Isopropyl alcohol:**
   1. **Lavage.**
   2. **Activated charcoal.**
   3. **Hemodialysis (severe cases manifested by hypotension and coma).**

R. **Methanol:**
   1. **Ethanol:**
      a. **Adult:** 0.6 g/kg, then 60–150 mg/kg/hr (*see* Ethylene glycol above).
   2. **Folate:** 1–2 mg/kg IV q 4–6 hr.
   3. **Bicarbonate** for severe metabolic acidosis.
   4. **Hemodialysis:** level >25 mg/dL.

S. **Opiates:**
   1. **Naloxone hydrochloride:**
      a. **Adult:** 2 mg IV q 2–5 min up to max. of 10–20 mg; may need to repeat initial reversal dose q 20–60 min or administer by continuous infusion to maintain effect (*see* Naloxone).
      b. **Pediatric:** 0.01 mg/kg IV bolus.

T. **Salicylates:**
   1. **Alkaline diuresis.**
   2. **Multidose activated charcoal.**
   3. **Hemodialysis** if severe.
   4. **Bicarbonate** for severe metabolic acidosis/urinary alkalinization.
   5. **Glucose** for hypoglycemia.
   6. **Vitamin K** 10 mg IM for hypoprothrombinemia.

U. **Theophylline:**
   1. **Multidose activated charcoal:** Theophylline undergoes enterohepatic circulation.
   2. **Charcoal hemoperfusion.**

V. **Warfarin:**
  1. **Fresh-frozen plasma 2–4 units.**
  2. **Vitamin K:** 10 mg IM or slowly IV (risk of anaphylaxis); may be repeated as clinically indicated q 4–6 hr up to max. of 50 mg.

BIBLIOGRAPHY

Goldfrank LR, Flomenbaum NE, Lewin NA, et al (ed): *Toxicologic Emergencies,* ed 5, Norwalk, 1994, Appleton and Lange.

Appendix I

SELECTED SERUM/PLASMA DRUG LEVELS

TABLE I–1.

Drug	Sample	Conventional Level	SI Units
Acetaminophen	Plasma	Toxic >5 mg/dL	>300 μmol/L
Amikacin	Serum	Peak/trough = 15–25/<10 μg/mL	
Carbamazepine	Plasma	4–10 mg/L	17–42 μmol/L
Chlorpromazine	Plasma	50–300 ng/mL	150–950 nmol/L
Chlorpropamide	Plasma	75–250 mg/L	270–900 μmol/L
Cyclosporin	Serum	125–300 μg/L	
Digoxin	Plasma	0.5–2.0 ng/mL	0.6–2.6 nmol/L
Disopyramide	Plasma	2–6 ng/L	6–18 μmol/L
Ethanol	Plasma	Legal <80 mg/dL	<17 mmol/L
		Toxic >100 mg/dL	>22 mmol/L
Ethosuximide	Plasma	40–110 mg/L	280–780 μmol/L
Gentamicin	Serum	Peak/trough = 5–8/<2 μg/ml	
Gold	Serum	300–800 μg/dL	15–40 μmol/L
Lidocaine	Plasma	1–5 mg/L	4.5–21.5 μmol/L
Lithium	Serum	0.5–1.5 mEq/L	0.5–1.5 mmol/L
Meprobamate	Plasma	Therapeutic <20 mg/L	<90 μmol/L
		Toxic >40 mg/L	>180 μmol/L
Nitroprusside thiocyanate	Plasma	Toxic >10 mg/dL	>1.7 mmol/L
Nortriptyline	Plasma	25–200 ng/mL	90–760 nmol/L
NAPA	Plasma	6–20 mg/L	
Pentobarbital	Plasma	20–40 mg/L	90–170 μmol/L
Phenobarbital	Plasma	2–5 mg/L	85–215 μmol/L
Phenytoin	Plasma	10–20 mg/L	40–80 μmol/L
Primidone	Plasma	6–10 mg/L	25–46 μmol/L
Procainamide	Plasma	4–8 mg/L	17–34 μmol/L
Propoxyphene	Plasma	Toxic >2 mg/L	>5.9 μmol/L
Quinidine	Plasma	1.5–5 mg/L	4.6–15.4 μmol/L
Salicylate	Serum	Toxic >20 mg/dL	>1.45 mmol/L
Theophylline	Plasma	10–20 mg/L	55–110 μmol/L
Tobramycin	Serum	Peak/trough = 5–8/<2 μg/mL	
Vancomycin	Serum	Peak/trough =30–40/ 5–10 μg/mL	

Appendix J

COMPARISON OF MUSCLE RELAXANTS

TABLE J-1

	Advantages	Disadvantages
Long-acting:		
Doxacurium	1. Hemodynamically very stable	1. Relatively slow onset of action
Metocurine	1. Long-acting	1. Predominantly renally excreted, of concern in patients with renal failure
	2. Less potential for hemodynamic instability than tubocurarine	
Pancuronium	1. Very inexpensive	1. Potential for tachycardia
	2. Preserves hemodynamic function	
Pipecuronium	1. Very hemodynamically stable	1. Expensive
		2. Slow onset of action
Tubocurarine	1. Inexpensive	1. Potential for histamine release.
	2. Long-acting	
Intermediate-acting:		
Atracurium	1. Minor hemodynamic alterations primarily from histamine release	1. Prolonged infusions in renal failure patients may produce significant serum laudanosine levels
	2. Unique metabolism not requiring renal or hepatic function	
Cisatracurium	1. Hemodynamically stable	1. Prolonged infusions in renal failure patients may produce significant serum laudanosine levels
	2. Unique metabolism not requiring renal or hepatic function	
Rocuronium	1. Rapid onset of action	1. Expensive
	2. Minimal hemodynamic effects	
	3. Predominantly biliary excretion; good in patients with renal failure	
Vecuronium	1. No hemodynamic effects	1. Expensive
	2. Predominantly biliary excretion; good in patients with renal failure	

TABLE J-1 (cont.)

	Advantages	Disadvantages
Short-acting:		
Mivacurium	1. Extremely short duration of action 2. Neither renal nor hepatic clearance	1. Potential for histamine release and hemodynamic instability with higher doses, required particularly when administered rapidly
Succinylcholine	1. Short-acting (<5 min) 2. Does not require renal or hepatic metabolism	1. May cause profound hyperkalemia 2. Prolonged action in patients with pseudocholinesterase deficiency 3. Potential for myalgias and myoglobinemia/myoglobinuria 4. May precipitate malignant hyperthermia 5. May cause arrhythmias.

Appendix K

PROTEASE INHIBITORS

Generic name	Saquinavir	Indinavir	Ritonavir
Trade name	Invirase	Crixivan	Norvir
Manufacturer	Roche	Merck	Abbott
Drug class	Hydroxy-ethylamine	Hydroxyamino-pentaneamide	Symmetry-based thiazole
In vitro $1C_{50}$	0.5–30 nM	25–100 nM	10–40 nM
Bioavailability	4% with food	60%–65%	60%–80%
Effect of food on bioavailability	↑	↓	↑
Protein binding	98%	60%	99%
Clearance	Hepatobiliary	Hepatobiliary	Hepatobiliary
Half-life	1.5–2 hr	1.5–2 hr	3–4 hr
Dose (mg) mg/day	600 tid 1800	800 tid 2400	600 bid 1200
How supplied	200 mg capsule	200 and 400 mg capsules	100 mg capsule
Main toxicities	GI	Hyperbilirubinemia, nephrolithiasis	Asthenia, GI, Headache, parasthesias (circumoral + peripheral)

Appendix L
VANCOMYCIN USE

Appropriate Vancomycin Uses (CDC Guidelines):

1. For treatment of serious infections due to β-lactam–resistant gram-positive organisms. Clinicians should be aware that vancomycin may be less rapidly bactericidal than β-lactam agents for β-lactam–susceptible staphylococci.
2. For treatment of gram-positive infections in patients with serious β-lactam allergy.
3. When antibiotic-associated colitis (AAC) fails to respond to metronidazole or if AAC is severe and potentially life threatening.
4. Prophylaxis, as recommended by the American Heart Association, for endocarditis following certain procedures in patients at high risk for endocarditis.
5. Prophylaxis for major surgical procedures involving implantation of prosthetic materials or devices at institutions with a high rate of infections due to methicillin-resistant *Staphylococcus aureus* (MRSA) or *Staphylococcus epidermidis* (MRSE).
6. **Treatment with vancomycin is reasonable as empiric therapy when MRSA, MRSE, or other coagulase-negative staphylococcus is suspected and/or until cultures are final.**

Inappropriate Vancomycin Uses (CDC Guidelines):

1. Routine surgical prophylaxis (unless life-threatening β-lactam allergy).
2. Empiric antimicrobial therapy for a febrile neutropenic patient, unless there is strong evidence at the outset that the patient has an infection due to gram-positive microorganisms, and the prevalence of infections due to MRSA in the hospital is substantial.
3. Treatment in response to a single blood culture positive for coagulase-negative staphylococci, if other blood cultures drawn in the same time frame are negative (i.e., contamination likely). Because contamination of blood cultures with skin flora may cause vancomycin to be administered inappro-

priately, phlebotomists and other personnel who obtain blood cultures should be trained properly to minimize microbial contamination of specimens.

4. Continued empiric use for presumed infections in patients whose cultures are negative for β-lactam–resistant gram-positive microorganisms.
5. Systemic or local prophylaxis for infection or colonization of indwelling central or peripheral intravascular catheters.
6. Selective decontamination of the digestive tract.
7. Eradication of MRSA colonization.
8. Primary treatment of antibiotic-associated colitis.
9. Routine prophylaxis for very-low-birth-weight infants.
10. Routine prophylaxis for patients on continuous ambulatory peritoneal dialysis or hemodialysis.
11. Treatment (chosen for dosing convenience) of infections due to β-lactam–sensitive gram-positive microorganisms in patients with renal failure.
12. Use of vancomycin solution for topical application or irrigation.

BIBLIOGRAPHY

MMWR 1995, 44:RR-12.

Appendix M

NUTRITIONAL FORMULAS

I. Intact-Protein Formulas

Product	Company	K cal/mL	Protein g/1000 K cal	Carbohydrate g/1000 K cal	Fiber	Fat g/1000 K cal	Osmolality	Sodium meq/1000 K cal	Potassium meq/1000 K cal	Calcium mg/1000 K cal
Diabetisource	Sandoz Nutrition	1.0	50	90	Yes	49	360	43	36	670
Ensure	Ross Products Division, Abbott Laboratories	1.06	35.2	137.2		35.2	470	34.8	37.9	500
Ensure with fiber	Ross Products Division, Abbott Laboratories	1.1	36	147	Yes	34	480	33.4	39.4	654
Ensure HN	Ross Products Division, Abbott Laboratories	1.06	42	133.6		33.6	470	33	37.8	715
Ensure Plus	Ross Products Division, Abbott Laboratories	1.5	36.6	133.2		35.5	690	30.6	33.1	470
Entrition 0.5	Clintec Nutrition Company	0.5	35	136		35	120	30.4	30.8	500
Entrition HN	Clintec Nutrition Company	1.0	44	114		41	300	36.7	40.5	770
Fibersource	Sandoz Nutrition	1.2	36	140	Yes	34	390	40	38	558
Fibersource HN	Sandoz Nutrition	1.2	45	133	Yes	34	390	40	38	558
Fiberlan	Elan Pharma	1.2	42	133	Yes	33	310	36.7	36.7	667
Glucerna	Ross Products Division, Abbott Laboratories	1.0	41.8	93.7	Yes	55.7	375	40.3	40	704
Glytrol	Clintec Nutrition Company	1.0	45	100	Yes	47.5	380	32.2	35.9	720

Product	Company	Phosphorus mg/1000 K cal	Magnesium mg/1000 K cal	Vit A IU/1000 K cal	Vit K µg/1000 K cal	Vit C meq/1000 K cal	Miscellaneous
I. Intact-Protein Formulas *(Continued.)*							
Diabetisource	Sandoz Nutrition	870	270	3350	67	200	Vegetable & fruit fiber 4.4g/1000 K cal
Ensure	Ross Products Division, Abbott Laboratories	500	200	2500	40	150	
Ensure with fiber	Ross Products Division, Abbott Laboratories	654	262	3269	46	196	Soy polysaccharide 13.1 g/1000 K cal
Ensure HN	Ross Products Division, Abbott Laboratories	715	286	3572	57	215	
Ensure Plus	Ross Products Division, Abbott Laboratories	470	189	2349	38	141	
Entrition 0.5	Clintec Nutrition Company	500	200	2500	100	150	
Entrition HN	Clintec Nutrition Company	770	308	3845	54	116	
Fibersource	Sandoz Nutrition	558	225	2750	40	167	Soy polysaccharide 8 g/1000 K cal
Fibersource HN	Sandoz Nutrition	558	225	2750	40	167	Soy polysaccharide 6 g/1000 K cal
Fiberlan	Elan Pharma	667	267	3333	67	120	Soy polysaccharide 12 g/1000 K cal
Glucerna	Ross Products Division, Abbott Laboratories	704	282	3520	57	212	Soy fiber 14.4 g/1000 K cal
Glytrol	Clintec Nutrition Company	720	286	4000	50	140	Gum arabic, pectin, soy polysaccharide; 15 g/1000 K cal

(Continued.)

I. Intact-Protein Formulas (Continued.)

Product	Company	K cal/mL	Protein g/1000 K cal	Carbohydrate g/1000 K cal	Fiber	Fat g/1000 K cal	Osmolality	Sodium meq/1000 K cal	Potassium meq/1000 K cal	Calcium mg/1000 K cal
Impact	Sandoz Nutrition	1.0	56	130		28	375	48	36	800
Impact with fiber	Sandoz Nutrition	1.0	56	140	Yes	28	375	48	36	800
Isocal	Mead Johnson	1.06	32	125		42	300	21.7	31.9	595
Isocal HN	Mead Johnson	1.06	42	117		42	300	38.1	38.5	800
Isolan	Elan Pharma	1.06	38	136		34	300	36.8	32.1	755
Isosource	Sandoz Nutrition	1.2	35.7	141		34	360	43.3	36.2	556
Isosource HN	Sandoz Nutrition	1.2	44	133		34	330	39.7	36.2	556
Isosource VHN	Sandoz Nutrition	1.0	62	130	Yes	29	300	57	41	800
Jevity	Ross Products Division, Abbott Laboratories	1.06	42	143	Yes	34	300	38.1	37.8	858
Magnacal	Sherwood Medical	2.0	35	125		40	590	21.8	16	500
Nepro	Ross Products Division, Abbott Laboratories	2.0	34.9	107.6		47.8	635	18.1	13.5	686
Nitrolan	Elan Pharma	1.24	48.4	129		32	310	30.6	30.6	645
Nutren 1.0	Clintec Nutrition Company	1.0	40	127		38	300–350	38.1	32	668
Nutren 1.0 with fiber	Clintec Nutrition Company	1.0	40	127	Yes	38	310–370	38.1	32	668

I. Intact-Protein Formulas (Continued.)

Product	Company	Phosphorus mg/1000 K cal	Magnesium mg/1000 K cal	Vit A IU/1000 K cal	Vit K μg/1000 K cal	Vit C meq/1000 K cal	Miscellaneous
Impact	Sandoz Nutrition	800	270	3350	67	80	High arginine, RNA, fish oil
Impact with fiber	Sandoz Nutrition	800	270	3350	67	80	High arginine, RNA, fish oil, soy & guar fiber
Isocal	Mead Johnson	500	200	2455	125	150	
Isocal HN	Mead Johnson	800	320	3962	100	235	
Isolan	Elan Pharm	755	302	3774	75.5	136	
Isosource	Sandoz Nutrition	556	224	2739	39.8	166	
Isosource HN	Sandoz Nutrition	556	224	2739	39.8	166	
Isosource VHN	Sandoz Nutrition	800	320	4000	80	240	Soy polysaccharide & guar; 10 g/000 K cal
Jevity	Ross Products Division, Abbott Laboratories	716	286	3572	58	214	Soy polysaccharide 13.6 g/1000 K cal
Magnacal	Sherwood Medical	500	200	2500	150	150	
Nepro	Ross Products Division, Abbott Laboratories	343	105	526	42	53	Renal formula
Nitrolan	Elan Pharma	645	258	3226	64.5	116	
Nutren 1.0	Clintec Nutrition Company	668	268	4000	50	140	
Nutren 1.0 with fiber	Clintec Nutrition Company	668	268	4000	50	140	Soy polysaccharide 14 g/1000 K cal

(Continued.)

I. Intact-Protein Formulas *(Continued.)*

Product	Company	K cal/mL	Protein g/1000 K cal	Carbohydrate g/1000 K cal	Fiber	Fat g/1000 K cal	Osmolality	Sodium meq/1000 K cal	Potassium meq/1000 K cal	Calcium mg/1000 K cal
Nutren 1.5	Clintec Nutrition Company	1.5	40	113		45	430–530	33.9	32	667
Nutren 2.0	Clintec Nutrition Company	2.0	40	98		53	720	28.3	24.6	670
NutriHep Diet	Clintec Nutrition Company	1.5	26.7	193		14	690	9.3	22.6	667
Nutri Vent	Clintec Nutrition Company	1.5	45	67		63	330–465	33.9	32	800
Osmolite	Ross Products Division, Abbott Laboratories	1.06	35.2	137.2		35.5	300	26.1	24.6	500
Osmolite HN	Ross Products Division, Abbott Laboratories	1.06	42	133.6		33.9	300	38.3	37.8	715
Probalance	Clintec Nutrition Company	1.2	45	130	Yes	34	350–450	27.7	33.3	1042
Promote	Ross Products Division, Abbott Laboratories	1.0	62.5	130		26	340	40.4	50.6	1200
Promote with fiber	Ross Products Division, Abbott Laboratories	1.0	62.5	139.4	Yes	28.2	370	56.5	50.6	1200
Pulmocare	Ross Products Division, Abbott Laboratories	1.5	41.7	70.4		62.2	475	38	29.5	704

I. Intact-Protein Formulas *(Continued.)*

Product	Company	Phosphorus mg/1000 K cal	Magnesium mg/1000 K cal	Vit A IU/1000 K cal	Vit K µg/1000 K cal	Vit C meq/1000 K cal	Miscellaneous
Nutren 1.5	Clintec Nutrition Company	667	268	4000	50	140	
Nutren 2.0	Clintec Nutrition Company	670	268	4000	50	140	
NutriHep Diet	Clintec Nutrition Company	667	267	3333	80	64	Hepatic formula; high in branched chain amino acids
Nutri Vent	Clintec Nutrition Company	800	320	4000	50	140	High fat
Osmolite	Ross Products Division, Abbott Laboratories	500	200	2500	40	150	
Osmolite HN	Ross Products Division, Abbott Laboratories	715	286	3572	58	215	
Probalance	Clintec Nutrition Company	833	333	3333	67	200	Soy polysaccharide and gum arabic; 8.3 g/1000 K cal
Promote	Ross Products Division, Abbott Laboratories	1200	400	5000	80	340	
Promote with fiber	Ross Products Division, Abbott Laboratories	1200	400	5000	80	340	Soy polysaccharide and oat fiber; 14.4 g/1000 K cal
Pulmocare	Ross Products Division, Abbott Laboratories	704	282	3520	56.7	211	High fat

(Continued.)

I. Intact-Protein Formulas (Continued.)

Product	Company	K cal/mL	Protein g/1000 K cal	Carbohydrate g/1000 K cal	Fiber	Fat g/1000 K cal	Osmolality	Sodium meq/1000 K cal	Potassium meq/1000 K cal	Calcium mg/1000 K cal
Replete	Clintec Nutrition Company	1.0	62.5	113		34	300–350	38.1	38.5	1000
Replete with fiber	Clintec Nutrition Company	1.0	62.5	113	Yes	34	310–390	38.1	38.5	1000
Resource	Sandoz Nutrition	1.06	35	140		35	430	36	39	500
Resource Plus	Sandoz Nutrition	1.5	37	130		35	600	37	35	470
Respalor	Mead Johnson	1.5	50	98		47	580	36.4	25.1	467
Suplena	Ross Products Division, Abbott Laboratories	2.0	15	128		48	600	17.1	14.3	693
Sustacal Basic	Mead Johnson	1.06	35.2	140		33.2	500	34.8	39	500
Sustacal Plus	Mead Johnson	1.5	41	127		39	650	24.6	25.2	567
Sustacal with fiber	Mead Johnson	1.06	43	132	Yes	33	480	29.5	33.6	792
Traumacal	Mead Johnson	1.5	55	95		45	490	34.2	23.8	500
TwoCal HN	Ross Products Division, Abbott Laboratories	2.0	41.7	108.2	Yes	45.3	690	28.4	31.2	526
Ultracal	Mead Johnson	1.06	42	116		42	310	38.1	38.9	800
Ultralan	Elan Pharma	1.5	40	135		33	540	34	32.7	667

I. Intact-Protein Formulas *(Continued.)*

Product	Company	Phosphorus mg/1000 K cal	Magnesium mg/1000 K cal	Vit A IU/1000 K cal	Vit K μg/1000 K cal	Vit C meq/1000 K cal	Miscellaneous
Replete	Clintec Nutrition Company	1000	400	4000	50	340	
Replete with fiber	Clintec Nutrition Company	1000	400	4000	50	340	Soy polysaccharide 14 g/1000 K cal
Resource	Sandoz Nutrition	500	200	2500	36	150	
Resource Plus	Sandoz Nutrition	470	210	2500	37	110	
Respalor	Mead Johnson	467	185	2310	37	139	
Suplena	Ross Products Division, Abbott Laboratories	364	105	526	42	53	Renal formula
Sustacal Basic	Mead Johnson	500	200	2520	62.4	92	
Sustacal Plus	Mead Johnson	567	227	2800	140	50.7	
Sustacal with fiber	Mead Johnson	660	265	3300	91.5	120	Soy fiber 5.6 g/1000 K cal
Traumacal	Mead Johnson	500	133	1666	84.7	98.7	
TwoCal HN	Ross Products Division, Abbott Laboratories	526	211	2632	43	158	
Ultracal	Mead Johnson	800	320	3962	64	236	Soy polysaccharide and oat fiber; 13.6 g/1000 K cal
Ultralan	Elan Pharma	667	267	3333	83.3	120	

(Continued.)

II. Peptide-Based Formulas

Product	Company	K cal/mL	Protein g/1000 K cal	Carbohydrate g/1000 K cal	Fiber	Fat g/1000 K cal	Osmolality	Sodium meq/1000 K cal	Potassium meq/1000 K cal	Calcium mg/1000 K cal
AlitraQ	Ross Products Division, Abbott Laboratories	1.0	52.5	165		15.5	575	43.5	30.7	733
Crucial	Clintec Nutrition Company	1.5	62.5	90		45	490	33.9	31.9	667
Peptamen	Clintec Nutrition Company	1.0	40	127		39	270–380	21.7	32.1	800
Peptamen VHP	Clintec Nutrition Company	1.0	62.5	104.5		39	300–430	24.3	38.4	800
Perative	Ross Products Division, Abbott Laboratories	1.3	51.2	136		29	425	34.8	34.1	667
Reabilan	Clintec Nutrition Company	1.0	31.5	131.5		40.5	350	30.4	32.1	500
Reabilan HN	Clintec Nutrition Company	1.33	44	119		40.5	490	32.6	32.1	500
Sandasource Peptide	Sandoz Nutrition Company	1.0	50	160		17	500	48	38	570
Vital HN	Ross Products Division, Abbott Laboratories	1.0	41.7	185		10.8	500	24.6	35.8	667

Product	Company	Phosphorus mg/1000 K cal	Magnesium mg/1000 K cal	Vit A IU/1000 K cal	Vit K μg/1000 K cal	Vit C meq/1000 K cal	Miscellaneous
II. Peptide-Based Formulas *(Continued.)*							
AlitraQ	Ross Products Division, Abbott Laboratories	733	267	3998	54	200	High glutamine, free amino acids, soy & whey, peptides, and intact protein
Crucial	Clintec Nutrition Company	667	267	4000	50	667	Casein peptides, high arginine, fish oil
Peptamen	Clintec Nutrition Company	700	400	4000	80	140	Whey peptides
Peptamen VHP	Clintec Nutrition Company	700	300	4000	80	340	Whey peptides
Perative	Ross Products Division, Abbott Laboratories	667	267	3333	53.3	200	Partially hydrolyzed casein, lactalbumin hydrolysate, high arginine, canola oil
Reabilan	Clintec Nutrition Company	500	250	2660	50	100	Casein & whey peptides, canola oil
Reabilan HN	Clintec Nutrition Company	500	250	2660	50	100	Casein & whey peptides, canola oil
Sandasource Peptide	Sandoz Nutrition Company	570	230	2860	46	170	Free amino acids, casein peptides, intact casein
Vital HN	Ross Products Division, Abbott Laboratories	667	267	3332	54	200	Powder, free amino acids, partially hydrolyzed whey, meat, soy

(Continued.)

Product	Company	K cal/mL	Protein g/1000 K cal	Carbohydrate g/1000 K cal	Fiber	Fat g/1000 K cal	Osmolality	Sodium meq/1000 K cal	Potassium meq/1000 K cal	Calcium mg/1000 K cal
III. Amino Acid Based Formulas										
Amin-Aid	R&D Laboratories	2.0	10	187		24	700	<7.5	<3	N/A
Criticare HN	Mead Johnson	1.06	36	208		4.7	650	25.8	31.9	500
Immun-aid	McGaw	1.0	80	120		22	460	25	27	500
Travasorb Renal	Clintec Nutrition Company	1.35	17	200		13	590	N/A	N/A	N/A
Vivonex TEN	Sandoz Nutrition Company	1.0	38	210		2.8	630	20	20	500
Vivonex Plus	Sandoz Nutrition Company	1.0	45	190		6.7	650	27	28	560

III. Amino Acid Based Formulas

Product	Company	Phosphorus mg/1000 K cal	Magnesium mg/1000 K cal	Vit A IU/1000 K cal	Vit K µg/1000 K cal	Vit C meq/1000 K cal	Miscellaneous
Amin-Aid	R & D Laboratories	N/A	N/A	N/A	N/A	N/A	Powder, essential amino acids plus histidine
Criticare HN	Mead Johnson	500	200	2453	125	150	Low fat, amino acids, hydrolyzed casein
Immun-Aid	McGaw	500	200	2665	40	60	Powder, lactalbumin, high glutamine, high arginine, high branched chain amino acids, RNA
Travasorb Renal	Clintec Nutrition Company	N/A	N/A	N/A	N/A	31.6	Powder, renal formula
Vivonex TEN	Sandoz Nutrition Company	500	200	2500	22	60	Powder, low fat
Vivonex Plus	Sandoz Nutrition Company	560	220	4200	44	67	Powder, low fat

Index